EXPLORING THE PSYCHO-SOCIAL IMPACT OF COVID-19

This comprehensive resource provides a one-stop information repository, exploring all psychological aspects of COVID-19. Divided into three sections, the book covers the psycho-social impact on society and individuals and our collective cooperative behaviour, as well as philanthropic efforts, coping strategies and technological interventions, and how lessons learned will help in preparedness for the future.

Including case studies and the latest research from diverse scientific studies across different regions, this book examines how psycho-social paradigms changed as a result of the pandemic and left their watermark on the human psyche. It also explores the coping strategies adopted to deal with this common aggressor and how the techniques varied in accordance with social, cultural, and geographical factors. The final section offers new insights for the future, highlighting the psychological infrastructure required, the type of preparedness and handling strategies necessary to mitigate the impact of any future biogenic pandemics.

Combining theory and practical application, this is a valuable reading for academics and researchers as well as practising psychologists, clinical psychologists, and lawmakers who are concerned with mental health.

Editors

Dr Rajesh Verma (PhD) is Assistant Professor and Student of Psychology at Feroz Gandhi Memorial Government College, Adampur, Haryana, India. He is an air veteran and academic gold medallist and completed his doctorate from MD University Rohtak. As a report writer, he worked on a DST-funded project on cognitive preparedness. His area of interest lies in indigenous psychology, cognitive psychology, social psychology, psychometrics, organising academic events, and content writing. Recently, he organised the ICSSR-sponsored National Conference on "Bhagavad Gita: An Eternal Repository of Multi-disciplinary Lessons for Mankind". He is tech-savvy, uploads psychology curriculum content-specific videos, and writes blogs regularly. He loves to interact with students.

Dr Uzaina (PhD, CPsychol) is a Practitioner Counselling Psychologist passionate about helping families and neurodiverse children. She holds critical positions as Research and Psychology Training Lead at Geniuslane in India and the United Kingdom. Additionally, she founded Psyche Vitality and is Co-Director of the Association of Child Brain Research and CDC Solutions India. Dr Uzaina's expertise lies in conducting diagnostic assessments and providing essential counselling and support to families. With nearly a decade of experience, she has dedicated herself to offering short-term and long-term counselling and psychotherapy services to adolescents, women, and families. She remains actively engaged in continuous research audits, furthering her commitment to advancing the field of psychology. She also takes great pride in delivering comprehensive training programmes to psychology trainees, sharing her knowledge and expertise with the next generation of professionals.

Co-Editors

Dr Gyanesh Kumar Tiwari (PhD) is Assistant Professor at Dr Harisingh Gour Vishwavidyalaya, Sagar, Madhya Pradesh, India. His research interests include forgiveness, positive body image, self-affirmation, self-compassion, eyewitness memory, metacognition, and the psychology of women. He is an active academician with extensive publications and projects. He also holds key roles in various organisations.

Prof. Leister Sam Sudheer Manickam (PhD) currently practises telepsychotherapy, is a trainer and supervisor of gestalt psychotherapy, and is engaged in independent research. He earned his master's degree in psychology from the University of Kerala. He did his clinical psychology training at the National Institute of Mental Health and Neuro Sciences, Bengaluru, India, and PhD from Columbia Pacific University, the United States. He served as Professor of Clinical Psychology and as Hon. Founder Director of Centre for Applied Psychological Studies, Thiruvananthapuram, India. Also, he served as Director of Training and Research, MHAT, Calicut, India. He had also served as Director of Wellness and Mental health at Trias Health Technologies, Bengaluru. He was formerly Professor of Clinical Psychology at JSS Academy of Higher Education and Research, Mysuru, India. He had taught at the Department of Psychiatry, Christian Medical College, Vellore, Tamil Nadu, India, and CSI Medical College Karakonam, Kerala, India. He was Visiting Fellow at the University of Birmingham, the UK, and is a gestalt psychotherapy trainer who had undergone training in different forms of therapy abroad. He is Fellow of several psychology and psychiatry associations in India, former General Secretary of the Indian Association of Clinical Psychologists, and initiator of the Indian Psychologists Network. He is the author of the book, *Integrative Psychotherapy: Indian Perspective* and has edited the book *COVID-19 Pandemic: Challenges and Responses of Psychologists from India*. He was awarded Excellence in International Scholarship by Division 17 of the American Psychology Association, the United States.

Dr Tushar Singh (D. Phil) is Professor of Psychology at the Department of Psychology, Banaras Hindu University, Uttar Pradesh, India. He obtained his D. Phil in Psychology from the University of Allahabad and served as Assistant Professor at Banaras Hindu University. His research focuses on understanding the miseries of and advocation for the rights of gender and social minorities, including but not limited to LGBTQ+, abused women, and children. He is also involved in academic administration and is associated with various national and international organisations in various capacities.

EXPLORING THE PSYCHO-SOCIAL IMPACT OF COVID-19

Global Perspectives on Behaviour, Interventions and Future Directions

Edited by Dr Rajesh Verma and Dr Uzaina

Co-Editors

Dr Gyanesh Kumar Tiwari,
Prof Leister Sam Sudheer Manickam,
Dr Tushar Singh

Routledge
Taylor & Francis Group

LONDON AND NEW YORK

Designed cover image: Getty Images

First published 2024

by Routledge

4 Park Square, Milton Park, Abingdon, Oxon OX14 4RN

and by Routledge

605 Third Avenue, New York, NY 10158

Routledge is an imprint of the Taylor & Francis Group, an informa business

British Library Cataloguing-in-Publication Data
A catalogue record for this book is available from the British Library

ISBN: 978-1-032-41274-0 (hbk)
ISBN: 978-1-032-41275-7 (pbk)
ISBN: 978-1-003-35720-9 (ebk)

DOI: 10.4324/9781003357209

Typeset in Times New Roman
by Apex CoVantage, LLC

CONTENTS

TABLES

FIGURES

CONTRIBUTORS

Amrita Deb is Associate Professor of Psychology in the Department of Liberal Arts, Indian Institute of Technology Hyderabad, India. Her research and teaching interests include positive psychology, clinical psychology, and personality psychology. She is specifically interested in psychological resilience and well-being outcomes among individuals who have undergone adverse mental health experiences.

Arundhathy Gopakumar is Masters's Student in Sports Psychology at the Central University of Rajasthan, Ajmer, Rajasthan, India. With a deep love for sports and a keen interest in the psychological aspects of athletic performance, she is dedicated to unravelling, understanding, and exploring the mind–sports association. Her core area of interest includes sports psychology, health, and well-being.

Annsweetta James is pursuing her master's degree in Sports Psychology from the Central University of Rajasthan. Having completed her undergraduate studies in B.Sc. Psychology, she developed a profound interest in unravelling the complexities of the human mind. Sports psychology and social psychology are the significant areas of her interest.

Dr Akancha Srivastava is Associate Professor at O.P. Jindal Global University. She completed her doctorate from the Defence Institute of Psychological Research in MoU with Bharathiar University Coimbatore, Coimbatore, Tamil Nadu, India. As a research fellow with the Defence Institute of Psychological Research (DIPR-DRDO), she worked on various defence-related projects involving various activities like conducting psychometric assessments, development of batteries, and experiments. She also worked with the Indian Institute of Management, Indore,

Madhya Pradesh, India. Her areas of interest are organisational behaviour, human resource management, and positive psychology. She has national and international publications to her credit.

Ashutosh Tewari is Management Professional who served as Senior Venture Coach at the Venture Development Centre of GITAM University. He spearheaded the establishment of an entrepreneurial ecosystem across a vibrant community of students and faculty members across three campuses in India. He had two decades of experience in IT Services, Management Consulting, and Supply Chain Industries. He is Certified Behaviour and Mentoring Analyst, which enriches his coaching and mentoring approach. He is passionate about research in the field of development studies and is particularly interested in examining Indian perspectives and is actively exploring themes related to sustainability and social innovation.

Bhavya Chhabra is Doctoral Fellow in the Faculty of Education and Psychology at Eotvos Lorand University, Budapest, Hungary. She received the Award of Master of Science in Mental Health Studies from King's College London. She was felicitated with a Gold Award for her exceptional volunteering services to promote positive change in the community. She has working experience with differently abled people at the South London and Maudsley Hospital, National Health Service, UK. She is also a reviewer of several peer-reviewed journals and has been invited to conferences to deliver talks and presentations.

Dr Bhawna Tushir is Assistant Professor at Christ University. With her extensive background in Malviyan and Gandhian philosophy, she has developed exceptional compassion and inclusivity that set her apart from her peers. Over the past five years, she has contributed her expertise to numerous universities, including the University of Delhi, Manipal University Jaipur, and Chaudhary Charan Singh University. In addition to her academic work, she has made significant contributions as a trainer and consultant, working with organisations such as India Vision Foundation, Christ Consultancy, and the Brain Behaviour Research Foundation of India. She is collaborating on an innovative research project with Banaras Hindu University and Mississippi State University, demonstrating her commitment to advancing knowledge in her field.

Dr Chetna Duggal is Associate Professor at the Tata Institute of Social Sciences (TISS), Mumbai, India. She has almost two decades of experience as a psychotherapist. She is Programme Coordinator for the Masters in Applied Psychology and Postgraduate Diploma in Supervision for Mental Health Practice and Psychotherapy and Counselling. She is Project Director of the School Initiative for Mental Health Advocacy. This initiative endeavours to promote the well-being of young people in schools and other institutes through advocacy, research, and capacity building. She also heads Rahbar, a field action project to promote training, supervision, and professional development for mental health practitioners. Her research interests include counselling, psychotherapy training, school mental health, religion, and spirituality.

Charu Joshi is an alumnus of Jamia Millia Islamia University, Delhi, India. She is practising Counselling Psychologist having extensive experience and specialises in individual and family therapy. Her core area of interest is social network analysis. She has worked on a project for the Ministry of Education titled "National Initiative of School Heads and Teachers Holistic Advancement" and studied the underlying processes and models that can build a long-term sustainable impact on classroom transactions. She is also Psychology Facilitator at 21K School, Bangalore, Karnataka, India.

Dr Divya Bhatia is Assistant Professor at O.P. Jindal Global University, Sonipat, Haryana, India. She is Associate Director of Research and Experimentation at the Emotion & Cognition Psychology Research Centre (E-Cog) at O.P. Jindal Global University. She obtained her PhD in behavioural neuroscience from Sapienza University, Rome, Italy. She is an accomplished academician and researcher who published in peer-reviewed journals and presented her work at international conferences. Her primary focus of research is working memory and cognition. She has successfully received several research grants, such as research start-up grants, joint mobility grants, and, more recently, Global Engagement Seed Grant.

Dr Deepak Pandiaraj is Assistant Professor and Director of the E-Cog (Emotion and Cognition) Research Centre at O.P. Jindal Global University. He had been associated with prestigious institutes such as IIT Bombay and National Metallurgical Laboratory, Chennai, as Research Fellow. His M.Phil. research was focused on the psychology of self-conscious emotion and doctoral research on philosophical psychology approaches to communication for social/self-transformation. He developed a self-decentring communication model and applied it to analyse film, fiction, and modern science. His current research pertains to "Heuristics in Decision making", "Phenomenology of Self-decentering", and "Logo-therapy in the Indian context".

Dr Garima Joshi is Assistant Professor at Christ University, Delhi. She obtained her doctorate in Clinical Neuropsychology from All India Institute of Medical Sciences, New Delhi, India. Her research interests lie in clinical neuropsychology, studying brain–behaviour relationships, and assessing cognitive functions in various clinical populations. She is working to develop effective interventions and treatment strategies for individuals with neurocognitive impairments. She actively engages in clinical practice, assessing and treating individuals with neurological and psychological disorders. She is also well-published in various national and international peer-reviewed journals.

Josbert Gyereh is from Ghana, completed his master's degree from the University of Chester, UK, supported by the Commonwealth Master's Scholarship, and is presently Nursing Assistant for Barts Health NHS Trust at St Bartholomew's Hospital in London. He has worked on an interdisciplinary study investigating how developmental psychology might be used in the criminal justice system. His work on systematic review at the University of Chester earned him a distinction. His areas of interest lie in systematic reviews and meta-analysis with a specialisation in advanced statistical skills in SPSS, jamovi, STATA, and R.

Mrinalini Mahajan is a New Delhi-based gold medallist Clinical Psychologist and Psychotherapist who completed her MPhil from the National Institute of Mental Health and Neurosciences, Bangalore, India. She had been a meritorious student throughout her academic pursuits securing a gold medal twice and a silver medal once. She has experience working with individuals with psychiatric difficulties and survivors of various forms of abuse. Her particular interest is working with individuals with trauma histories, which aligns with her research interest. She believes in acknowledging and appreciating the role of social justice, intersectionality, and sociopolitical frameworks in mental health.

Dr Meenakshi Shukla is Assistant Professor of Psychology at the University of Allahabad, Prayagraj, India, and obtained her PhD from Banaras Hindu University, Varanasi, Uttar Pradesh, India. She has received a fellowship from the University Grants Commission of India and a Commonwealth Split-site (PhD) Scholarship for her doctorate. Her research interests involve exploring the relationship of emotions and emotional disorders with health, and she has published extensively in reputed journals and presented research papers at national and international conferences. She is a member of several national and international academic bodies such as the Indian Science Congress Association, American Psychological Association, International Association of Applied Psychology, and Association for Psychological Science.

Maneela Sirisety is Doctoral Scholar working on "Psychosocial factors underlying mob behaviour in India" at Rashtriya Raksha University, Gujarat, India. Her research interests are transdisciplinary, transnational, and translational. She has working experience in prominent institutions in India, such as UNESCO MGIEP and IIM Visakhapatnam. She also has experience working with national and international non-profit organisations. Her working areas are social psychology and personality, cyberpsychology, media psychology, geriatrics, positive psychology, and entrepreneurship.

Dr Nidhi Mishra is Assistant Professor at the Gandhi Institute of Technology and Management, Visakhapatnam. She completed her Doctorate from the University of

Allahabad, Prayagraj, Uttar Pradesh, India. She has worked in national and international research projects focusing on health and well-being, identity and collective experiences, lived experiences of stigmatised and marginalised groups, ageing, and inclusive education. She has working experience in psycho-social gerontology. She was previously involved in the United Nations Population Funds project on Building Knowledge Base on Ageing in India. She has represented India in the United Nations International Program in Policy Formulation, Planning, Implementation and Monitoring of the Madrid International Plan of Action on Ageing in Malta. She founded and managed Senior Express – an online initiative to promote active ageing in India.

Dr Neethu Pathiyan Satheesh is currently working as Assistant Professor in the Department of Sports Psychology, Central University of Rajasthan. She has completed her PhD in Applied Psychology from Pondicherry University, Kalapet, Pondicherry, India. Her core research areas are environmental psychology, sports psychology, and health and well-being. She has published articles in national and international journals and edited books for international publishers. She received the Prof. Deepak Bhatt Award and Dr Barbara Hanfstingl InSPA Award.

Niti Upadhyay is Research Scholar pursuing her PhD in Psychology from Banaras Hindu University. She is currently investigating the relationship of mindfulness with mental health and the role of decentring, non-attachment and emotion regulation difficulties in explaining the mindfulness–mental health relationship in her doctoral endeavour. Her research focuses on understanding mindfulness' mechanism(s) on mental health. She is working on making an absolute model of mindfulness and mental health relationship to help plan strategies and interventions to reduce mental health problems and enhance mental health. She is currently working on a funded project related to mindfulness.

Ritika Chokhani is a Mumbai-based Researcher and Clinical Psychologist and completed her M.Sc. with Inlaks scholarship from University College London. She is Research Coordinator on a project to update the National Guidelines on Psychosocial Support and Mental Health in Disasters in India through the Tata Institute of Social Sciences (TISS) and the National Disaster Management Authority (NDMA) of India. She is an experienced mental health professional. Her core area of interest is mental health and psychotherapy. According to her, mental health is to be informed and guided by principles of social justice and people's own lived experiences and know-how.

Dr Ravi Shanker Datti is Assistant Professor at the Department of Applied Psychology, GITAM School of Gandhian Studies, Visakhapatnam, Andhra Pradesh, India. He completed his Doctorate in Health Psychology from Andhra University. He had served as Capacity Building Officer for the Global Fund project. He started his career in teaching at the Department of Psychology at Adikavi Nannaya

University, Rajahmundry, Andhra Pradesh, India, and headed the department for seven years. Beck Institute trains him as Cognitive Behavioural Therapist. He had delivered a series of lectures at James Madison University, Virginia. Further, he has extended his research collaboration on Cyberpsychology with URAL Federal University, Russia.

Shruti Dua is Assistant Professor at Rukmini Devi Institute of Advanced Studies, Delhi, India. She graduated in Psychology from the University of Delhi. She is a practising student counsellor focusing on students' personal, academic, and professional lives. She is an experienced counsellor oriented towards dealing with human behaviour dynamics. She has presented her research works at various international and national conferences. Previously, she worked at O.P. Jindal Global University, where she was involved in research projects and taught elective courses.

Subhash Meena is working as Assistant Professor of Psychology at the University of Delhi, Delhi. He is an accomplished writer who has published research papers and articles in national and international journals and presented research papers at national and international conferences. He is on the editorial board of *Vasant Sahastradhara: An Interdisciplinary Journal*. He is actively associated with several academic bodies, such as the Indian Academy of Applied Psychology, the Somatic Ink Blot Society, and the International Society for Research and Development. He received the "Young Scientist Award" in 2014 from the Indian Academy of Applied Psychology (IAAP), Ahmedabad, Gujarat, India.

Dr Sadananda Reddy obtained his Doctoral Degree from the NIMHANS, and his work centred on "Development and Feasibility Testing of a Supported Education Program for Students with Mental Health Issues". His work focused on Pathways to Psychiatric Care in Children and Adolescents with First Episode Psychosis. He is also Research Fellow in the IMPACT project, NIHR, funded through the University of York. He also worked as Psychiatric Social Worker at the National Institute of Mental Health in Neurosciences. He received an ICSSR grant for a project entitled "Exploring the Mental Health Help Seeking Practices and Policies Among Higher Educational Institutions in Bangalore: A Qualitative Study".

Shikha Soni is Doctoral Research Scholar in Psychology at the Indian Institute of Technology Hyderabad, Hyderabad, Telangana, India. She completed her M.Phil. in Clinical Psychology from the Central Institute of Psychiatry, Ranchi, India, and is registered with the Rehabilitation Council of India. She has been trained in psychological testing like psycho diagnostics, intelligence tests, and neuropsychology and therapies like cognitive behaviour therapy, behaviour therapy, supportive therapy, and marital/family therapy. Her research interests bridge the areas of positive, social, personality, and clinical psychology. She is currently researching the area of positive adaptation to loss through the unique lens of life stories.

Vijeyata Chauhan is a research scholar who completed her master's degree from Banaras Hindu University and is presently pursuing her M.Phil. in Clinical Psychology from Gautam Buddha University, Uttar Pradesh, India. She has experience working as a counselling psychologist with Salaam Baalak Trust, New Delhi, India, and an NGO focusing on street children in and around the national capital region. She has presented a couple of research papers at international conferences. Her academic interest lies in developing indigenous mental health interventions for the local population and bridging the gap between science and spirituality.

FOREWORD

The pandemic of COVID-19, after shaking the entire humanity, has forced modern man walking on the path of progress to rethink the risks involved in the journey of development. Coronavirus had suddenly engulfed most of the countries of Asia, Europe, and North America and affected many states of India as well. Unfortunately, no country was fully prepared to face such a disaster. This highly contagious and deadly virus had severely affected personal and social lives by disrupting the rhythm and pace of life globally. With the passage of time, the number of patients affected by it increased tremendously. Everyone's life was getting disturbed under the shadow of this terror. This invisible virus gave rise to an infectious disease – its medium or carrier could be any person or object already infected. It was so subtle that it could not be directly experienced and inferred only by its manifestations. It could be detected only by a special type of diagnostic test. Its symptoms were also not visible initially in many patients and appeared quite late. The difficulty was that its symptoms were similar to unhealthy conditions like the common cold, cold, runny nose, cough, difficulty in breathing and fever, which attack the body system together. The World Health Organization termed it an "epidemic". The disease's transmission mode was through coughing, sneezing, shaking hands, and coming in contact with a surface where the virus is present. That's why it spread quickly and became fatal if proper medical help did not reach in time. It had adversely impacted national economies and jeopardised various developmental projects at global levels. It forced countries to redefine their economic and political equations with other countries. Against this backdrop, *Exploring the Psycho-Social Impact of COVID-19: Global Perspectives on Behaviour, Interventions and Future Directions*, jointly edited by Verma, Uzaina, Singh, Tiwari, and Manickam, is a welcome contribution to health psychology. It offers the state of psychological knowledge about health-related challenges faced by humanity in coping with COVID-19. Drawing upon the findings from diverse scientific studies across different regions, they furnish evidence about the psycho-social cost of this epidemic in terms of psycho-social and psychophysiological challenges faced by the people, including grief and bereavement. The contributions to this volume bring together the variability in the pattern of prosocial behaviour and the effectiveness of interventions, including cognitive behavioural therapy (CBT), spirituality, and positive adaptation in the context of a pandemic. Finally, the volume examines the issue of vaccine reluctance and the potential of digital health technologies and infrastructure.

Indeed, the situation created by the virus was unique and unprecedented in many respects. The course of events leading to contact with the virus was of unavoidable nature. The person coming in contact with an infected person in any manner became the carrier of infection. Hence, the process of infection went on uninterruptedly. In such a situation, breaking the spread link became an ultimate challenge, and the possibility of virus infection substantially increased. The nature of the problem was further complicated by the high degree of similarity of this disease with cold and fever. Symptoms similar to cough, cold, and fever made it like pneumonia, and lung infection became fatal. Due to poor immunity in the case of diabetes and heart disease, etc., this infection increased the difficulties of the sick. It was not easy to detect, and, interestingly, people avoided its disclosure, although infected people recovered by getting proper treatment on time. Therefore, it was not in anyone's interest to ignore the disease by acting with preconceived notions. But, the prejudices did operate, and the story of the struggle to overcome this complex health issue took many turns. The virus was new to humanity, and, in the initial stages, no definite medicine for a clear line of treatment was available. Without a vaccine or a definitive drug, the only way to contain the infection was prevention, that is to prevent human-to-human contact. Keeping this in mind, the decision was taken to impose a lockdown. The decision to lock down was extremely difficult and painful; yet, there was no other way to save lives.

Due to this, the work of businesses; traffic operations; and running of educational institutions, courts, parliament, and legislative assembly all came to a standstill. It had a detrimental effect on the daily routine of common people. The migrant daily wage labourers were forced to leave the cities for their villages. Despite the extreme difficulties, people accepted the lockdown, and thankfully the efforts yielded good results. But the sparse events of not complying with social distancing norms were also witnessed. The possibility of infection increased rapidly because more contact started pouring in continuously from different regions. Due to such irresponsible behaviour, controlling the infection became a real problem. The government had to make tough decisions to deal with this worrying situation.

The collective war of humanity against COVID-19 was unprecedented. The fear of infection was intense as no one knew when and how someone will come into its grip. Everyday things were arranged to be managed through online modes such as "booking" and e-paying, and the material was delivered. People were continuously hooked to their TV sets for updates within the walls of their homes. The lifestyle was new, and the unexpected change disrupted people's lives. People of different age groups and professions were asked to redefine their habitual ways and familiar roles and to switch to newer ways. In times of uncertainty, the experience of social isolation and social distance was causing anxiety, fatigue, and stress. Symptoms of depression were also visible in many people.

Along with emotional confusion, feelings of insecurity also intensified in the people. Cases of disturbances in eating habits and sleep patterns were registered with e-platforms, although each person appeared to be reacting differently to the onset of this sudden situation. The availability of vaccines became a great relief. The same, however, was initially resisted. However, with sincere efforts of government agencies and large-scale campaigns, the vaccine was accepted, saving people's lives.

The reviews of studies reported in *Exploring the Psycho-Social Impact of COVID-19* suggest that health operates in a matrix of sociocultural and contextual factors. The health-related challenges, therefore, have multiple routes. Combating COVID-19 as an invisible enemy requires courage, hope, contentment, and a flexible mindset. Solving the challenge by recognising, organising, and redefining the experience in a new way and adopting a creative approach often lead to a sense of meaning. How we react to these difficult times also depends on how we perceive the situation and how proactively and cautiously we face the upcoming challenges. In difficult times, seeking the meaning of life becomes necessary by accepting the changed life conditions and organising life free from fear and anxiety. Parents are role models for children, so it is necessary to talk to children, asking them to relax, avoid the sea of information and rumours floating on social media, and rely on reliable information. One should also learn to work with contentment and patience with a sense of cleanliness and personal hygiene. People need to protect themselves and help their neighbours. To this end, a balanced diet, regular routine, and physical exercise must be maintained so that the body's immune system remains strong. There is no substitute for restraint, patience, and self-control.

The health of the elderly and children requires special attention. It is necessary that instead of narrowing our lives, we should be ready to expand and fight problems with patience. While the COVID-19 pandemic had plagued everyone's life, it cleared the illusions prevailing in our lives, about which we all were getting very confident. The present volume illustrates that health is the greatest asset and that a relationship of mutual dependence and complementarity between human beings and nature can nurture it. It also underscores the value of systematic interventions at individual and societal levels to restore and promote health. Rich in scope, the present volume highlights the role of psycho-social processes and contextual factors in shaping health outcomes in complex happenings in highly ambiguous and challenging times. It will be received well by the students, scholars, and practitioners in the area of health psychology and health behaviour.

Girishwar Misra, PhD, FNAPsy,
Special Issue Editor Psychological Studies (Springer)
Former National Fellow (ICSSR)
Ex-Vice Chancellor, Mahatma Gandhi Antarrashtriya Hindi Vishwavidyalaya,
Wardha (Maharashtra), India
Ex-Head and Professor, Department of Psychology, University of Delhi

PREFACE

The last few days of the year 2019 witnessed something strange and unprecedented. A virus (novel coronavirus) whose origin is still debated typically entered the human bio-network. The virus pragmatically paralysed the globe within three months and confined people within the walls of their homes. It was nothing less than a total upheaval laden with uncertainty, helplessness, and, more importantly, hopelessness. Finally, a global pandemic led by COVID-19, a novel coronavirus, was declared. The impact of COVID-19 was multidimensional, sparking a cascade of extensive consequences across almost all domains of human life, where the fear factor was one of the major players in the killing of people. It was estimated that more people died due to physiological complications consequent to psychological complications than physiological complications alone, which led to the significance of exploring the psychological impact of the virus.

Exploring the Psycho-Social Impact of COVID-19: Global Perspectives on Behaviour, Interventions and Future Directions is a unique combination of systematic reviews of studies done during this time, which covers all three components, that is the impact of the virus, evidence-based psychological interventions, and lessons learnt for future preparedness. This book is aimed to provide a comprehensive and academically rigorous examination of coronavirus impact. It contains an analysis of studies, which delves deep into the intricate web of emotions, thoughts, and behaviours that have emerged in human beings in the wake of the pandemic. This book endeavours to provide a comprehensive and academically rigorous exploration of the psychological dimensions of the COVID-19 pandemic, encompassing the profound effects on individuals. *Exploring the Psycho-Social Impact of COVID-19* results from extensive research and the latest scientific findings.

The book comprises ten chapters, each containing findings from many scientific studies. This way, it is not exaggerated to say that the book is a macrocosm of global findings which added a pool of knowledge to understand the multifaceted nature of the psychological impact of COVID-19. It focuses on how the tech-baby [virus] gripped susceptible populations, leading to extreme measures by regulators such as social isolation, total lockdown, and acute mobility restrictions to contain the great spread. These measures impacted the population in the form of loneliness, dark stress, fear of the unknown, and fear of contagion from the known experienced by individuals.

It is not the first time that the world has faced a pandemic of such a scale. However, this time, the response pattern of governments and the general population has certain unique features, such as addressing psychological needs, collective and cooperative behaviour, philanthropic efforts, technological interventions, and preparedness. The book delves deep into the interventions and coping mechanisms humanity employs to mitigate the death toll arising from the virus. It explains how the pandemic reminded the efficacy of prosocial behaviour and philanthropy in circumventing and mitigating the impact of virus-led crises on fellow human beings. The book examines the efficacy of Digital Infrastructure for Psychological Support and other online support groups in dealing with tech-baby-related complications. The studies are collated in a way that explores the role of cognitive behavioural therapy in navigating people in these challenging times. Through this book, we seek to provide a roadmap for healing and resilience in the face of adversity.

Considering the fragility of the human psyche, we included the lessons gleaned from the pandemic for future generations, including the indelible mark on the collective psyche of the generation who helplessly witnessed the gross destruction that had a lasting impact. The lessons learnt are expected to equip us all to deal with future challenges of a similar scale. The learnings from the first-hand experience of going through the pandemic are expected to prepare us for the development of more targeted and effective interventions in advance.

Exploring the Psycho-Social Impact of COVID-19 is expected to serve as a valuable scholarly resource for students, academicians, researchers, mental health practitioners, policymakers, and individuals curious to understand the psychological impact of the pandemic on the general population. It is an attempt to synthesise and present the existing knowledge in a scholarly and accessible manner. This academic effort initiates further research by stimulating and encouraging multidisciplinary collaboration.

We sincerely acknowledge the contribution of psychologists, mental health professionals, academicians, researchers, scholars, and healthcare professionals who have worked extensively on the psychological dimensions of COVID-19. Their contributions provided the base for this project, and we hope it will continue to shape the collective understanding of the psychological impact of the pandemics. We hope this book serves as a piece of scholarly evidence of the power of psychology in enhancing the quality of life of human beings.

Editors,
Dr Rajesh Verma and Dr Uzaina
Co-Editors,
Dr Gyanesh Kumar Tiwari, Prof. Leister Sam Sudheer Manickam,
and Dr Tushar Singh

ACKNOWLEDGEMENTS

Writing a book is a collaborative effort that involves the dedication and support of numerous individuals. *Exploring the Psycho-Social Impact of COVID-19: Global Perspectives on Behaviour, Interventions and Future Directions* would not have been possible without the contribution and encouragement of many remarkable people we would like to acknowledge with heartfelt gratitude.

First and foremost, we sincerely appreciate this edited book's contributors, whose insightful contributions have enriched every chapter. Their expertise, research, and commitment to shedding light on the psychological aspects of the COVID-19 pandemic have been truly invaluable.

We express our deepest thanks to our publisher for believing in the significance of this work and supporting us throughout the publication process. Your guidance and professionalism have been instrumental in shaping this book.

We thank the peer reviewers who provided valuable feedback and constructive criticism, helping us refine and improve the content, making it more comprehensive and meaningful.

Our heartfelt appreciation goes to all the healthcare professionals, researchers, and frontline workers who worked tirelessly to combat the pandemic. Your unwavering dedication and sacrifice have been a constant source of inspiration.

We are immensely grateful to our families and friends for their unwavering support, understanding, and encouragement during the countless hours spent researching, writing, and editing this book.

Lastly, we thank all the readers who will engage with this book. We hope that the insights and knowledge presented within these pages will contribute to a deeper understanding of the psychological impact of COVID-19 and pave the way for better interventions and future insights.

Thank you, each and every one of you, for your invaluable contributions to *Exploring the Psycho-Social Impact of COVID-19: Global Perspectives on Behaviour, Interventions and Future Directions*. Your support has been the driving force behind this endeavour, and we are truly grateful for the opportunity to present this work to the world.

With warm regards,
The Editors

SECTION 1

Impact

1

CORONAVIRUS

The Dreaded Avatar That Surprised Humanity

Rajesh Verma

COVID-19, the dreaded alphanumeric abbreviation, has been associated with comprehensive psycho-physical consequences. Coronavirus disease (COVID-19) is an infectious disease caused by the SARS-CoV-2 virus (WHO, 2019) that proved to be a significant health stressor (Brooks et al., 2020). It profoundly affected total health, left a trail of new events, made typical medical science technical words part of common parlance, modified human behaviour to the extent of uprooting social norms, and, more importantly, surprised humanity (Clemente-Suarez et al., 2020). The paradigms of human interaction were overhauled to more unique forms. The psycho-biological footprints of COVID-19 are still lying inexpressive in the cognitive landscape of humanity. The psychological impact was to the extent that a new form of pandemic-specific phobia, that is coronaphobia (Arora et al., 2020), has emerged in psychological literature. The primary difficulty lies in the uniqueness of the virus structure, impact, and targeted human body organs. The scientific community was in a fix because it was a novel strain of coronavirus (Goyal et al., 2020) to humans. The situation was more like fighting an invisible enemy in the darkness without armour and arms.

The transmission rate was the highest, and it took just 11 weeks (Verma, 2023) to engulf 213 countries (Ojha et al., 2020) in its grip. Considering the faster rate of transmission and no cure in sight, WHO on 30 January 2020 declared the outbreak to be a public health emergency of international concern (PHEIC) and, later on 11 March 2020, upgraded it to the scale of pandemic. The declaration of the outbreak as a pandemic led to the more often manifestation of negative emotions (Clemente-Suarez et al., 2020), suicide (Mamun et al., 2020; Goyal et al., 2020), and suicide ideation (Lee, 2020), and pessimism was at the top of the cognition among the general population. It was the first pandemic post-ICT and AI era, leading to a social-media-mandated infodemic (Hao & Basu, 2020). Interestingly, the same

DOI: 10.4324/9781003357209-2

technology was instrumental in implementing the measures designed to contain the spread (Pandey et al., 2021). It was a biomedical catastrophe (Verma, 2023) designed to inflict a heavy pressure on global health infrastructure and likely to increase the global health burden. COVID-19, the pandemic of digital times, necessitated a zero-mobility situation of lockdown and social isolation to contain its spread. The lockdowns and social isolation took their psychological toll. Verma (2023, p. 218) made an exciting revelation: "For the first time in human history, various government and non-government agencies realised the importance of mental health and responded quite well with building up mental health infrastructure".

The evidence suggests that psychophysiological complications were prevalent not only among COVID-19 patients but also among those who were not afflicted. The most common mental health challenges (Bhuiyan et al., 2020) faced by individuals during the pandemic include psychological distress (Zhang et al., 2020), anxiety, depression (47 studies examined the prevalence of anxiety and depression) (Schou et al., 2021), sleep disorders (Xiong et al., 2021) post-traumatic stress symptoms (Rudroff et al., 2020), and other psychosomatic manifestations (Yang et al., 2020). At the initial stage, the organic menace was handled with the traditional approach of looking at the outbreak from a physiological perspective. However, the larger perspective, the combination of psychological and physiological aspects, was ignored even by WHO. Later specific studies found that psychological complications were responsible for enhanced morbidity. The psychological toll of the virus has been exacerbated by factors such as the constant fear of infection (Shanafelt et al., 2020); isolation; and strict mobility measures such as complete lockdowns, and excessive media reporting (Pedrosa et al., 2020). Media, particularly electronic media, took centre stage and became mainstream information feeders creating an information-explosion-type situation. The information explosion (Booth, 1996) made the situation challenging. Arora et al. (2020) call the relentless information flow "infodemia". During the lockdowns, people felt relaxed at the initial stage, as in the case of vacations, but later began to manifest a chain of symptoms typical to mental health disorders (Clemente-Suarez et al., 2020). One of the most significant factors in developing mental health issues was witnessing others suffering, fear of infection of loved ones (Shanafelt et al., 2020), and death of others due to infection. The death of loved ones, which was sudden and unexpected (Goveas & Shear, 2020), engendered death anxiety (Corpuz, 2021), hopelessness (Lee, 2020), and helplessness. The sudden onset of the pandemic caught humanity unprepared. It hammered the cognitive piece of the human body, leading to a perception that life is trivial, temporary, and unworthy of living. These recurring ideas generated a host of negative emotions in those infected with COVID-19, caregivers, the general population who were glued to the e-screen for news updates, and frontline healthcare professionals. The negative emotions have a link with various neurological complications (Egbert et al., 2020), including encephalopathy, cerebrovascular events (strokes), and Guillain–Barre syndrome (31 cases of GBS are related to COVID-19 (Rahimi, 2020). Neurological manifestations, such as cognitive impairments (Schou et al., 2021; Zhou et al., 2020) and emotional disturbances, can result in psychophysiological consequences. Furthermore, individuals experiencing "long COVID" or post-acute sequelae of SARS-CoV-2 infection have reported persistent mental health issues, highlighting an important intersection between physical and mental well-being. The healthcare providers on the frontline (Pedrosa et al., 2020), too, have been subjected to immense stress, facing unprecedented challenges in managing patient care and being at a higher risk of developing mental health issues. The pandemic has brought into focus the importance of understanding and addressing the psychological complications experienced by individuals worldwide. Prevalence rates of anxiety (35%), depression (35%) (Hu et al., 2020; Arslan et al., 2020; Dubey et al., 2020; Barron et al., 2021), post-traumatic stress disorder (PTSD) (Bao et al., 2020), and other mental health issues have been alarmingly high, necessitating urgent action to integrate mental health support into the global pandemic response. By acknowledging the profound impact of the pandemic on mental well-being, healthcare systems and policymakers can work towards providing comprehensive and accessible mental health services to mitigate the psychophysiological burden of COVID-19 and promote resilience among affected populations. The pandemic is, of course, extremely challenging. Still, it has opened the gates for a few new opportunities. These sentiments are echoed by Murthy (2014) while referring to the Bhopal Gas Tragedy of 1984 in his concluding remarks, "Disasters are a challenge in every country, for the affected populations as well as the mental health professionals, and they represent special challenges and opportunities in developing countries".

Opportunities Offered by the COVID-19 Pandemic

COVID-19 offered various psychological, social, economic, scientific, political, and technological opportunities. However, addressing social, economic, scientific, political, and technological type of opportunities is beyond the scope of this text. I am interested in discussing only the psychological opportunities available to humanity in this section.

- Coping with indigenous strategies (homemade masks, using Mahua flower extract as a potential sanitiser[1]), that is people were forced to look for solutions within their immediate environs.
- Overcoming the irrationality attached to the fear of contracting the virus [coronaphobia] (Arora et al., 2020).
- Strengthening resilience (lessons from the first and second waves mitigated the impact of the third wave).
- Adjustment and adaptation (learning to live without physical, social contacts).
- Coping with cognitive fatigue (modifying the belief system with indigenous relaxation strategies such as *Vipassana Dhyan*, Pranayama, *Sudarshan Kriya*, *Kapaal Bhaanti*, and *Yoga*).

- Isolation management (Yoga, meditation, and strengthened faith in gurus and deities).
- Strengthening of interpersonal [family] bonds (proximity of family members reinforced the genetic support system, upholding the social support theory of Cohen & Wills, 1985).
- Psychological preparedness (psycho-education (Vieta, 2005) and readiness for new challenges.
- Behaviour modifications (importance of hygiene) {regular hand washing, elbow sneezing, sanitising hands, shifting to new ways of greeting (*Namaste*), and avoiding handshake}.
- Handling uncertainty {psycho-education (Vieta, 2005)}.
- Distress tolerance {Unconditional acceptance (Bhattacharjee & Ghosh, 2022)}.

Against the backdrop of an all-out attack of coronavirus on humanity and consequent widespread death and psychological destruction (Malik et al., 2020; Kaurani et al., 2020; Singh et al., 2021; Singh et al., 2020), the present volume offers scientific insight gleaned from 196 studies published in English from 2019 to 2022. The book has been designed to present the synthesised findings from the research specific to COVID-19.

Why Reviews?

COVID-19 emerged as a significant research topic and generated substantial scientific literature. According to Teixeira da Silva et al. (2020), 23,634 unique documents were published between 1 January and 30 June 2020. The International Association of Scientific, Technical and Medical Publishers (2020, June 24) reports, "Scientific research papers on COVID-19 have been downloaded more than 150 million times since the international publishing community provided free access to tens of thousands of articles".

Before explaining the rationale for incorporating reviews in the book, let us first examine the brief introduction of different reviews used in the present volume.

Systematic Review

The primary objective of a systematic review is to synthesise the existing scientific literature on a specific research statement, question, subject, or topic. Reviews tend to provide clarity and valuable insights to the readers (Sataloff et al., 2021). Reviews, particularly systematic reviews, provide qualitative and quantitative outputs. Considering the scale and widespread impact of the COVID-19 pandemic, a considerable amount of scientific literature has emerged. The availability of a large amount of scientific literature related to COVID-19 makes it difficult for the reader and other stakeholders, such as policymakers, healthcare professionals (Evans, 2004), and academicians, to select the appropriate research for practice and application. Excess information made the situation complicated. Evans (2004, p. 8) rightly pointed out that "this complexity can serve as a barrier to research utilisation". It was impossible to collate and subsequently record all available scientific literature in one volume. To overcome this, systematic review approach was found most suitable.

Scoping Review

Scoping reviews are literary tools to dig deeper into emerging areas in a specific field or subject. The literary synthesisers include in their scope all forms of articles, not just peer-reviewed ones (Levac et al., 2010). Mak and Thomas (2022) suggest that scoping review provides a potential gap in the literature and scope for future research. The scale of the COVID-19 pandemic was massive in terms of spread, death, destruction, and impact; it caught up and inflicted damage to everything related to human beings. In light of COVID-19 and its impact, it was imperative to document the findings in one volume for quicker and easy reference; for this, scoping review offered scope to include even grey literature (Maggio et al., 2020) in its manifold, which has the potential to maintain relevancy and validity of the present book.

Narrative Review

A narrative review is another literature-synthesising tool based on collecting scientific evidence, commonly called the collative strategy. Descriptiveness is the primary strength of narrative review, providing a qualitative summary through a scientific perspective. It encompasses a qualitative component, which makes it prone to subjective and selection biases. However, the very nature of the narrative review is flexible, relatively less rigorous, and systematic than other review approaches. Though the qualitative literature on COVID-19 was lesser in quantity, authors who adopted this approach found nine articles worth reviewing. The idea to include a narrative review is based on the all-encompassing approach of the present volume.

Thematic Analysis

The thematic analysis approach's central thrust is identifying patterns or, in other words, under-laying themes in qualitative structured and unstructured data (Braun & Clarke, 2006; Daly et al., 1997; Saldana, 2009). The qualitative data includes interviews, focus groups, surveys, textual documents, and open-ended questions' responses. The authors of Chapter 7 used thematic analysis to identify the potential unperceived set of patterns hidden within the observed data set. It is, of course, a blessing in disguise for the book. The chapter offers one of the widely used data analysis approaches for the readers of the volume. With this data analysis approach, the book has become an amalgamation of the most used data-synthesising approaches.

The reviews provide meta-findings, that is findings from the various findings to form literary milestones for researchers and scientific writers. Identifying research gaps, presenting research mobility trends, collating theoretical frameworks, establishing quality assessment paradigms, and re-assessing the contemporary literature devoted to a specific subject or topic are some of the essential functions and purposes of various scientific reviews. The reviews serve as tools for organising and presenting the current research, ultimately driving the academic progression and facilitating decision-makers for evidence-based decision-making. Therefore, to keep this volume relevant for all academic tastes, the editorial team included all those studies' approaches [reviews] that attempted to synthesise the scientific literature on COVID-19 in the most suitable and convincing style for the readers. I am pretty sure that we have succeeded in this original endeavour.

Volume Characteristics

The present volume comprises chapters based on systematic reviews (5, 55%), narrative reviews (1, 11%), scoping review (1, 11%), thematic analysis (1, 11%), and systematic literature reviews (1, 11%) (Table 1.1, Figures 1.1 and 1.2). One chapter (7th) is based on an independent study where the authors used thematic analysis. The population (total sample – 21,69,633) ages are within the range of 12 to 89 years. The period for the studies to be included in the review protocols was from 2019 onwards.

TABLE 1.1 Summary

Chapter No.	Review Type	No. of Studies Reviewed	Total Sample	Focal Variable in the Backdrop of COVID-19
2	Systematic review	28	46,048	Psycho-physical complications
3	Systematic review	26	Not reported	Prosocial behaviour
4	Systematic review	17	2,701	Cognitive behaviour therapy
5	Narrative review	9	Not reported	Spiritual process
6	Scoping review	15	3,944	Grief and bereavement
7	Thematic analysis	Independent study	10	Positive adaptation
8	Systematic review	54	21,14,783	Vaccine reluctance
9	Systematic literature review	37	Not reported	Digital health technologies
10	Systematic review	9	2,147	Digital infrastructure providing psychological support
	Total	196	21,69,633	

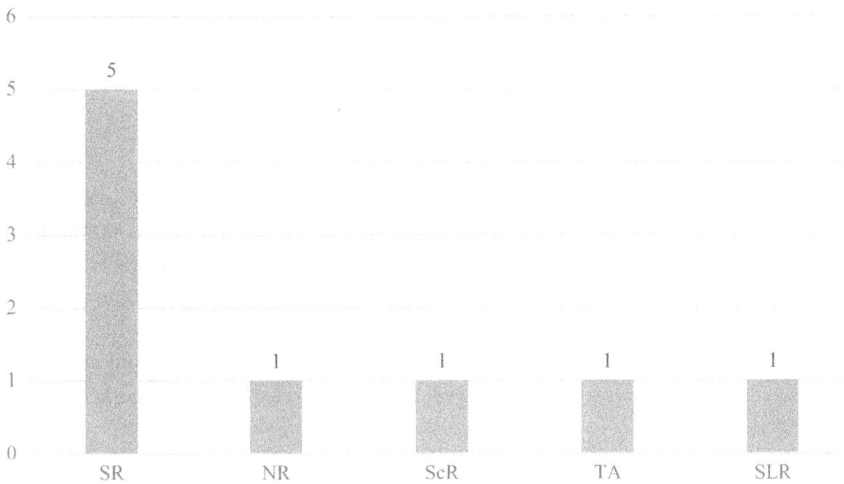

FIGURE 1.1 Different review types

Abbreviations: SR, systematic review; NR, narrative review; ScR, scoping review; TA, thematic analysis; SLR, systematic literature review.

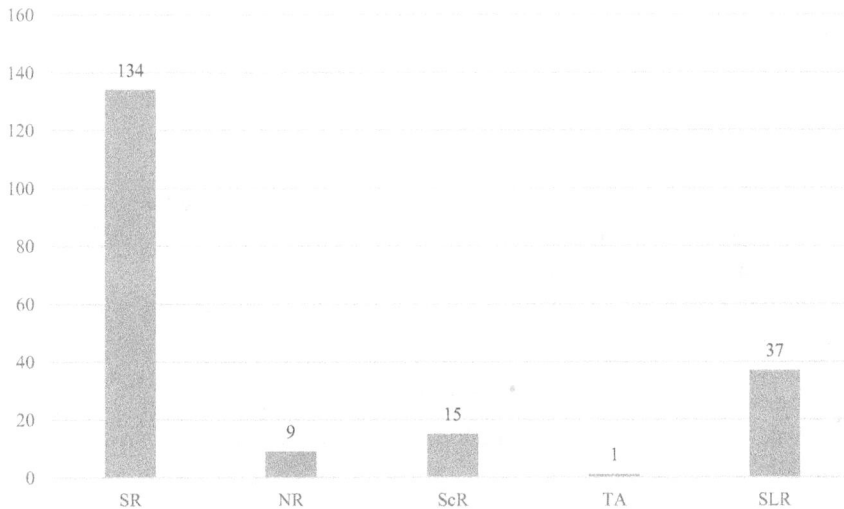

FIGURE 1.2 Number of studies included in different review types

Brief Summary of Contents

The book's title, "Exploring the Psycho-Social Impact of COVID-19: Global Perspectives on Behaviour, Interventions and Future Directions", is an all-encompassing, comprehensive, and multidimensional exploration of the psychological paradigms associated with the COVID-19 pandemic. The three elements, namely, "Psycho-Social Impact (PS-Impact), Interventions and Future Directions" in the title portray the scope and contents of the book.

Psycho-Social Impact (PS-Impact)

PS-impact refers to how deeply COVID-19 and its subsidiary dreaded institutions penetrated the core of the psycho-social landscape of individuals and communities. The purpose of studying the PS-impact of COVID-19 is associated with wide-ranging impact, encompassing behavioural, cognitive, and social responses to the pandemic. The section has been designed to explore the psycho-social morbidity, genesis or aggravation of mental disorders such as anxiety, depression, stress, irrational fear (phobia), grief, and apparent changes in interpersonal interaction and behaviours.

Interventions

It implies exploring the various coping strategies such as behavioural, mindful, and social media coping (Barron et al., 2021); scientific programmes; and interventions implemented to address the psychological challenges posed by the pandemic. It could include discussions on therapeutic approaches, mental health support, crisis helplines, online counselling, and other initiatives to mitigate adverse psychological effects.

Future Directions

This part of the title indicates that lessons learnt for handling any future pandemic go beyond the current state and delve into predictions and considerations for the future. The chapters written from this perspective encompass potential long-term psychological impacts, strategies for building resilience, and insights for preparing for similar crises in the future.

The impact of COVID-19 transcended physical health leading to a spiralling effect on various health dimensions, including psychological, social, economic, spiritual, and educational. Some of these dimensions covered in the book are mentioned in Table 1.2.

Conclusion

The book's contents indicate an interdisciplinary approach to understanding how the pandemic has affected and continues to affect individuals and societies. It covers the psychophysiological complications, helping others to ease their needs and mitigate their challenges through prosocial behaviour; well-established, evidence-based standard interventions, such as CBT [i & o]; spirituality; behavioural and

TABLE 1.2 Major health dimensions covered in the book*

Health Dimension	Dimension Type			Factors/Interventions/Strategies/Outcomes
	Psychological	Physiological	Digital	
Fatigue	–	✓	–	Higher rates visible across studies
PTSD	✓	–	–	Higher rates visible across studies
Anxiety	✓	–	–	Higher rates visible across studies
Depression	✓	–	–	Higher rates visible across studies
Burnout and stress	✓	–	–	Higher rates visible across studies
Insomnia	✓	–	–	Higher rates visible across studies
Prosocial behaviour and mental health	✓	–	–	A significant association between the two
[i & o]** Cognitive behavioural therapy	✓	–	–	Instrumental in mitigating the severity of mental health-related symptoms
Chronic insomnia	✓	✓	–	Higher rates
Mindfulness	✓	–	–	Instrumental in reducing anxiety and depression scores
Spirituality	✓	–	–	Component of total health, likely to prove crucial in providing holistic health services
Grief and bereavement	✓	–	–	Psychological interventions such as Yoga, active listening, self-care, adaptation to new circumstances, mindfulness, heart-healing reading, gratitude expression, emotional validation, information sharing, psycho-education, bad news communications, felicitating loss accepting, group-based sessions, managing loss through structured writing, focused loss, desensitisation, closure and revaluation, forest bathing, visualisation

(Continued)

TABLE 1.2 (Continued)

Health Dimension	Dimension Type			Factors/Interventions/Strategies/Outcomes
	Psychological	Physiological	Digital	
Positive adaptation to fear and anxiety	✓	✓	–	Strategies used for positive adaptation include Yoga, web-based interventions, and acceptance of situations that might help in positive emotions.
Vaccine reluctance	✓	✓	–	Majorly demographic and psycho-social factors such as gender- and age-influenced vaccine reluctance.
Digital Health	–	–	✓	Ayushman Bharat Digital Mission, virtual visits, mobile health, wearable technology, digital therapeutics, artificial intelligence, and other digital platforms played essential and influential roles in comprehensive health management.
Digital Infrastructure for Psychological Support (DIPS)	–	–	✓	Virtual Yoga, mHealth, mindfulness-based mobile application (anxiety and depression), CORE application (BPD, MDD, schizophrenia), Foundations app, I-EAET, video-conferencing platform.
Bipolar Disorders, Major Depressive Disorders, Somatic Symptom Disorders, Eating Disorders, Schizophrenia, Stress, Anxiety, Depression	✓	–	–	Managed through virtual platforms

*Source: Respective authors of chapters in this book.

**i stands for Internet-based CBT and o stands for offline CBT.

emotional dimensions such as grief and bereavement; adaptation in the new normal scheme from the positive perspective; reluctance to pro-active virus-containing measures (vaccine); and virtual platforms for delivering psychological services popularly known as digital infrastructure for psychological support (DIPS).

Various psychophysiological complications can be attributed to COVID-19, including anxiety and depression, PTSD, cognitive impairments, sleep disturbances, chronic physical and cognitive fatigue, respiratory distress, cardiovascular effects, phobia, fears, grief, stress and stress-related complications, and other psychological distresses. It is essential for individuals experiencing any of these complications to seek appropriate medical and psychological support. Additionally, ongoing research is needed to fully understand the psychophysiological effects of COVID-19 and develop effective interventions.

Prosocial behaviour is not unique to human beings; it is found in animals too. Prosocial behaviour is a core component of human nature, which has an essential role in mental health, building a social network and strengthening interpersonal bonds, and it is one of the cohesive factors in building communities. Personal satisfaction-cum-deep-contentment, societal expectation, evolutionary adaptation, empathy, and reciprocity are crucial features associated with the manifestation of prosocial behaviour. The idea of Karma in Indian thought reinforces belief in prosocial behaviour. Evidence suggests that society responded with prosocial behaviour to the pandemic with unprecedented passion. Altruism, philanthropism, dedication, [formation of] mutual aid networks, and unconditional help have emerged as essential forms of prosocial behaviour during the pandemic. The large number of prosocial behavioural responses is probably the result of the internal drive of mutual solidarity and a sense of unity for the community's well-being.

Mental health is a crucial issue and has been adequately recognised during the infodemic-led pandemic. Interventions are the end action plans designed to modify clients' thought processes, behaviours, and response patterns. CBT is one of the scientific, structured, and evidence-based psychotherapeutic approaches. CBT effectively manages cognition and behaviour when delivered through competent professionals and in gradual sessions. CBT in both internet-based and face-to-face modes was instrumental in managing COVID-19-related psycho-behavioural symptoms of anxiety, depression, stress, insomnia, and PTSD. Evidence suggests that CBT proved effective in enhancing clients' self-esteem, significantly improving mental health conditions.

Adhyaatm, a Sanskrit word that roughly translates into "spiritual" in English, is a compound word with deep meaning and extensive connotative applications. *Adhyaatm* means *"Svayam ka Adhyayan"*, that is studying or knowing self by self-reflective enquiry and experience. It is a subjective and nuanced idea on the tapestry of the human mind developed by self-studying Indian civilisation. The association of self (*Atman*) with supreme consciousness (*Brahman*) is the core philosophical thought of *Adhyaatm*. The uncertainty and unhoped death of loved ones due to COVID-19 perplexed the fragile human thought process. The coronavirus' impact was so huge that even the idea of existence was questioned at one point in time. To remain relevant in times of crisis, COVID patients, caregivers, health workers, and all other stakeholders turned inwards to seek the refuge of spirituality. The evidence suggests that engaging in spiritual practice helped in better coping with challenges thrown up by COVID-19. It helped in the acceptance of the situation, finding purpose in life, a sense of belongingness, strengthening faith and resilience, and reducing psychological distress symptoms.

The comprehensive loss caused by the coronavirus triggered multifaceted grief and bereavement (G&B). The COVID-19-led G&B was unique owing to the following terms:

- Families suffered from the day of diagnosis and subsequent hospitalisation.
- Excessive worries due to multiple factors such as isolation, shortage of medicine, higher cost, lower survival rate, and hyper-phobia attached to different health paradigms.
- Sudden and unexpected loss and high restrictions to say parting goodbye in person and limited funerals and mourning rituals.

These factors enhanced the complexity of the G&B process ending with higher levels of emotional distress and psychological disturbance. Evidence suggests that G&B was addressed using interventions such as counselling micro-skills, CBT, paradigms of positive psychology, Yoga, mindfulness, body-based techniques, eye movement desensitisation therapy, psycho-education, and a community support system. During the first and second waves, the interventions were delivered through a virtual platform, while post-COVID-19, the delivery mode was face-to-face. Findings indicated that interventions were instrumental in mitigating the G&B symptomatology and fostering resilience in adversity.

One of the evolutionary survival strategies of the animal kingdom is adaptation to the immediate environment. Humans have an advantageous edge over other species by having consciousness and consciousness-accrued decision-making and problem-solving abilities. Positive adaptation (PA) is one of the consciousness-mandated coping strategies in the psychological armoury of humans. The positive adaptation post-crisis reflects the multifaceted phenomenon. The psychological, spiritual, cultural, social, and biological factors are the components of this phenomenon. PA has assisted individuals with previous psycho-physical morbidities to make better life decisions, respond effectively to challenges, enhance mental health prospects, and inform adaptive adjustment.

Usually, a vaccine requires a decade (Broom, 2020) for full operationalisation. Thanks to technology, the COVID-19 vaccine was developed in record time, that is less than a year at an unprecedented pace. WHO says, "Vaccination is one of the cheapest and most effective ways of preventing disease". However, there are several hurdles to total vaccination, and refusal to vaccinate is one of them. According to the apex health body WHO, "it has been one of the ten biggest health threats facing the world". Demographic factors such as gender, age, socio-economic status, education, and religion (Kibongani et al., 2022) were found to be significant contributors to vaccine hesitancy. Others were misinformation, negative attitudes towards vaccines, negative emotions related to vaccines, conspiracy, paranoia (Nazli et al., 2022), vaccine risk perceptions, uncritical usage of social media, and infodemic (Romate et al., 2022). Evidence suggests that vaccine reluctance and hesitancy are a global phenomenon significantly influenced by psycho-demographical factors.

Digital Infrastructure Providing Psychological Support (DIPS), coined by the author (Verma, 2023), is a digital technology-led platform where psychological services are delivered virtually. The present generation was relatively fortunate to witness the COVID-19 pandemic during digital technology. Digital technology has engendered a parallel virtual world. Fortunate in terms of easy accessibility of information, virtual meetings with loved ones, working from the comforts of home, on-the-roll entertainment, educational services and other opportunities available through it. The virtual infrastructure that came up during the pandemic was in the form of various psychological distress helplines (telehealth), mobile-based applications, web-based virtual delivery platforms, video conferencing, and specialised websites. More than 21 states, union territories, organisations, and institutions (Verma, 2023) of India started psychological distress helplines. The popularity of DIPS was attributable to the maintenance of anonymity, easy accessibility, 24×7 availability, convenience, ability to deliver at drawing rooms, customised interventions, and overcoming physical boundaries. DIPS helped mitigate the pandemic's negative impact and provided mental health support. Evidence suggests that DIPS was instrumental in enhancing total well-being across the globe.

Acknowledgement

The author would like to express his sincere gratitude to all authors who contributed chapters to this book. Further, he acknowledges the contribution of his wife, Dr Sujit Verma, in preparing this manuscript.

Conflict of Interest

There was no conflict of interest.

Funding

The author received no funding from any source for this work.

Note

1 The efficacy of Mahua flower extract as a potential sanitiser has not been established scientifically.

References

Arora, A., Jha, A. K., Alat, P., & Das, S. S. (2020). Understanding coronaphobia. *Asian Journal of Psychiatry*, *54*, 102384. https://doi.org/10.1016/j.ajp.2020.102384

Arslan, G., Yıldırım, M., Tanhan, A., Buluş, M., & Allen, K.-A. (2020). Coronavirus stress, optimism-pessimism, psychological inflexibility, and psychological health: Psychometric properties of the coronavirus stress measure. *International Journal of Mental Health and Addiction*. https://doi.org/10.1007/s11469-020-00337-6

Bao, Y., Sun, Y., Meng, S., Shi, J., & Lu, L. (2020). 2019-nCoV epidemic: Address mental health care to empower society. *The Lancet*, *395*(10224), e37–e38. https://doi.org/10.1016/S0140-6736(20)30309-3

Barron, M. E., Singhal, D., Vijayaraghavan, P., Seshadri, S., Smith, E., & Dixon, P. (2021). Health anxiety, coping mechanisms and COVID-19: An Indian community sample at week 1 of lockdown. *PLoS One*, *16*(4), e0250336. https://doi.org/10.1371/journal.pone.0250336

Bhattacharjee, A., & Ghosh, T. (2022). COVID-19 pandemic and stress: Coping with the new normal. *Journal of Prevention and Health Promotion*, *3*(1), 30–52. https://doi.org/10.1177/26320770211050058

Bhuiyan, A. K. M. I., Sakib, N., Pakpour, A. H., Griffiths, M. D., & Mamun, M. A. (2020). COVID-19-related suicides in Bangladesh due to lockdown and economic factors: Case study evidence from media reports. *International Journal of Mental Health Addiction*. https://doi.org/10.1007/s11469-020-00307-y

Booth, A. (1996). In search of the evidence: Informing effective practice. *Journal of Clinical Effectiveness*, *1*(1), 25–29.

Braun, V., & Clarke, V. (2006). Using thematic analysis in psychology. *Qualitative Research in Psychology*, *3*(2), 77–101. https://doi.org/10.1191/1478088706qp063oa

Brooks, S. K., Webster, R. K., Smith, L. E., Woodland, L., Wessely, S., Greenberg, N., & Rubin, G. J. (2020). The psychological impact of quarantine and how to reduce it: Rapid review of the evidence. *The Lancet*, *395*(10227), 912–920. https://doi.org/10.1016/S0140-6736(20)30460-8

Broom, D. (2020, June 2). 5 charts that tell the story of vaccines today. *World Economic Forum*. Retrieved from www.weforum.org/agenda/2020/06/vaccine-development-barriers-coronavirus/

Clemente-Suarez, V. J., Dalamitros, A. A., Beltran-Velasco, A. I., Mielgo-Ayuso, J., & Tornero-Aguilera, J. F. (2020). Social and psychophysiological consequences of the COVID-19 pandemic: An extensive literature review. *Frontiers in Psychology*, *11*, 580225. https://doi.org/10.3389/fpsyg.2020.580225

Cohen, S., & Wills, T. A. (1985). Stress, social support, and the buffering hypothesis. *Psychological Bulletin*, *98*(2), 310–357. https://doi.org/10.1037/0033-2909.98.2.310.

Corpuz, J. C. G. (2021). Loss, grief and healing: Accompaniment in time of COVID-19. *Journal of Public Health (Oxford, England)*, *43*(2), e336–e337. https://doi.org/10.1093/pubmed/fdab041

Daly, J., Kelleher, A., & Gliksman, M. (1997). *The public health researcher: A methodological approach* (pp. 611–618). Oxford University Press.

Dubey, S., Biswas, P., Ghosh, R., Chatterjee, S., Dubey, M. J., & Chatterjee, S. (2020). Psychosocial impact of COVID-19. *Diabetes and Metabolic Syndrome*, *14*, 779–788.

Egbert, R. A., Cankurtaran, S., & Karpiak, S. (2020). Brain abnormalities in COVID-19 acute/subacute phase: A rapid systematic review. *Brain, Behavior, and Immunity*, *89*, 543–554. https://doi.org/10.1016/j.bbi.2020.07.014

Evans, D. (2004). The systematic review report. *Collegian, 11*(2), 8–11. https://doi.org/10.1016/s1322-7696(08)60448-5

Goveas, J. S., & Shear, M. K. (2020). Grief and the COVID-19 pandemic in older adults. *The American Journal of Geriatric Psychiatry: Official Journal of the American Association for Geriatric Psychiatry, 28*(10), 1119–1125. https://doi.org/10.1016/j.jagp.2020.06.021

Goyal, K., Chauhan, P., Chhikara, K., Gupta, P., & Singh, M. P. (2020). Fear of COVID 2019: First suicidal case in India!. *Asian Journal of Psychiatry, 49*, 101989. https://doi.org/10.1016/j.ajp.2020.101989

Hao, K., & Basu, T. (2020). The coronavirus is the first true social media "infodemic". *MIT Technology Review*. Retrieved from www.technologyreview.com/2020/02/12/844851/the-coronavirus-is-the-first-true-social-media-infodemic/

Hu, Y., Chen, Y., Zheng, Y., You, C., Tan, J., Hu, L., Zhang, Z., & Ding, L. (2020). Factors related to mental health of inpatients with COVID-19 in Wuhan, China. *Brain, Behavior, and Immunity*. https://doi.org/10.1016/j.bbi.2020.07.016

International Association of Scientific, Technical and Medical Publishers. (2020, June 24). *COVID-19 research downloaded more than 150 million times, Reports STM*. Retrieved from www.prnewswire.co.uk/news-releases/covid-19-research-downloaded-more-than-150-million-times-reports-stm-824020806.html

Kaurani, P., Batra, K., & Hooja, H. R. (2020). Psychological impact of COVID-19 lockdown (phase 2) among Indian general population: A cross-sectional survey. *International Journal of Scientific Research, 9*(8), 2277–8179. https://doi.org/10.36106/ijsr/2439876

Kibongani, V. A., Scavone, C., Catalan-Matamoros, D., & Capuano, A. (2022). Vaccine hesitancy among religious groups: Reasons underlying this phenomenon and communication strategies to rebuild trust. *Frontiers in Public Health, 10*, 824560. https://doi.org/10.3389/fpubh.2022.824560

Lee, S. A. (2020). Coronavirus Anxiety Scale: A brief mental health screener for COVID-19 related anxiety. *Death Studies, 44*, 393–401. https://doi.org/10.1080/07481187.2020.1748481

Levac, D., Colquhoun, H., & O'Brien, K. K. (2010). Scoping studies: Advancing the methodology. *Implement Science, 5*(69). https://doi.org/10.1186/1748-5908-5-69

Maggio, L. A., Larsen, K., Thomas, A., Costello, J. A., & Artino, A. R. (2020). Scoping reviews in medical education: A scoping review. *Medical Education, 55*(6), 689–700. https://doi.org/10.1111/medu.14431.

Mak, S., & Thomas, A. (2022). An introduction to scoping reviews. *Journal of Graduate Medical Education, 14*(5), 561–564. https://doi.org/10.4300/JGME-D-22-00620.1

Malik, V. S., Poonam, & Bahmani, R. K. (2020). Effect of COVID-19 lockdown on mental health and family relationship in north Indian people: Lockdown and you. *Shodh Sarita, 7*(27), 76–84.

Mamun, M. A., Bodrud-Doza, M., & Griffiths, M. D. (2020). Hospital suicide due to non-treatment by healthcare staff fearing COVID-19 infection in Bangladesh? *Asian Journal of Psychiatry, 54*, 102295. https://doi.org/10.1016/j.ajp.2020.102295

Murthy, R. S. (2014). Mental health of survivors of 1984 Bhopal disaster: A continuing challenge. *Industrial Psychiatry Journal, 23*(2), 86–93.

Nazli, S. B., Yigman, F., Sevindik, M., & Deniz Ozturan, D. (2022). Psychological factors affecting COVID-19 vaccine hesitancy. *Irish Journal of Medical Science, 191*(1), 71–80. https://doi.org/10.1007/s11845-021-02640-0

Ojha, R., Gupta, N., Naik, B., Singh, S., Verma, V. K., Prusty, D., & Prajapati, V. K. (2020). High throughput and comprehensive approach to develop multiepitope vaccine against minacious COVID-19. *European Journal of Pharmaceutical Sciences, 151*, 105375. https://doi.org/10.1016/j.ejps.2020.105375 PMID:32417398

Pandey, V., Misra, N., Greeshma, R., Astha, A., Jeyavel, S., Lakshmana, G., Rajkumar, E., & Prabhu, G. (2021). Techno trend awareness and its attitude towards social connectedness and mitigating factors of COVID-19. *Frontiers in Psychology, 12*, 637395. https://doi.org/10.3389/fpsyg.2021.637395 PMID:34113286

Pedrosa, A. L., Bitencourt, L., Froes, A. C. F., Cazumba, M. L. B., Campos, R. G. B., de Brito, S. B. C. S., & Simões e Silva, A. C. (2020). Emotional, behavioral, and psychological impact of the COVID-19 pandemic. *Frontiers in Psychology, 11*. https://doi.org/10.3389/fpsyg.2020.566212

Rahimi, K. (2020). Guillain-Barre syndrome during COVID-19 pandemic: An overview of the reports. *Neurological Sciences: Official Journal of the Italian Neurological Society and of the Italian Society of Clinical Neurophysiology, 41*(11), 3149–3156. https://doi.org/10.1007/s10072-020-04693-y

Romate, J., Rajkumar, E., Gopi, A., Abraham, J., Rages, J., Lakshmi, R., Jesline, J., & Bhogle, S. (2022). What contributes to COVID-19 vaccine hesitancy? A systematic review of the psychological factors associated with COVID-19 vaccine hesitancy. *Vaccines, 10*(11), 1777. https://doi.org/10.3390/vaccines10111777

Rudroff, T., Fietsam, A. C., Deters, J. R., Bryant, A. D., & Kamholz, J. (2020). Post-COVID-19 fatigue: Potential contributing factors. *Brain Sciences, 10*(12), 1012. https://doi.org/10.3390/brainsci10121012

Saldana, J. (2009). *The coding manual for qualitative researchers*. Sage.

Sataloff, R. T., Bush, M. L., Chandra, R., Chepeha, D., Rotenberg, B., Fisher, E. W., Goldenberg, D., Hanna, E. Y., Kerschner, J. E., Kraus, D. H., Krouse, J. H., Li, D., Link, M., Lustig, L. R., Selesnick, S. H., Sindwani, R., Smith, R. J., Tysome, J., Weber, P. C., & Welling, D. B. (2021). Systematic and other reviews: Criteria and complexities. *Journal of Otolaryngology, 50*(1), 41. https://doi.org/10.1186/s40463-021-00527-9

Schou, T. M., Joca, S., Wegener, G., & Bay-Richter, C. (2021). Psychiatric and neuropsychiatric sequelae of COVID-19 – A systematic review. *Brain, Behaviour, and Immunity, 97*, 328–348. https://doi.org/10.1016/j.bbi.2021.07.018

Shanafelt, T., Ripp, J., & Trockel, M. (2020). Understanding and addressing sources of anxiety among health care professionals during the COVID-19 pandemic. *JAMA, 323*, 2133–2134. https://doi.org/10.1001/jama.2020.5893

Singh, A., Gupta, K., & Yadav, V. K. (2021). Adopting e-learning facilities during COVID-19: Exploring perspectives of teachers working in Indian public-funded elementary schools. *International Journal of Primary, Elementary and Early Years Education*, 1–15.

Singh, V., Poonam, & Behmani, R. K. (2020). Influence of food pattern on life of people during COVID-19 lockdown. *International Journal of Creative Research, 8*(7), 4922–4941.

Teixeira da Silva, J. A., Tsigaris, P., & Erfanmanesh, M. (2020). Publishing volumes in major databases related to COVID-19. *Scientometrics, 126*, 831–842. https://doi.org/10.1007/s11192-020-03675-3

Verma, R. (2023). Responding to COVID-19: A case of psychological response centers. In R. K. Kovid & V. Kumar (Eds.), *Cases on emerging market responses to the COVID-19 pandemic* (pp. 216–243). IGI Global. https://doi.org/10.4018/978-1-6684-3504-5

Vieta, E. (2005). Improving treatment adherence in bipolar disorder through psychoeducation. *The Journal of Clinical Psychiatry, 66*(1), 24–29.

WHO. (2019, December 5). *Immunization*. Retrieved from www.who.int/news-room/facts-in-pictures/detail/immunization

Xiong, Q., Xu, M., Li, J., Liu, Y., Zhang, J., Xu, Y., & Dong, W. (2021). Clinical sequelae of COVID-19 survivors in Wuhan, China: A single-centre longitudinal study.

Clinical Microbiology and Infection: The Official Publication of the European Society of Clinical Microbiology and Infectious Diseases, 27(1), 89–95. https://doi.org/10.1016/j.cmi.2020.09.023

Yang, H., Wang, C., & Poon, L. C. (2020). Novel coronavirus infection and pregnancy. *Ultrasound Obstetrician Gynecology, 55*, 435–437. https://doi.org/10.1002/uog.22006

Zhang, J., Litvinova, M., Liang, Y., Wang, Y., Wang, W., Zhao, S., Wu, Q., Merler, S., Viboud, C., Vespignani, A., Ajelli, M., & Yu, H. (2020). Changes in contact patterns shape the dynamics of the COVID-19 outbreak in China. *Science, eabb8001*. https://doi.org/10.1126/science.abb8001

Zhou, H., Lu, S., Chen, J., Wei, N., Wang, D., Lyu, H., Shi, C., & Hu, S. (2020). The landscape of cognitive function in recovered COVID-19 patients. *Journal of Psychiatric Research, 129*, 98–102. https://doi.org/10.1016/j.jpsychires.2020.06.022

2

PREVALENCE OF PSYCHOPHYSIOLOGICAL COMPLICATIONS OF COVID-19

A Systematic Review

Meenakshi Shukla, Niti Upadhyay and Josbert Gyereh

Introduction

With the remission of the coronavirus pandemic, which took the world by jolt in 2019, the scientific community is now more focused on its aftermath. If the past viral pandemics (for instance, SARS-CoV-1 and MERS) have been any indication, the neuropsychiatric complications can persist several months after the patient has reportedly recovered, affecting general well-being, daily life functioning, and cognitive activity (Boldrini et al., 2021; del Rio et al., 2020). The pathological sequelae of COVID-19, termed "post-acute COVID-19 syndrome", have been defined as complications continuing after COVID-19, emerging/lasting beyond four weeks from the first time the symptoms appeared (Nalbandian et al., 2021). Research focusing on this syndrome has identified several respiratory, haematological, renal, as well as neuropsychiatric presentations among "recovered" COVID-19 patients (also called "long-haulers") (Carfì et al., 2020; Nalbandian et al., 2021), especially those who were hospitalised. For instance a study involving 143 coronavirus patients reported that a mere 12.6% of the patients were completely asymptomatic after a mean time of two months since the inception of symptoms (Carfì et al., 2020).

Healthcare workers (HCWs), comprising not only physicians and nursing staff but also the medical support staff, such as the human resources team, medical residents, trainees, interns, and medical technical assistants, is another group that has been severely affected due to the pandemic (Choi et al., 2020). Multiple lines of research converge in concluding that this group has faced poor psychological well-being, in particular, because of the overwhelming workload, limited availability of protective kits, fear of catching and transmitting the infection, loneliness, and stigma (Choi et al., 2020; Pappa et al., 2020). However, most such studies have concentrated on the general population or patients suffering from the coronavirus infection and less on recovered patients or HCWs. Even fewer publications

DOI: 10.4324/9781003357209-3

have looked at the level of psychophysiological complications they experienced, with less focus on the post-pandemic phase. It is imperative to study the psycho-physiological complications of both these neglected groups and compare how the psychological impact of directly experiencing COVID-19 infection (among recovered patients) and indirectly experiencing the infection by treating infected patients (among HCWs) varies. Studying and comparing psychophysiological complications among recovered patients and HCWs are important as their well-being and mental health are intertwined. While treating patients affected with coronavirus places an increased risk of such complications among HCWs, HCWs suffering from these psychophysiological ramifications would adversely affect the treatment of coronavirus patients, which could lead to greater severity of post-recovery complications in patients. Further, long-haulers can easily overburden the healthcare system, which already took a major hit during the pandemic (Menges et al., 2021). Thus, the present systematic review addressed the following enquiries:

1   Which major psychophysiological complications appear post-COVID-19, that is among recovered COVID-19 patients?
2   What were the common psychophysiological complications experienced by HCWs in contact with COVID-19 patients?
3   What is the prevalence of psychophysiological complications among recovered patients of COVID-19 and HCWs, and how do these complications differ across these two most keenly affected groups as a result of the pandemic?

Given the immensely high number of people affected with COVID-19 the world over, it is the need of the hour to review systematically and document evidence indicating the nature and prevalence of psychophysiological complications among recovered patients and HCWs. Further, with the recent resurgence of coronavirus cases in China, with about 65 million cases per week (India Today World Desk, 2023), the burden of HCWs would likely be further compounded. Addressing this could help plan mental healthcare and preventive measures in subsequent pandemics and inform intervention and rehabilitation program design to assist the patients and HCWs.

Method

The review protocol was registered on PROSPERO (Registration no.: CRD42022363505). The reporting of the review has been done in agreement with the PRISMA guidelines.

Eligibility Criteria

Online records were investigated for studies published between 2019 and 2022. The databases accessed were MEDLINE, PubMed, PsychInfo (last assessed: 30 September 2022), ProQuest, APA PsychArticles (last assessed: 4 October 2022),

TABLE 2.1 Eligibility criteria for studies included in the review

Categories	Inclusion Criteria	Exclusion Criteria
Participants	• HCWs dealing directly/indirectly with COVID-19 patients • Recovered coronavirus patients discharged from the hospital/ICU or identified as recovered COVID-19 patients. • Assessment of psychophysiological complications is done at least a month after but not later than a year after discharge.	• HCWs dealing with patients affected by other physical/mental health conditions (apart from COVID-19). • Studies with uninfected participants or those identified as having pre-diagnosed mental health conditions focusing only on medical conditions like respiratory and pulmonary linked to COVID-19.
Type of studies	• Longitudinal, cross-sectional, cohort, and case-control studies, as well as qualitative studies • Published in English • Published between 2019 and 2022	• Studies involving interventions, randomised-controlled trials, systematic reviews, or meta-analyses
Outcome	• Studies focusing on the prevalence and types of psychophysiological complications among HCWs • Studies describing psychophysiological complications among recovered COVID-19 patients	• Studies describing the general quality of life, physical problems, etc., among HCWs during the pandemic • Studies describing only physical health outcomes among recovered patients of COVID-19

Scopus, Cochrane Controlled Trials Register (last assessed: 7 and 8 October 2022, respectively). The inclusion and exclusion criteria for the studies are depicted in Table 2.1.

Search Strategy

Studies for potential inclusion were identified after exploring the electronic databases mentioned earlier. The two databases' search results were largely irrelevant to the review objectives. The search string was: (Psychophysiological stresses) **OR** (Burnout) **OR** (Sleep disturbance) **OR** (Psychological distress) **AND** (COVID-19) **OR** (2019 novel coronavirus) **OR** (Coronavirus) **OR** (Pandemic) **OR** (Corona) **OR** (SARS-CoV-2) **AND** (Psychophysiological complications) **OR** (Psychophysiological difficulties) **OR** (Psychophysiological problems) **AND** (Follow-up) **OR** (Discharge) **OR** (Post-discharge) **OR** (Long-term effect) **OR** (Post-intensive care). The search string was adjusted to suit the wildcard and truncation of the various databases, where necessary.

Selection Process

Two authors independently read the title and abstract of the shortlisted studies to screen studies. In case of any discrepancy regarding a study, mutual discussion in the presence of the third author was employed to arrive at a unanimous conclusion.

Data Collection Process and Data Items

The outcomes for which data were sought were the various psychophysiological complications among healthcare professionals and hospital-discharged and/or re-covered COVID-19 patients. Secondary outcomes like the proportion of HCWs and COVID-19 patients reporting psychophysiological complications and a compara-tive exploration of the differences in such complications across HCWs and recov-ered patients were also explored. Before extracting the data, a data extraction table contained the following categories: authors, year, study design, population type, sample size, main complications, percent sample affected, measures used, and study outcomes. This table was pretested for suitability and completeness. For this, two authors independently extracted the data on 20% of the studies, verified by the third author. Following these, two authors independently extracted the data, and the third author randomly selected 50% of the studies to verify the extracted data.

Risk of Bias and Quality Assessment

To minimise the risk of bias, two review authors (J.G. and M.S.) independently reviewed the full text of each paper to be included in the review. Any disagreement was resolved by the third author (N.U.). The risk of bias in the studies was evalu-ated independently by two authors using the Cochrane Risk of Bias Tool. Any dif-ferences were resolved with discussions involving the third author.

Quality assessment of studies meeting the criteria for inclusion was done via the Joanna Briggs Institute (JBI) Critical Appraisal Tools (JBI, 2011). To ensure bias-free quality assessment, two authors (M.S. and N.U.) independently analysed each study, and the average of the quality rating score assigned by the two authors formed the final quality rating of the study. Data was extracted only from studies rated moderate-to-high quality (see Table 2.2). Data extraction for the final short-listed studies was done by two authors (M.S. and N.U.).

Data Synthesis

Identified psychophysiological complications of recovered patients and HCWs were summarised in a tabular format and compared. Their prevalence was esti-mated by calculating pooled prevalence across studies that mentioned the percent-age/number of HCWs/patients reporting psychophysiological complications to compare the complications across groups. The significance of the difference in the proportion of recovered patients and HCWs for complications common to both was calculated using chi-square test.

Results

Study Selection

Twenty-eight studies were included (N = 46,048). The procedure used for selecting studies is illustrated in the PRISMA flowchart in Figure 1.1. Nine studies reported patient samples (n = 2,211; range: 73–495). Nineteen studies reported HCW samples (n = 43,837; range: 59–10,051). Studies included populations from Australia, Italy, China, Canada, the United States (n = 5, 4, 3, 2, 2, respectively), Mexico, Iran, Malaysia, the Netherlands, Switzerland, Spain, Germany, France, Cyprus, and Brazil (n = 1 each). Cravero et al. (2021) included participants from the United States, China, Saudi Arabia, and Taiwan. Another study by Couarraze et al. (2021) included participants from 44 countries hailing from Europe, America, Africa, and Asia. The characteristics of the chosen studies are presented in Table 2.2.

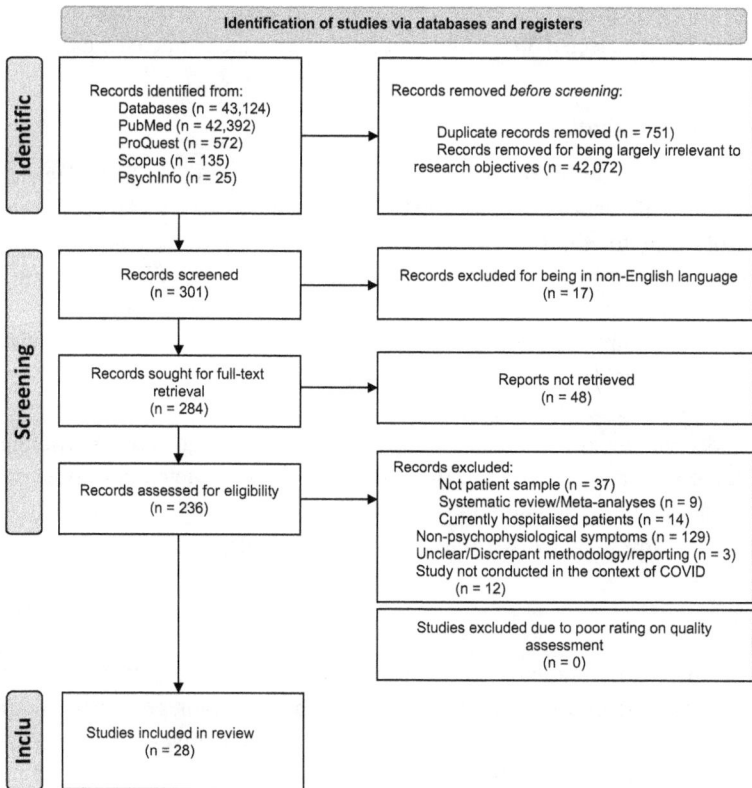

FIGURE 2.1 Illustration of the study search, identification and screening process

TABLE 2.2 Summary characteristics of studies

Author(s)	Year	Design	Population Type	Sample Size	Main Complications and Percent Cases Affected (Where Available or Calculable from Data)	Measures	Outcomes	Quality Assessment Score*
Mazza et al.	2022	Prevalence study	Patients	495	Fatigue (22%, 27%, 30%, 34% for 1, 3, 6, and 12 months, respectively)	Fatigue Severity Scale	Fatigue worsened over time.	5
Zhou et al.	2022	Face-to-face survey		73	PTSD	Impact of Event Scale-Revised (IES-R)	PTSD correlated inversely with physical health condition in recovered individuals.	7
Beck et al.	2021	Prospective observational cohort		126	Anxiety:17.5%, depression: 7.9%, PTSD: 8.7%	Hospital Anxiety and Depression Scale (HADS), IES-R	Anxiety, depression, and PTSD were reported 30 days post-discharge.	7
Bellan et al.	2021	Prospective cohort		238	PTSD:17.2%	IES-R	PTS symptoms were reported four months post-discharge.	5
Bonazza et al.	2021	Cross-sectional		261	PTSD: 36.4%, anxiety: 28%, depression: 17%	IES-R, HADS	High levels of PTS and anxiety present post-discharge.	6
Ju et al.	2021	Survey		114	PTSD: 36%	IES-6	PTSD is common one-month post-discharge.	5

(Continued)

TABLE 2.2 (Continued)

Author(s)	Year	Design	Population Type	Sample Size	Main Complications and Percent Cases Affected (Where Available or Calculable from Data)	Measures	Outcomes	Quality Assessment Score*
Spencer-Segal et al.	2021	Prospective cohort		114	Post-Traumatic Stress (PTS): 24.6%, anxiety: 11.3%, depression: 8.7%	Memory Impairment Screen-Telephone (MIS-T), Patient Health Questionnaire-9 (PHQ-9), Generalised Anxiety Disorder-7 (GAD-7), PTSD Checklist (PCL-2), UCLA, Three-Item Loneliness Scale	Compared to non-COVID hospitalised patients, COVID-hospitalised ones experienced higher anxiety, PTS, and loneliness post-discharge.	9

Author	Year	Study design		N	Outcomes measured	Measurement tools	Findings	
Vlake et al.	2021	Observational cohort		294	PTSD (one month: 16%; three months:13%), anxiety (one month: 29%; three months: 20%), depression (one month: 32%; three months: 24%)	IES-R, HADS	Psychological distress and poor health-related quality of life experienced by patients post-discharge.	9
Zhu et al.	2020	Retrospective cohort		432	Anxiety: 28.70%	Zung's anxiety scale	Confirmed and probable clinical anxiety was consistent among recovered cases.	5
Armstrong et al.	2022	Longitudinal survey	HCWs	558	Burnout, stress	Perceived Stress Scale (PSS), Shirom—Melamed Burnout Measure (SMBM)	Burnout among hospital employees was high. Resilience correlated negatively with burnout and stress.	5
Deschodt-Arsac et al.	2022	Descriptive Exploratory Pilot study		31	Anxiety, HRV	HADS, Brief COPE	High anxiety in HCWs was reflected in vagal and HRV indicators.	5
Dominguez-Espinosa et al.	2022	Cross-sectional online survey		201	Burnout	Burnout Index, EDO – 23-item version	Medical residents subjected to daily medical pressures feel emotional exhaustion.	6
Vieira et al.	2022	Cross-sectional		153	Burnout: 11.1%	MBI	Burnout was present, and resilience was a protective factor.	8

(Continued)

TABLE 2.2 (Continued)

Author(s)	Year	Design	Population Type	Sample Size	Main Complications and Percent Cases Affected (Where Available or Calculable from Data)	Measures	Outcomes	Quality Assessment Score*
Abdoli et al.	2021	Survey		321	Depression, anxiety, stress, insomnia: 86.3%	Depression, Anxiety, and Stress Scale (DASS-21), Athens Insomnia Scale (AIS)	Full-time frontline HCWs had higher probability of insomnia and poor general health.	5.5
Chow et al.	2021	Cross-sectional		200	Anxiety: 36.5%, depression: 29.5%	HADS	Scores for anxiety and depression failed to approach the cut-off.	6
Couarraze et al.	2021	Online survey		10,051	Stress	Analogue scale	HCWs have a higher risk of high stress than other workers.	6
Cravero et al.	2021	Survey		1,148	Burnout: 38.76%	Maslach Burnout Inventory (MBI)	Exposure to COVID-19 patients increased physician trainees' burnout.	4
Di Mattei et al.	2021	Online survey		1,055	Anxiety:29.31%, Insomnia: 10.57%, PTS, burnout, depression: 27.79%	DASS:21, Insomnia Severity Index, IES-R, MBI	COVID ward staff reported increased anxiety, PTSD, insomnia, anger, and burnout than non-COVID ward workers.	6

Author	Year	Study type	N	Findings	Instruments	Conclusion	Score
Harry	2021	Survey	249	Perceived stress, burnout, insomnia: 61.0%, anxiety: 57.4%, depression: 39.0%, PTSD: 35.7%	PSS, Oldenburg Burnout Inventory (OBI: 16), Retrospective Insomnia, Depression, Anxiety, and Trauma Scale (R-DATS-5)	Nurses experienced moderate burnout, stress, and mental distress.	8
Holton et al.	2021	Survey	668	Depression:13.02%, anxiety:10.63%, stress:12.42%	DASS-21	HCWs experienced poor psychological well-being.	6
Kapetanos et al.	2021	Epidemiological	381	Anxiety:26.6%, depression: 18.11%, stress:15%, burnout: 12.3%	DASS-21, MBI	HCWs had relatively high prevalence of psychophysiological symptoms.	7
Khan et al.	2021	Online survey	302	Burnout:68%	MBI	Prevalence of burnout was high among HCWs.	6
Martínez-López, et al.	2021	Survey	296	Burnout:6.4%	MBI	Burnout among HCWs was quite low.	6
Nanmi et al.	2021	Qualitative survey	118	Burnout	MBI	Not only elevated burnout, but also resilience, in HCWs.	5

(Continued)

TABLE 2.2 (Continued)

Author(s)	Year	Design	Population Type	Sample Size	Main Complications and Percent Cases Affected (Where Available or Calculable from Data)	Measures	Outcomes	Quality Assessment Score*
Schneider et al.	2021	Survey		3,293	Anxiety:20%, depression: 21%	PHQ-2, GAD-2	Anxiety and depression strongly correlated with moral distress.	5.5
Smallwood, Pascoe, Karimi, and Willis	2021	Online survey		7,846	Anxiety, depression, PTSD, burnout	GAD-7, PHQ-9, IES-6, MBI	Moral distress related with greater odds of psychophysiological complications.	5
Smallwood, Karimi et al.	2021	Online survey		7,846	Anxiety:59.8%, burnout: 70.9%, depression:57.3%	GAD-7, IES-6, MBI, PHQ-9	Significant mental health problems were noted in frontline HCWs.	5
Smallwood, Pascoe, Karimi, Bismark et al.	2021	Online survey		7,846	Anxiety, depression, burnout, PTSD	GAD-7, IES-6, MBI, PHQ-9	Workplace interruptions associated with worse consequences for HCWs.	6

Note: *Systematic reviews and cohort studies' checklists (11 criteria each) – score of 5–6: moderate quality; ≥ 7: high quality. Prevalence and quasi-experimental studies (9 criteria each) – score of 4–5: moderate quality. Cross-sectional studies' checklist (8 criteria each) – score of 4: moderate quality; ≥ 5: high quality.

Risk of Bias Assessment

Among the 28 studies included, more than half the studies (n = 16) had high selection bias while 13 studies had low selection bias or unclear risk of bias. Twelve studies contained limited information regarding allocation concealment while 17 indicated low risk of allocation concealment. In terms of reporting of outcomes, just four studies provided insufficient information to allow judgement, while a majority (n = 15) had low selective reporting bias. Yet, there were nine studies with high bias of selective reporting. Other sources of bias were either low or unclear from the information reported in the method section of the studies. Thus, overall, the risk of bias is judged to be low since the measures, demographics, statistical analyses, and results were reported in detail for most studies.

Nature and Prevalence of Psychophysiological Complications

As depicted in Table 2.2, the most common complications reported by recovered patients were PTSD/PTS, anxiety, depression, and fatigue. In contrast, the major psychophysiological complication among HCWs was burnout. Other significant complications were anxiety, depression, PTSD/PTS, insomnia, and stress.

Table 2.3; reports the pooled prevalence across studies for the psychophysiological complications reported by patients and HCWs as well as the total (patients + HCWs) group. As evident from Table 2.3, several patients reported fatigue

TABLE 2.3 The pooled prevalence of psychophysiological complications across studies

Types of Participants	Psychophysiological Complications	Total No. of Studies	Total No. of People Affected	Total Sample	Percentage
Patients	Fatigue	1	54	158	34.17
	PTSD	7	277	1,036	26.74
	Anxiety	5	255	1,076	23.70
	Depression	4	102	644	15.84
Healthcare	Burnout	6	6,191	10,126	61.14
Workers	Anxiety	7	6,050	13,692	44.19
(HCWs)	Depression	7	5,792	13,692	42.30
	PTSD	1	89	249	35.74
	Insomnia	3	536	1,625	32.98
	Stress	2	140	2,049	6.83
Total	Burnout	6	6,191	10,126	61.14
(Patients +	Anxiety	12	6,305	14,768	42.69
HCWs)	Depression	11	5,894	14,336	41.11
	Fatigue	1	54	158	34.17
	Insomnia	3	536	1,625	32.98
	PTSD	8	366	1,285	28.48
	Stress	2	140	2,049	6.83

(34.17%), PTSD/PTS (26.74%), anxiety (23.70%), and depression (15.84%). On the contrary, a majority of HCWs reported burnout (61.14%), followed by anxiety (44.19%), depression (42.30%), PTSD/PTS (35.74%), and insomnia (32.98%). A small percentage of HCWs also reported stress (6.83%).

Further, for the common psychophysiological complications among recovered patients and HCWs, we assessed if the differences between the proportions of the two groups reporting such complications were significant. Using the chi-square test, we found a significantly higher proportion of HCWs experiencing anxiety ($\chi^2 = 171.17$, $p < .0001$), depression ($\chi^2 = 177.86$, $p < .0001$), and PTSD ($\chi^2 = 7.98$, $p < .01$) compared to recovered patients.

Discussion

This review highlights the major psychophysiological complications appearing in two groups that is among recovered COVID-19 patients and HCWs. In the patient group, the most identified complications were fatigue, PTSD/PTS, anxiety, and depression; in the HCWs, these were burnout, anxiety, depression, PTSD/PTS, insomnia, and stress. Anxiety, depression, and PTSD/PTS were the common psychophysiological symptoms present in the two groups. Fatigue was specific only to the patient group, which was among the most prevalent complications across the two groups. Chronic fatigue has emerged as the hallmark symptom of long-COVID syndrome and is the most common reason for medical attention being sought by recovered COVID patients (Sharma et al., 2022). It involves excessive tiredness that interferes with daily activities and does not dissipate with sufficient rest and sleep. Anxiety, depression, and PTSD (prevalent among recovered patients as per our systematic review) are considered potential contributors to such fatigue (Brooks et al., 2020). Burnout and stress were found exclusively among HCWs, which is understandable as the increase in workload and the fear of contracting the infection among the HCWs would be likely to create burnout and stress (Armstrong et al., 2022).

Pooled prevalence indicated that fatigue was the most commonly reported complication post-recovery. A high prevalence of fatigue found among the recovered patients is supported by a recent review (Sandler et al., 2021), which reports persistent fatigue among a substantial number of recovered patients. However, the prevalence of fatigue was lesser than that reported in the general populace during the pandemic (43.7%; Leung et al., 2022). The reports of anxiety, depression, and PTSD in recovered patients are in agreement with the conclusions of meta-analyses (Ahmed et al., 2020; Rogers et al., 2020) on recovered COVID patients.

Approximately one-third of HCWs also reported insomnia. This number closely parallels the prevalence of insomnia reported in HCWs in a review of meta-analyses (Sahebi et al., 2021), which reports it to be 36.36% during the pandemic. This is most likely the results of work overload and extreme stress due to the pandemic (Zou et al., 2021). Previous coronavirus studies (Netland et al., 2008) and post-mortem brain investigations of coronavirus patients (Paniz-Mondolfi et al., 2020) show that coronavirus may pass the blood–brain barrier, eliciting immune responses. Such responses are linked to mood and sleep issues (Dantzer, 2018; Cespuglio et al., 2021).

High levels of burnout noted among HCWs may be connected to psychological vigilance and concern over high death rates (Ehrlich et al., 2020), perceptions of low workplace support (Du et al., 2020), and fearing contagion (Smallwood, Pascoe, Karimi, & Willis, 2021). Compared to the general population (Krishnamoorthy et al., 2020), recovered patients in our review were found to have lesser prevalence of anxiety (26% vs. 23.70%) and depression (24% vs. 15.84%) but a higher prevalence of PTSD (15% vs. 26.74%). The HCWs, however, had an enormously higher prevalence of anxiety, depression, PTSD, and insomnia (44.19% vs. 26%, 42.30% vs. 24%, 35.74% vs. 15%, and 32.98% vs. 7%, respectively) than the general population (Krishnamoorthy et al., 2020). A significantly higher proportion of HCWs experienced anxiety, depression, and PTSD compared to the recovered patients in our systematic review despite the patient group having directly experienced the physical and mental repercussions of the coronavirus infection. This suggests that interventions targeting improvement in mental health and well-being should be comparatively more focused on HCWs than recovered patients.

Despite a number of studies reporting psychophysiological complications among HCWs and patients post-COVID-19, the findings have not been absolutely consistent. For instance among HCWs, Chow et al. (2021) reported lower-than-cut-off scores for anxiety and depression. Martínez-López et al. (2021) reported quite low rates of burnout (6.4%) among HCWs. These discrepant findings indicate that the manifestation of psychophysiological complications among recovered patients and HCWs may be influenced by other unaccounted (possibly psycho-social) factors.

The findings of the present systematic review should be interpreted with caution. Noteworthily, nearly all the included research employed self-report measures to assess psychophysiological complications, which cannot be considered as reliable as clinical assessment. Moreover, the pooled prevalence for different psychophysiological complications was calculated only from the studies where such data was available. The prevalence of the various psychophysiological complications reported was also not analysed as a function of duration post-recovery or with respect to demographic factors since wide variations existed among studies on these factors. For instance the duration of assessment of psychophysiological complications post-recovery among patients varied from a month to a year. Future studies may aim to look into the stratified assessment of prevalence, considering different psycho-social and COVID-19-related factors.

Findings from this systematic review are likely to have important implications for rehabilitation services and healthcare organisations. Given the particular types of psychophysiological complications among patients and HCWs, it would be helpful to design distinct rehabilitative programmes for recovered patients and HCWs.

A combination of pharmacotherapy, neurorehabilitation, physiotherapy, neuropsychological, neuropsychological treatment, and psychological services may prove useful in alleviating the most common complications like anxiety, depression, PTSD, fatigue, and insomnia. With periodic resurgence in new cases of COVID, it would be indeed effective if telerehabilitation and telepsychiatry could be provided to HCWs and patients. In their charter, the World Health Organization (2020) has implored governments to focus on improving both the physical and mental health of HCWs as only the safe and healthy HCWs can ensure the safety of patients. Our systematic review has utility in this regard as it highlights the aspects of HCWs' health that require immediate attention.

Conclusion

This systematic review found the psychophysiological profiles of COVID-19 recovered patient group and HCWs. We can infer from the overall pooling of the prevalence of psychophysiological complications present in both groups that the nature and prevalence of these symptoms differ across the two groups because fatigue was the most exclusively identified complication in the patient group. Burnout and stress, on the other hand, were only found in HCWs. The common psychophysiological symptoms shared by the two groups included anxiety, depression, and PTSD/PTS; however, these complications were reported by a significantly higher proportion of HCWs than recovered patients. In order to better manage the psychophysiological consequences of COVID-19, rehabilitation facilities should be equipped with close multidisciplinary collaboration between different healthcare professionals and specialists, as well as the development of multifaceted strategies and specific intervention programmes.

References

Abdoli, N., Farnia, V., Jahangiri, S., Radmehr, F., Alikhani, M., Abdoli, P., Davarinejad, O., Dürsteler, K. M., Brühl, A. B., Sadeghi-Bahmani, D., & Brand, S. (2021). Sources of sleep disturbances and psychological strain for hospital staff working during the COVID-19 pandemic. *International Journal of Environmental Research and Public Health, 18*(12), 6289. https://doi.org/10.3390/ijerph18126289

Ahmed, H., Patel, K., Greenwood, D. C., Halpin, S., Lewthwaite, P., Salawu, A., Eyre, L., Breen, A., O'Connor, R., Jones, A., & Sivan, M. (2020). Long-term clinical outcomes in survivors of severe acute respiratory syndrome and Middle East respiratory syndrome coronavirus outbreaks after hospitalisation or ICU admission: A systematic review and meta-analysis. *Journal of Rehabilitation Medicine, 52*(5), jrm00063. https://doi.org/10.2340/16501977-2694

Armstrong, S. J., Porter, J. E., Larkins, J. A., & Mesagno, C. (2022). Burnout, stress and resilience of an Australian regional hospital during COVID-19: A longitudinal study. *BMC Health Service Research, 22*, 1115. https://doi.org/10.1186/s12913-022-08409-0

Beck, K., Vincent, A., Becker, C., Keller, A., Cam, H., Schaefert, R., Reinhardt, T., Sutter, R., Tisljar, K., Bassetti, S., Schuetz, P., & Hunziker, S. (2021). Prevalence and factors associated with psychological burden in COVID-19 patients and their relatives: A prospective observational cohort study. *PLoS One, 16*(5), e0250590. https://doi.org/10.1371/journal.pone.0250590

Bellan, M., Soddu, D., Balbo, P. E., Baricich, A., Zeppegno, P., Avanzi, G. C., Baldon, G., Bartolomei, G., Battaglia, M., Battistini, S., Binda, V., Borg, M., Cantaluppi, V., Castello, L. M., Clivati, E., Cisari, C., Costanzo, M., Croce, A., Cuneo, D., De Benedittis, C., . . . Pirisi, M. (2021). Respiratory and psychophysical sequelae among patients with COVID-19 four months after hospital discharge. *JAMA Network Open, 4*(1), e2036142. https://doi.org/10.1001/jamanetworkopen.2020.36142

Boldrini, M., Canoll, P. D., & Klein, R. S. (2021). How COVID-19 affects the brain. *JAMA Psychiatry, 78*(6), 682–683. https://doi.org/10.1001/jamapsychiatry.2021.0500

Bonazza, F., Borghi, L., di San Marco, E. C., Piscopo, K., Bai, F., Monforte, A. D., & Vegni, E. (2021). Psychological outcomes after hospitalization for COVID-19: Data from a multidisciplinary follow-up screening program for recovered patients. *Research in Psychotherapy (Milano), 23*(3), 491. https://doi.org/10.4081/ripppo.2020.491

Brooks, S. K., Webster, R. K., Smith, L. E., Woodland, L., Wessely, S., Greenberg, N., & Rubin, G. J. (2020). The psychological impact of quarantine and how to reduce it: Rapid review of the evidence. *The Lancet, 395*(10227), 912–920. https://doi.org/10.1016/S0140-6736(20)30460-8

Carfì, A., Bernabei, R., Landi, F., & Gemelli against COVID-19 Post-Acute Care Study Group (2020). Persistent symptoms in patients after acute COVID-19. *JAMA, 324*(6), 603–605. https://doi.org/10.1001/jama.2020.12603

Cespuglio, R., Strekalova, T., Spencer, P. S., Román, G. C., Reis, J., Bouteille, B., & Buguet, A. (2021). SARS-CoV-2 infection and sleep disturbances: Nitric oxide involvement and therapeutic opportunity. *Sleep, 44*(3), zsab009. https://doi.org/10.1093/sleep/zsab009

Choi, K. R., Heilemann, M. V., Fauer, A., & Mead, M. (2020). A second pandemic: Mental health spillover from the novel coronavirus (COVID-19). *Journal of the American Psychiatric Nurses Association, 26*(4), 340–343. https://doi.org/10.1177/1078390320919803

Chow, S. K., Francis, B., Ng, Y. H., Naim, N., Beh, H. C., Ariffin, M. A. A., Yusuf, M. H. M., Lee, J. W., & Sulaiman, A. H. (2021). Religious coping, depression and anxiety among healthcare workers during the COVID-19 pandemic: A Malaysian perspective. *Healthcare (Basel, Switzerland), 9*(1), 79. https://doi.org/10.3390/healthcare9010079

Couarraze, S., Delamarre, L., Marhar, F., Quach, B., Jiao, J., Avilés Dorlhiac, R., Saadaoui, F., Liu, A. S., Dubuis, B., Antunes, S., Andant, N., Pereira, B., Ugbolue, U. C., Baker, J. S., COVISTRESS Network, Clinchamps, M., & Dutheil, F. (2021). The major worldwide stress of healthcare professionals during the first wave of the COVID-19 pandemic – The international COVISTRESS survey. *PLoS One, 16*(10), e0257840. https://doi.org/10.1371/journal.pone.0257840

Cravero, A. L., Kim, N. J., Feld, L. D., Berry, K., Rabiee, A., Bazarbashi, N., Bassin, S., Lee, T. H., Moon, A. M., Qi, X., Liang, P. S., Aby, E. S., Khan, M. Q., Young, K. J., Patel, A., Wijarnpreecha, K., Kobeissy, A., Hashim, A., Houser, A., & Ioannou, G. N. (2021). Impact of exposure to patients with COVID-19 on residents and fellows: An international survey of 1420 trainees. *Postgraduate Medical Journal, 97*(1153), 706–715. https://doi.org/10.1136/postgradmedj-2020-138789

Dantzer, R. (2018). Neuroimmune interactions: From the brain to the immune system and vice versa. *Physiological Reviews, 98*(1), 477–504. https://doi.org/10.1152/physrev.00039.2016

del Rio, C., Collins, L. F., & Malani, P. (2020). Long-term health consequences of COVID-19. *JAMA, 324*(17), 1723–1724. https://doi.org/10.1001/jama.2020.19719

Deschodt-Arsac, V., Berger, V., Khlouf, L., & Arsac, L. M. (2022). Degraded psychophysiological status in caregivers and human resources staff during a COVID-19 peak unveiled by psychological and HRV testing at workplace. *International Journal of Environmental Research and Public Health, 19*(3), 1710. https://doi.org/10.3390/ijerph19031710

Di Mattei, V. E., Perego, G., Milano, F., Mazzetti, M., Taranto, P., Di Pierro, R., De Panfilis, C., Madeddu, F., & Preti, E. (2021). The "healthcare workers' wellbeing (Benessere Operatori)" project: A picture of the mental health conditions of Italian healthcare workers during the first wave of the COVID-19 pandemic. *International Journal of Environmental Research and Public Health, 18*(10), 5267. https://doi.org/10.3390/ijerph18105267

Dominguez-Espinosa, A. D. C., Montes de Oca-Mayagoitia, S. I., Sáez-Jiménez, A. P., de la Fuente-Zepeda, J., & Monroy Ramírez de Arellano, L. (2022). The moderating role of sociodemographic and work-related variables in burnout and mental health levels of Mexican medical residents. *PLoS One, 17*(9), e0274322. https://doi.org/10.1371/journal.pone.0274322

Du, R. H., Liang, L. R., Yang, C. Q., Wang, W., Cao, T. Z., Li, M., Guo, G. Y., Du, J., Zheng, C. L., Zhu, Q., Hu, M., Li, X. Y., Peng, P., & Shi, H. Z. (2020). Predictors of mortality for patients with COVID-19 pneumonia caused by SARS-CoV-2: A prospective cohort study. *The European Respiratory Journal, 55*(5), 2000524. https://doi.org/10.1183/13993003.00524-2020

Ehrlich, H., McKenney, M., & Elkbuli, A. (2020). Protecting our healthcare workers during the COVID-19 pandemic. *The American Journal of Emergency Medicine, 38*(7), 1527–1528. https://doi.org/10.1016/j.ajem.2020.04.024

Harry, S. (2021). *Predictors of burnout for frontline nurses in the COVID-19 pandemic: Well-being, satisfaction with life, social support, fear, work setting factors, psychological impacts, and self-efficacy for nursing tasks.* Teachers College, Columbia University.

Holton, S., Wynter, K., Trueman, M., Bruce, S., Sweeney, S., Crowe, S., Dabscheck, A., Eleftheriou, P., Booth, S., Hitch, D., Said, C. M., Haines, K. J., & Rasmussen, B. (2021). Psychological well-being of Australian hospital clinical staff during the COVID-19 pandemic. *Australian Health Review: A Publication of the Australian Hospital Association, 45*(3), 297–305. https://doi.org/10.1071/AH20203

India Today World Desk. (2023, May 23). *China braces for new wave of XBB Covid variant, could see 65 million cases weekly.* Retrieved from https://www.indiatoday.in/coronavirus-outbreak/story/china-braces-for-massive-covid-wave-could-see-65-million-cases-weekly-2384352-2023-05-25

JBI. (2011). *Joanna Briggs Institute reviewers' manual.* University of Adelaide.

Ju, Y., Liu, J., Ng, R. M. K., Liu, B., Wang, M., Chen, W., Huang, M., Yang, A., Shu, K., Zhou, Y., Zhang, L., Liao, M., Liu, J., & Zhang, Y. (2021). Prevalence and predictors of post-traumatic stress disorder in patients with cured coronavirus disease 2019 (COVID-19) one month post-discharge. *European Journal of Psychotraumatology, 12*(1), 1915576. https://doi.org/10.1080/20008198.2021.1915576

Kapetanos, K., Mazeri, S., Constantinou, D., Vavlitou, A., Karaiskakis, M., Kourouzidou, D., Nikolaides, C., Savvidou, N., Katsouris, S., & Koliou, M. (2021). Exploring the factors associated with the mental health of frontline healthcare workers during the COVID-19 pandemic in Cyprus. *PLoS One, 16*(10), e0258475. https://doi.org/10.1371/journal.pone.0258475

Khan, N., Palepu, A., Dodek, P., Salmon, A., Leitch, H., Ruzycki, S., Townson, A., & Lacaille, D. (2021). Cross-sectional survey on physician burnout during the COVID-19 pandemic in Vancouver, Canada: The role of gender, ethnicity and sexual orientation. *BMJ Open, 11*(5), e050380. https://doi.org/10.1136/bmjopen-2021-050380

Krishnamoorthy, Y., Nagarajan, R., Saya, G. K., & Menon, V. (2020). Prevalence of psychological morbidities among general population, healthcare workers and COVID-19 patients amidst the COVID-19 pandemic: A systematic review and meta-analysis. *Psychiatry Research*, *293*, 113382. https://doi.org/10.1016/j.psychres.2020.113382

Leung, H. T., Gong, W. J., Sit, S. M. M., Lai, A. Y. K., Ho, S. Y., Wang, M. P., & Lam, T. H. (2022). COVID-19 pandemic fatigue and its sociodemographic and psycho-behavioral correlates: A population-based cross-sectional study in Hong Kong. *Science Reports,* 12, 16114. https://doi.org/10.1038/s41598-022-19692-6

Martínez-López, J. Á., Lázaro-Pérez, C., Gómez-Galán, J. (2021). Burnout among direct-care workers in nursing homes during the COVID-19 pandemic in Spain: A preventive and educational focus for sustainable workplaces. *Sustainability*, *13*, 2782. https://doi.org/10.3390/su13052782

Mazza, M. G., Palladini, M., Villa, G., De Lorenzo, R., Rovere Querini, P., & Benedetti, F. (2022). Prevalence, trajectory over time, and risk factor of post-COVID-19 fatigue. *Journal of Psychiatric Research*, *155*, 112–119. https://doi.org/10.1016/j.jpsychires.2022.08.008

Menges, D., Ballouz, T., Anagnostopoulos, A., Aschmann, H. E., Domenghino, A., Fehr, J. S., & Puhan, M. A. (2021). Burden of post-COVID-19 syndrome and implications for healthcare service planning: A population-based cohort study. *PLoS One*, *16*(7), e0254523. https://doi.org/10.1371/journal.pone.0254523

Nalbandian, A., Sehgal, K., Gupta, A., Madhavan, M. V., McGroder, C., Stevens, J. S., Cook, J. R., Nordvig, A. S., Shalev, D., Sehrawat, T. S., Ahluwalia, N., Bikdeli, B., Dietz, D., Der-Nigoghossian, C., Liyanage-Don, N., Rosner, G. F., Bernstein, E. J., Mohan, S., Akinpelumi, A. B.,. . . Wan, E. Y. (2021). Post-acute COVID-19 syndrome. *Nature Medicine*, *27*(4), 601–615. https://doi.org/10.1038/s41591-021-01283-z

Nanni, E. (2021). Investigating physician assistant burnout amidst the COVID-19 global pandemic: A qualitative survey response from practicing PAs in Canada: Burnout among Canadian PA during COVID. *The Journal of Canada's Physician Assistants*, *3*(8), 1–18. https://doi.org/10.5203/jcanpa.v3i8.909

Netland, J., Meyerholz, D. K., Moore, S., Cassell, M., & Perlman, S. (2008). Severe acute respiratory syndrome coronavirus infection causes neuronal death in the absence of encephalitis in mice transgenic for human ACE2. *Journal of Virology*, *82*(15), 7264–7275. https://doi.org/10.1128/JVI.00737-08

Paniz-Mondolfi, A., Bryce, C., Grimes, Z., Gordon, R. E., Reidy, J., Lednicky, J., Sordillo, E. M., & Fowkes, M. (2020). Central nervous system involvement by severe acute respiratory syndrome coronavirus-2 (SARS-CoV-2). *Journal of Medical Virology*, *92*(7), 699–702. https://doi.org/10.1002/jmv.25915

Pappa, S., Ntella, V., Giannakas, T., Giannakoulis, V. G., Papoutsi, E., & Katsaounou, P. (2020). Prevalence of depression, anxiety, and insomnia among healthcare workers during the COVID-19 pandemic: A systematic review and meta-analysis. *Brain, Behavior, and Immunity*, *88*, 901–907. https://doi.org/10.1016/j.bbi.2020.05.026

Rogers, J. P., Chesney, E., Oliver, D., Pollak, T. A., McGuire, P., Fusar-Poli, P., Zandi, M. S., Lewis, G., & David, A. S. (2020). Psychiatric and neuropsychiatric presentations associated with severe coronavirus infections: A systematic review and meta-analysis with comparison to the COVID-19 pandemic. *The lancet. Psychiatry*, *7*(7), 611–627. https://doi.org/10.1016/S2215-0366(20)30203-0

Sahebi, A., Abdi, K., Moayedi, S., Torres, M., & Golitaleb, M. (2021). The prevalence of insomnia among health care workers amid the COVID-19 pandemic: An umbrella review of meta-analyses. *Journal of Psychosomatic Research*, *149*, 110597. https://doi.org/10.1016/j.jpsychores.2021.110597

Sandler, C. X., Wyller, V. B. B., Moss-Morris, R., Buchwald, D., Crawley, E., Hautvast, J., Katz, B. Z., Knoop, H., Little, P., Taylor, R., Wensaas, K. A., & Lloyd, A. R. (2021). Long COVID and post-infective fatigue syndrome: A review. *Open Forum Infectious Diseases*, *8*(10), ofab440. https://doi.org/10.1093/ofid/ofab440

Schneider, J. N., Hiebel, N., Kriegsmann-Rabe, M., Schmuck, J., Erim, Y., Morawa, E., Jerg-Bretzke, L., Beschoner, P., Albus, C., Hannemann, J., Weidner, K., Steudte-Schmiedgen, S., Radbruch, L., Brunsch, H., & Geiser, F. (2021). Moral distress in hospitals during the first wave of the COVID-19 pandemic: A web-based survey among 3,293 healthcare workers within the German Network University Medicine. *Frontiers in Psychology*, *12*, 775204. https://doi.org/10.3389/fpsyg.2021.775204

Sharma, P., Bharti, S., & Garg, I. (2022). Post COVID fatigue: Can we really ignore it? *The Indian Journal of Tuberculosis*, *69*(2), 238–241. https://doi.org/10.1016/j.ijtb.2021.06.012

Smallwood, N., Karimi, L., Bismark, M., Putland, M., Johnson, D., Dharmage, S. C., Barson, E., Atkin, N., Long, C., Ng, I., Holland, A., Munro, J. E., Thevarajan, I., Moore, C., McGillion, A., Sandford, D., & Willis, K. (2021). High levels of psychosocial distress among Australian frontline healthcare workers during the COVID-19 pandemic: A cross-sectional survey. *General Psychiatry*, *34*(5), e100577. https://doi.org/10.1136/gpsych-2021-100577

Smallwood, N., Pascoe, A., Karimi, L., Bismark, M., & Willis, K. (2021). Occupational disruptions during the COVID-19 pandemic and their association with healthcare workers' mental health. *International Journal of Environmental Research and Public Health*, *18*(17), 9263. https://doi.org/10.3390/ijerph18179263

Smallwood, N., Pascoe, A., Karimi, L., & Willis, K. (2021). Moral distress and perceived community views are associated with mental health symptoms in frontline health workers during the COVID-19 pandemic. *International Journal of Environmental Research and Public Health*, *18*(16), 8723. https://doi.org/10.3390/ijerph18168723

Spencer-Segal, J. L., Smith, C. A., Slavin, A., Sampang, L., DiGiovine, D., Spencer, A. E., Zhang, Q., Horowitz, J., & Vaughn, V. M. (2021). Mental health outcomes after hospitalization with or without COVID-19. *General Hospital Psychiatry*, *72*, 152–153. https://doi.org/10.1016/j.genhosppsych.2021.07.004

Vieira, L. S., Machado, W. L., Dal Pai, D., Magnago, T. S. B. S., Azzolin, K. O., & Tavares, J. P. (2022). Burnout and resilience in intensive care nursing professionals in the face of COVID-19: A multicenter study. Burnout e resiliência em profissionais de enfermagem de terapia intensiva frente à COVID-19: estudo multicêntrico. *Revista latino-americana de enfermagem*, *30*, e3589. https://doi.org/10.1590/1518-8345.5778.3589

Vlake, J. H., Wesselius, S., van Genderen, M. E., van Bommel, J., Boxma-de Klerk, B., & Wils, E. J. (2021). Psychological distress and health-related quality of life in patients after hospitalization during the COVID-19 pandemic: A single-center, observational study. *PLoS One*, *16*(8), e0255774. https://doi.org/10.1371/journal.pone.0255774

World Health Organization. (2020, September 17). *Keeping health workers safe to keep patients safe*. Retrieved April 16, 2023, from www.who.int/news/item/17-09-2020-keep-health-workers-safe-to-keep-patients-safe-who

Zhou, K., Chi, H., Wang, J., Zheng, Y., Pan, J., Yu, D., Xu, J., Zhu, H., Li, J., Chen, S., Zhao, X., Wu, X., Shen, B., Tung, T. H., & Luo, C. (2022). Physical condition, psychological status, and posttraumatic stress disorder among recovered COVID-19 subjects: A mediation analysis. *Frontiers in Psychiatry*, *13*, 918679. https://doi.org/10.3389/fpsyt.2022.918679

Zhu, S., Gao, Q., Yang, L., Yang, Y., Xia, W., Cai, X., Hui, Y., Zhu, D., Zhang, Y., Zhang, G., Wu, S., Wang, Y., Zhou, Z., Liu, H., Zhang, C., Zhang, B., Yang, J., Feng, M., Ni, Z.,

Chen, B., . . . Reinhardt, J. D. (2020). Prevalence and risk factors of disability and anxiety in a retrospective cohort of 432 survivors of Coronavirus Disease-2019 (COVID-19) from China. *PLoS One*, *15*(12), e0243883. https://doi.org/10.1371/journal.pone.0243883

Zou, X., Liu, S., Li, J., Chen, W., Ye, J., Yang, Y., & Ling, L. (2021). Factors associated with healthcare workers' insomnia symptoms and fatigue in the fight against COVID-19, and the role of organizational support. *Frontiers in Psychiatry*, *12*, 652717. https://doi.org/10.3389/fpsyt.2021.652717

3

PROSOCIAL BEHAVIOUR DURING THE COVID-19 PANDEMIC

A Systematic Review

Neethu Pathiyan Satheesh, Annsweetta James and Arundhathy Gopakumar

Introduction

In December 2019, the first report of coronavirus and associated disease (COVID-19) was made in Wuhan, China. Numerous people died due to the virus, which had spread to most parts of the world by 2020. The implementation of nationwide lockdowns, quarantines, travel bans, store and department closures, and curfews disrupted people's social lives in a way that had never been seen before. As a result, widespread unemployment, economic deprivation, and reduced productivity were experienced. Moreover, COVID-19 poses a threat to the health and psychological well-being of people. Despite crisis and uncertainty, human behaviour has shown impressive prosocial characteristics. Studies have shown that prosocial behaviours tend to increase during times of crisis (Zaki, 2020). Even though the virus affected how people were separated, altruistic behaviours persisted in explicit and implicit forms. From caring for infected people, doctors, and frontline workers to reducing the virus spread by wearing masks and keeping interpersonal distance, citizens contributed their efforts to prosocial work (Dinić & Bodroza, 2021). Infected patients volunteered for research, contributing to the war against the virus in other altruistic acts. These protective practices had global benefits, fighting the pandemic's causes and consequences.

An Important question that arose during this crisis is how and why people exhibit prosocial behaviour during emergencies. Prosocial behaviour has been studied extensively across several times of crises. As social beings, humans are inclined to help their fellows during emergencies. Studies conducted in Louisiana after Hurricane Katrina and in China after an earthquake in Sichuan reported impressive incidences of generosity from a wide range of people towards the ones affected by the disasters (Rodríguez & Aguirre, 2006; Rao et al., 2011). Similar activities

DOI: 10.4324/9781003357209-4

can be seen during the COVID-19 pandemic across the world, with people joining the frontline healthcare team, donating blood, organs, money and resources, and much more. Drury et al. (2019) reported that one of the primary reasons that people help each other is a sense of identity that promotes unanimity and collectivism, and that is why we observe solidarity and generosity more than selfishness during crises. In the self-categorisation theory (Turner et al., 1987), it is said that unity among group members is strengthened by identifying and categorising themselves as group members and acting in accordance with it.

Even when the fundamental importance of altruistic acts was recognised and practised, antisocial and misanthropic acts were prevalent in society. People undermined and ignored the social distancing rules, and essential resources were scarce due to stockpiling (Columbus, 2021). There was also increased xenophobia and discrimination, especially against East-Asian nations (Reny & Barreto, 2022). This gives another perspective where individuals become less prosocial during emergencies due to the competition for rare resources. Studies conducted by Hsiang et al. (2013) and Brancati in 2007 have shown that times of crisis can bring out selfish and antisocial behaviour in people.

From a developmental and psychological viewpoint, it is necessary to understand the most critical factors that drive human life in this constantly changing environment. Prosocial behaviours were evident in society in different possible ways, starting from wearing a mask to protect oneself and the people around, maintaining social distance, prioritising personal hygiene to volunteering to help in the frontline, dealing with the affected, providing financial and other resources to individuals, etc. (Dinić & Bodroza, 2021). An individual's decision to engage in prosocial behaviours in emergencies comes with a sense of belongingness and responsibility towards the society (Hellmann et al., 2021).

This systematic review aims to analyse prosocial behaviour shown during the COVID-19 pandemic and assess the positive outcomes, therapeutic effects, and different types of prosocial behaviour. The present review focuses on studies conducted across the world during the outbreak of the virus. Longitudinal, cross-sectional studies, online and offline survey methods, and experiments were analysed for this review. Important findings emerged from these studies as they determine a crucial aspect of humanity: the need and significance of helping and cooperating. In any crises like the pandemic, natural calamities, or economic deprivation, prosocial behaviours are the most critical factors to fight the situation.

Methods

The study was designed on the basis of the recommendation and structure of other systematic reviews (Castro-Piñero et al., 2010; Esteban-Cornejo et al., 2015) and PRISMA guidelines (Moher et al., 2009).

TABLE 3.1 Main search terms used for finding relevant studies

Databases	Search Strategy	Limits	Filters
PubMed	Altruism during Covid 19, Prosocial during Covid 19, and	Publication date: 01/12/2019 to 31/08/2022	235 items filtered
PsycArticles	Covid 19 studies in psychology	Studies on humans	11 items filtered
Scientific Reports		English language	35 items filtered
PLoS One			1,660 items filtered
Scopus			Nine items filtered
Heliyon			17 items filtered
Wiley			48 items filtered
Frontiers in Psychology			137 items filtered
ResearchGate			100 items filtered
Google Scholar			993 items filtered

Search Strategy

Electronic literature searches were performed using PubMed, PsycArticles, Scopus, Scientific Reports, *PLoS One, Heliyon*, Wiley, *Frontiers in Psychology*, Research-Gate, and Google Scholar databases, including publications from December 2019 to August 2022. The keywords used include: altruism during Covid 19, prosocial behaviour during Covid 19, and COVID-19 studies in psychology. Over 30 articles and publications were read and reviewed, and bibliographies of relevant articles were reviewed for further information. Table 3.1 shows the main search terms used for finding relevant studies.

Study Selection Criteria

The following selection criteria were applied:

1 Studies were considered for inclusion if they provided quantitative or qualitative data on prosocial behaviour exhibited during the pandemic.
2 Cross-sectional, longitudinal, survey, or experimental designs were used.
3 Studies in the English language with all ethnic origins were included.

Review Methods

The relevance of the abstracts of the identified publications to the selection criteria was checked following computerised searches. Articles were rejected if they failed to meet the study requirements determined from the abstract. The whole article was evaluated when an abstract could not be dismissed entirely. Three independent reviewers pulled papers that might be eligible for consideration (N.P.S., A.J., A.G.). The reviewers examined every title and abstract, and disagreements were settled at a consensus meeting.

Results and Discussion

General Findings

Table 3.1 displays the findings of the systematic review procedure. Thirty articles were retrieved after duplicates, and those excluded at the title or abstract level were eliminated. For the systematic review, 26 studies were included on the basis of selection criteria. Out of the 26 studies found by the research strategy, 24 were quantitative, and 2 were qualitative. A thorough examination of the studies revealed that eight studies are cross-sectional (Haller et al., 2022; Noël & Dardenne, 2022; Al Dhaheri et al., 2021; Shillington et al., 2022; Byrne et al., 2021; Thu et al., 2021; Feng et al., 2020), five were experimental (Miles et al., 2022; Varma et al., 2022; Barragan et al., 2021; Abel & Brown, 2020; Grimalda et al., 2021), one was a systematic review (Jones et al., 2021), eight studies have employed survey methods (Hellmann et al., 2021; Cho et al., 2022; Dinić & Bodroza, 2021; Kislyakov & Schmeleva, 2021; Zhu et al., 2022; Gijzen et al., 2020; Columbus, 2021; Vieira et al., 2021), one study followed a between-subjects design (Andrews et al., 2022), one was a latent class analysis (Aresi et al., 2022), one intervention method was included (Kabir et al., 2021) and one study was a qualitative content analysis (Tekin et al., 2021).

Types of Prosocial Behaviour

As stated in Table 3.2, 11 studies examined the prosocial behaviour displayed throughout the pandemic. A study with a between-subjects design examined how reading narrative (story-like) versus expository (factual recounting) messages affected readers' beliefs about the need to protect vulnerable populations during pandemics. The study discovered that reading narratives strengthened readers' intentions to engage in prosocial behaviours (such as social distancing) through transportation (Andrews et al., 2022). Out of the four studies that used the survey method to understand the different prosocial behaviours seen during the pandemic, one study suggested that older adults demonstrated considerable prosocial behaviours (donating clothes, delivering food or medications, lending or donating money, donating blood) towards isolated people and significant others (Cho et al., 2022). Another study revealed that compliance with protective measures (wearing gloves, washing hands, wearing masks, social distancing) was an indicator of prosocial and unselfish forms of behaviour (Dinić & Bodroza, 2021). One of the studies found that prosocial orientation was manifested in several behavioural strategies (volunteering, caring for others – proactive strategy, charity, and

TABLE 3.2 Characteristics of the analysed studies

Authors and Variables	Study Design/ Duration	Sample/Age/Country	Psychological Measures	Results
Haller et al. (2022). Prosocial behaviour, well-being.	Cross-sectional, two months	Random sampling, adults (30s), 60 countries	Mental Health Continuum – Short Form (MHCS-SF), PANAS, Prosocial Scale for Adults (PSA). Oslo 3-Item Social Support Scale (OSSS-3), Psy-flex, Perceived Stress Scale	Prosocial behaviour was shown to be associated with better well-being consistently across regions. Considering the predictors of prosocial behaviour, high levels of perceived social support, positive affect, and psychological flexibility are strongly associated with perceived stress. Similarity across regions was shown in the psycho-social and sociodemographic predictors of prosocial behaviour.
Jones et al. (2021). Impact of COVID-19 on mental health in adolescents	Systematic Review from 2019 to 2021	Adolescents, 12–18 years, global	–	The study found that home quarantining, parent–child discussions, social support, and positive coping skills influenced adolescent mental health positively during the pandemic.
Noël and Dardenne (2022). Greenspace attendance, perceived crowdedness, perceived beauty and prosocial behaviour	A cross-sectional, online survey, ten minutes	Snowball sampling, 12–28 years, French-speaking Belgium	Perceived value orientation scale	The study identified the interaction between green space attendance and perceived crowdedness of the green space and its association with increased prosociality.
Al Dhaheri et al. (2021). Mental health and quality of life	Cross-sectional, one month	Random sampling, adults, Middle East and North Africa (Mena region)	Event Scale-Revised (IES-R), Perceived Support Scale (PSS)	The COVID-19 pandemic had a mild psychological impact on people, and it also positively impacted mental health awareness and family support among adults.

Study	Method	Sampling	Measures	Results
Miles et al. (2022). Prosocial behaviour, mental health and emotional well-being	Experimental, three weeks	Random sampling, adults, the United States and Canada	Prosocial acts, self-focused acts, track activities	The study did not find any difference between those in the prosocial condition and those in the neutral or self-focused conditions during the intervention or follow-up, and no difference was found in the prosocial effects for those who had been negatively affected socially or economically by the pandemic.
Hellmann et al. (2021). Prosocial Behaviour, Responsibility and Vulnerability	The online study, 20 min	Random sampling, 31 years, Germany	Social Value Orientations Slider Measure (SVO) perceived vulnerability, perceived responsibility	Results showed that different dimensions of responsibility are associated with different actors (self, recipient, politicians). The study also found that prosocial behaviour increased when the perceived models (politicians) were responsible for helping.
Tekin et al. (2021). Altruistic and prosocial behaviour during the COVID-19 pandemic	Qualitative content analysis, 24 weeks	—	—	Research results found that (a) senior citizens, (b) individuals with disabilities and satisfactory health conditions, (c) marginalised communities and the working class, and (d) frontline workers mostly received primary support. Psychological, socio-emotional, and material support are the three types of support received. They also found that support comes from (a) volunteers, (b) different organisations, and (c) advantaged groups. The reasons behind prosocial behaviours were allyship, community sharing or humanity identity, and expressing gratitude.

(Continued)

TABLE 3.2 (Continued)

Authors and Variables	Study Design/ Duration	Sample/Age/Country	Psychological Measures	Results
Varma et al. (2022). Prosocial behaviour, positive emotion	Online experiment, one month	Random sampling, 26 years	COVID-19 impact questionnaire, Stanford Sleepiness Scale (SSS)	Results indicated that participants purchased for themselves or someone else COVID-19-related or unrelated items. Prosocial behaviour leads to social connectedness, empathy, and positive affect. It was also noted that the psychological benefits are more extensive when the generous acts are unrelated to COVID-19.
Andrews et al. (2022). Healthcare workers' helping behaviours	Between-subjects design, 2019–21	Purposive sampling, 37–38 years	Narrative and expository methods	Participants in the narrative (vs expository) condition reported greater transportation into the message. They also observed the indirect effects of narrative messages on several dimensions through increased message transportation.
Cho et al. (2022). Ageing, empathy, prosocial behaviours	Survey method, 2021	Random sampling, 18–89 years, the United States	Toronto Empathy Questionnaire (TEQ)	The study's results indicated that empathy and age were positively related to increased prosocial behaviour during the pandemic. Increasing age was associated with greater prosocial behaviours towards close others such as family and friends.
Shillington et al. (2022). Prosocial behaviour	Cross-sectional, four months	Random sampling, Canadian adults, Canada	Prosocialness Scale for Adults (PSA)	The study shows no significant differences in prosocial behaviour between adults' lives in urban and rural locations. Prosocial behaviour during the early months of the pandemic was high among Ontarians in both urban and rural areas.

Study	Method	Sampling	Measure	Results
Aresi et al. (2022). Prosocial behaviour during collective quarantine conditions	Latent class analysis, 2020 lockdown (March)	Snowball sampling, adults, Italy	The Italian version of the Sense of Community Responsibility Scale (SoC-R), Community Advancing Resilience toolkit	Results revealed four classes of prosocial behaviours: money donors, online and offline helpers, online health information sharers, and neighbour helpers.
Barragan et al. (2021). Cooperative health behaviours	Online experiment, 64 days	Random sampling, 18–86 years, global	—	Results found that the identification with all humanity is a psychological construct that promotes cooperative health behaviour and help-oriented concern for others during the pandemic.
Byrne et al. (2021). Prosocial behaviour, volunteering	A cross-sectional survey, one month	Purposive sampling, Adults, the UK	Level of agreement scale	The study revealed that the decision to volunteer depends on possessing the necessary skills, the nature of volunteering roles offered, and seniority.
Thu et al. (2021). Prosocial behaviour	Cross-sectional study, 19 days	Snowball sampling, 16 years and above, Vietnam	Prosocial experience scale by Alvis and Shook	Results revealed that the prevalence of high prosocial behaviours was 75.3%.
Kabir et al. (2021). Prosocial behaviour of wearing masks	Intervention, 2021	Adults, Bangladesh, Japan	—	Numerical results reveal a diverse and rich social dilemma structure that is hidden behind the mask – wearing was a dilemma.
Dinić and Bodroza (2021). Protective behaviours as prosocial behaviours	Survey method, one month	Random sampling, 19–72 years, Serbia	COVID-19-protective behaviours' scale, empathy towards persons in forced isolation scale, the fear scale from the PANAS, The Selfishness Questionnaire (SQ), the Prosocial Tendencies Measure (PTM),	The study revealed that compliance with protective measures was an indicator of prosocial and unselfish forms of behaviour. The study findings have practical implications for shaping public messages and can help to endorse health-responsible behaviours efficiently.

(Continued)

TABLE 3.2 (Continued)

Authors and Variables	Study Design/ Duration	Sample/Age/Country	Psychological Measures	Results
Kislyakov and Schmeleva (2021). Prosocial behaviour strategies	Online survey, one month	Purposive sampling, 17–25 years, Russia	PVQ-21 scale,	The study found that prosocial orientation may manifest in several behavioural strategies during the pandemic.
Zhu et al. (2022). Traveller prosocial behaviour	Online survey, 2020	Random sampling, adults, China	Items from scales for ascription of responsibility, personal norm, social norm, prosocial behavioural intentions, and anticipated feelings of pride and guilt	Based on the outcome, corresponding managerial implications for heritage tourism practitioners and some meaningful references for future researchers to endorse prosocial and sustainable heritage tourism products were explained.
Gijzen et al. (2020). Mental health and well-being	Online survey, one week	Random sampling, 18–91 years, Dutch	Loneliness scale, Short Warwick–Edinburgh Mental Wellbeing Scale (SWEMWBS)	The study revealed the positive association between social loneliness and stable mental health by emphasising the significance of meaningful relationships.
Abel and Brown (2020). Effect of Public and private role models	Experimental design, early April 2020	Random sampling, 37 years, the United States	—	The result found that positive private role models lead to more prosocial behaviour because they increase norms of trust. At the same time, negative public role models increase the sense of responsibility among individuals, which encourages them to engage in more prosocial behaviours.
Columbus (2021). Honesty-humility, beliefs, and prosocial behaviour	Survey Method, 3 minutes	Random sampling, 34.25 years, the UK	HEXACO-100	Results suggest that when exposed to a social dilemma, people high in Honesty-Humility parameter are seen to be more willing to give up individual benefits.

Study	Design	Sample	Measures	Findings
Grimalda et al. (2021). Increased altruism	Two online experiments, the first wave of the pandemic	Random sampling, adults, the United States and Italy	—	The study found that the exposure to COVID-19 increased donations compared to those not exposed. For targets of giving, they also found that donors mostly helped at the local level. Social identity was seen to have influenced charity choice in both countries.
Feng et al. (2020). Altruism and mental health	Cross-sectional online survey, 30 minutes	Random sampling, 17–21, China	Self-Report Altruism Scale (SR), PANAS, Generalised Anxiety Disorder Scale, Patient Health Questionnaire Depression Scale (PHQ-9)	Results implied that the more negative effects were found in individuals with high altruism than those with low altruism, indirectly increasing their anxiety and depressive symptoms.
Vieira et al. (2021). Perceived threat and acute anxiety, altruism	Online survey, four weeks	Random sampling, adults, the United States	Self-Report Altruism Scale (SRA), Prosocial Behavioural Intentions Scale (PBIS), self-reported feelings and thoughts about the pandemic, Depression Anxiety Stress Scale (DASS-21)	Study results revealed a strong association between experiencing acute anxiety and high physiological arousal during the pandemic and engaging in altruistic behaviours. These findings support the relationship between defensive and altruistic motivation in humans.
Han et al. (2021). Preventive health behaviour and prosocial behaviour during the pandemic	Data from cross-sectional and longitudinal study, one month	Random sampling, adults, 23 countries	Three items for trust in the government, three items for preventive health behaviours, and four items for prosocial behaviours	The study found that higher trust in the government about COVID-19 control is significantly related to higher adoption of health behaviours and prosocial behaviours.

helping a stranger) during the pandemic (Kislyakov & Shmeleva, 2021). A different study found that in travellers, problem awareness, attribution of responsibility, and anticipated feelings of pride contributed to practising prosocial behaviours (Zhu et al., 2022). A cross-sectional study shows no significant differences between adults in urban and rural areas in prosocial behaviour. The participants scored high on items (empathy with those who are in need), and they viewed kindness as a vital factor in their COVID-19 pandemic experience (Shillington et al., 2022). One study showed that medical students deciding to volunteer depended on various motivating and barrier factors (moral obligation, family, social commitment, and others' safety) and whether they had the necessary skills to help (Byrne et al., 2021). A study showed that a high prevalence of prosocial behaviour was associated with an increased trust in institutions (Thu et al., 2021). An intervention study showed that wearing a mask is prosocial behaviour and has more advantages than non-mask-wearers. It was supported by an evolutionary explanation (Kabir et al., 2021).

Another latent class analysis showed four classes of prosocial behaviours: money donors, online and offline helpers, online health information sharers, and neighbour helpers (Aresi et al., 2022). One online experiment result revealed that the identification with whole humanity is a psychological construct that promotes cooperative health behaviour and help-oriented concern for others during the pandemic (Barragan et al., 2021).

Therapeutic Effects

Three cross-sectional studies analysed the therapeutic effects of prosocial behaviour, out of which one study revealed that prosocial behaviour was related to better well-being across regions. A study by Haller et al. (2022) identified the association of perceived social support, psychological flexibility, positive affect, and perceived stress with prosocial behaviour (Haller et al., 2022). One of the studies' social orientation scores revealed the interaction between green space attendance and perceived crowdedness of green space, suggesting that attending low-crowded green space is associated with increased prosocial behaviour (Noël & Dardenne, 2022).

A study by Al Dhaheri et al. (2021) showed that the COVID-19 pandemic had a mild psychological impact on people. It also positively impacted family support and mental health awareness among adults. A systematic review by Jones et al. (2021) found that positive coping skills, social support, parent–child discussions, and home quarantining positively influenced adolescent mental health during the pandemic. An experimental study by Miles et al. (2022) did not find any difference during intervention or follow-up between individuals in the prosocial condition and self-focused or neutral acts. Similarly, no difference was found in the prosocial effects between those negatively affected emotionally or socially by the pandemic. An online study by Hellmann et al. (2021) found that different dimensions of responsibility are associated with different actors (self, recipient, politicians). The study also found that prosocial behaviour increases when individuals view themselves and perceived models (politicians) as accountable to help.

A qualitative content analysis by Tekin et al. (2021) found that older individuals, people with disabilities and fine health conditions, marginalised communities and working class, and frontline workers received primary support during the virus outbreak. The study identified three types of support: psychological, socio-emotional, and material. They also found that support came from various sources: (a) volunteers, (b) different organisations, and (c) advantaged groups. Moreover, they found that allyship, sharing a community/humanity identity, and showing gratitude were prominent reasons for prosocial behaviour.

Varma et al. (2022) conducted an online experiment which revealed that participants showed prosocial behaviour by purchasing for themselves or someone else COVID-19-related items (including personal protective equipment or PPE) or unrelated items like food and writing supplies. Prosocial behaviour is associated with higher levels of empathy, social connectedness, and positive affect. The study found more considerable psychological benefits when the generous acts were unrelated to COVID-19.

Positive Outcomes

Seven studies that analysed the positive outcomes included a study by Gijzen et al. (2020), which found a significant positive association between social loneliness and stable mental health. The study also emphasised the importance of meaningful relationships. An experimental study by Abel and Brown (2020) found that positive private role models increase the norms of trust, and negative public role models can increase a sense of responsibility among individuals, encouraging them to exhibit more prosocial behaviours. In another study conducted by Columbus (2021) that used a survey method, it was revealed that when exposed to a social dilemma, people high in Honesty and Humility parameter are seen to be more willing to give up individual benefits for collective benefits.

Two online experiments conducted by Grimalda et al. (2021) reported that individuals exposed to COVID-19 donated more than those not exposed. With regard to the targets of giving donations, they found that donors primarily benefited the local level. Feng and colleagues (2020) conducted a cross-sectional online survey; the results show that more negative altruism was found in individuals with high altruism than those with low altruism. Negative altruism indirectly increases the individual's anxiety and depressive symptoms. Online survey results implied a strong association between acute anxiety and higher physiological arousal during the pandemic and engaging in altruistic behaviours. These findings support the relationship between humans' defensive and altruistic motivation (Vieira et al., 2021). Data from a double design study consisting of one cross-sectional and one longitudinal study by Han et al. (2021) suggested that higher trust in the government with regard to COVID-19 control is significantly associated with higher adoption of health behaviours and prosocial behaviours.

Conclusion

This systematic review investigated prosocial behaviour during the time of the COVID-19 pandemic. Studies from January 2020 to August 2022 were obtained from ten databases. Out of over 30 articles reviewed, 16 studies met the inclusion criteria. According to the research method, seven were cross-sectional, five were experimental, eight used a survey method, one followed a between-subjects design, one was a systematic review, one was latent class analysis, one was an intervention study, one was qualitative content analysis, and one included a double design of the cross-sectional and longitudinal study.

COVID-19 was one of the most significant health emergencies humans have faced in generations, and people suffered severe repercussions for their physical, mental, and social well-being. This systematic review focuses on the positive be-haviours displayed during the pandemic. It emphasises on the prosocial behaviours observed during the pandemic, the therapeutic effects of prosocial behaviour, and the positive outcomes of self-directed prosocial behaviour.

The review revealed that several prosocial behaviours, like social distancing, were prevalent during the pandemic (Andrews et al., 2022). Some studies also showed that other activities, such as donating money, checking in with isolated patients, and delivering food or medications, were observed during that time (Cho et al., 2022). Compliance with protective measures such as wearing gloves and masks and washing hands was also considered prosocial (Dinić & Bodroza, 2021). These studies implied that kindness is a crucial component that helps humanity thrive in crises such as the pandemic.

Studies have found that therapeutic effects of prosocial behaviour were associ-ated with better well-being across regions. It was observed that perceived social support is highly correlated with prosociality (Haller et al., 2022). Prosocial acts such as procuring personal protective equipment and purchasing food and supplies led to increased levels of empathy and social connectedness that had influenced people positively in physical and psychological realms.

Due to the personal experiences of exposure to the virus, donations, volunteer-ing, and other prosocial acts were beneficial to crisis management at the local and global levels (Feng et al., 2020). Social distancing and isolation had positive rela-tions with mental health and stressed the importance of meaningful relationships. Other positive outcomes included increased trust in the government, which led to higher adoption of healthy behaviours and prosociality (Han et al., 2021).

Despite having witnessed several prosocial activities during the pandemic, which helped manage the crisis to a great extent, it had devastating effects on several spheres of life. The present systematic review throws light on the brighter

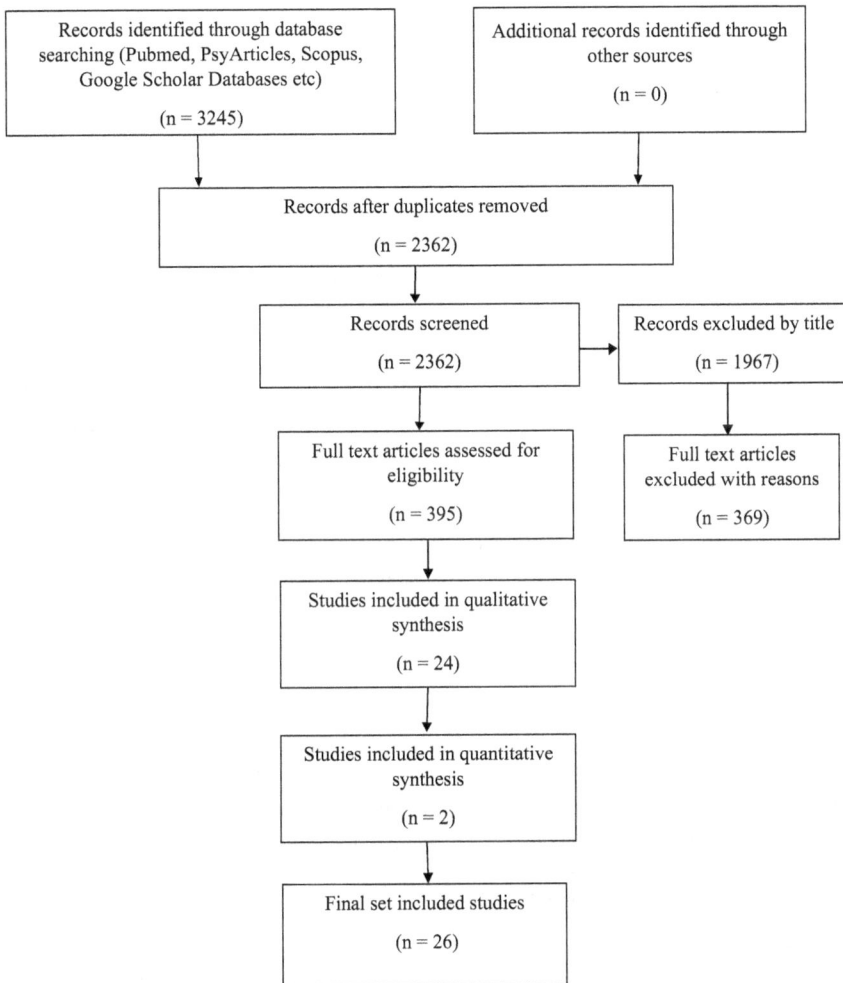

FIGURE 3.1 PRISMA flow diagram

side of humanity, which is paramount during difficult times of life. It also draws attention to more research focusing on the positive and damaging effects of tough times and helps us prepare for unforeseen events such as COVID. A few studies have been conducted to understand people's prosocial behaviour during the pandemic. A considerable increase has been found in the prosocial activities of people despite other contradictory factors. It is a crucial humane quality of people to be cooperative and helpful during crises, and studies have repeatedly proven the same.

References

Abel, M., & Brown, W. (2020). *Prosocial behavior in the time of COVID-19: The effect of private and public role models (IZA Discussion Papers No. 13207)*. IZA Institute of Labor Economics.

Al Dhaheri, A. S., Bataineh, M. A. F., Mohamad, M. N., Ajab, A., Al Marzouqi, A., Jarrar, A. H., Habib-Mourad, C., Abu-Jamous, D. O., Ali, H. I., Al Sabbah, H., & Hasan, H. (2021). Impact of COVID-19 on mental health and quality of life: Is there any effect? A cross-sectional study of the MENA region. *PLoS One, 16*(3). https://doi.org/10.1371/journal.pone.0249107

Andrews, M. E., Mattan, B. D., Richards, K., Moore-Berg, S. L., & Falk, E. B. (2022). Using first-person narratives about healthcare workers and people who are incarcerated to motivate helping behaviors during the COVID-19 pandemic. *Social Science & Medicine, 299*, 114870.

Aresi, G., Procentese, F., Gattino, S., Tzankova, I., Gatti, F., Compare, C., Marzana, D., Mannarini, T., Fedi, A., Marta, E., & Guarino, A. (2022). Prosocial behaviours under collective quarantine conditions. A latent class analysis study during the 2020 COVID-19 lockdown in Italy. *Journal of Community & Applied Social Psychology, 32*(3), 490–506. https://doi.org/10.1002/casp.25712

Brancati, D. (2007). Political aftershocks: The impact of earthquakes on intrastate conflict. *Journal of Conflict Resolution, 51*(5), 715–743.

Byrne, M. H., Ashcroft, J., Wan, J. C., Alexander, L., Harvey, A., Schindler, N., Brown, M. E., & Brassett, C. (2021). Examining medical student volunteering during the COVID-19 pandemic as a prosocial behavior during an emergency. *medRxiv*, 2021–2027. https://doi.org/10.1101/2021.07.06.21260058

Castro-Piñero, J., Artero, E. G., España-Romero, V., Ortega, F. B., Sjöström, M., Suni, J., & Ruiz, J. R. (2010). Criterion-related validity of field-based fitness tests in youth: A systematic review. *British Journal of Sports Medicine, 44*(13), 934–943.

Cho, I., Daley, R. T., Cunningham, T. J., Kensinger, E. A., & Gutchess, A. (2022). Aging, empathy, and prosocial behaviors during the COVID-19 pandemic. *The Journals of Gerontology: Series B, 77*(4), e57–e63.

Columbus, S. (2021). Honesty-humility, beliefs, and prosocial behaviour: A test on stockpiling during the COVID-19 pandemic. *Collabra: Psychology, 7*(1). https://doi.org/10.1525/collabra.19028

Dinić, B. M., & Bodroža, B. (2021). COVID-19 protective behaviours are forms of prosocial and unselfish behaviours. *Frontiers in Psychology*, 1128. https://doi.org/10.3389/fpsyg.2021.647710

Drury, J., Carter, H., Cocking, C., Ntontis, E., Tekin Guven, S., & Amlôt, R. (2019). Facilitating collective psychosocial resilience in the public in emergencies: Twelve recommendations based on the social identity approach. *Frontiers in Public Health, 7*, 141.

Esteban-Cornejo, I., Tejero-Gonzalez, C. M., Sallis, J. F., & Veiga, O. L. (2015). Physical activity and cognition in adolescents: A systematic review. *Journal of Science and Medicine in Sport, 18*(5), 534–539.

Feng, Y., Zong, M., Yang, Z., Gu, W., Dong, D., & Qiao, Z. (2020). When altruists cannot help: The influence of altruism on the mental health of university students during the COVID-19 pandemic. *Globalisation and Health, 16*, 1–8. https://doi.org/10.1186/s12992-020-00587-y

Gijzen, M., Shields-Zeeman, L., Kleinjan, M., Kroon, H., van der Roest, H., Bolier, L., Smit, F., & de Beurs, D. (2020). The bittersweet effects of COVID-19 on mental health: Results of an online survey among a sample of the Dutch population five weeks after relaxation of lockdown restrictions. *International Journal of Environmental Research and Public Health, 17*(23), 9073. https://doi.org/10.3390/ijerph17239073

Grimalda, G., Buchan, N. R., Ozturk, O. D., Pinate, A. C., Urso, G., & Brewer, M. B. (2021). Exposure to COVID-19 is associated with increased altruism, particularly at the local level. *Scientific Reports, 11*(1), 18950.

Haller, E., Lubenko, J., Presti, G., Squatrito, V., Constantinou, M., Nicolaou, C., Papacostas, S., Aydın, G., Chong, Y. Y., Chien, W. T., & Cheng, H. Y. (2022). To help or not to help? Prosocial behavior, its association with wellbeing, and predictors of prosocial behavior during the coronavirus disease pandemic. *Frontiers in Psychology, 12*, 6518. https://doi.org/10.3389/fpsyg.2021.775032

Han, Q., Zheng, B., Cristea, M., Agostini, M., Bélanger, J. J., Gützkow, B., Kreienkamp, J., Leander, N. P., & PsyCorona Collaboration. (2021). Trust in government regarding COVID-19 and its associations with preventive health behaviour and prosocial behaviour during the pandemic: A cross-sectional and longitudinal study. *Psychological Medicine, 53*(1), 149–159.

Hellmann, D. M., Dorrough, A. R., & Glöckner, A. (2021). Prosocial behavior during the COVID-19 pandemic in Germany. The role of responsibility and vulnerability. *Heliyon, 7*(9), 1–11.

Hsiang, S. M., Burke, M., & Miguel, E. (2013). Quantifying the influence of climate on human conflict. *Science, 341*(6151), 1235367.

Jones, E. A., Mitra, A. K., & Bhuiyan, A. R. (2021). Impact of COVID-19 on mental health in adolescents: A systematic review. *International Journal of Environmental Research and Public Health, 18*(5), 2470. https://doi.org/10.3390/ijerph18052470

Kabir, K. A., Risa, T., & Tanimoto, J. (2021). Prosocial behavior of wearing a mask during an epidemic: An evolutionary explanation. *Scientific Reports, 11*(1), 12621. https://doi.org/10.1038/s41598-021-92094-2

Kislyakov, P. A., & Shmeleva, E. A. (2021). Strategies of prosocial behavior during the COVID-19 pandemic. *The Open Psychology Journal, 14*(1), 266–272.

Miles, A., Andiappan, M., Upenieks, L., & Orfanidis, C. (2022). Using prosocial behavior to safeguard mental health and foster emotional wellbeing during the COVID-19 pandemic: A registered report of a randomised trial. *PLoS One, 17*(7). https://doi.org/10.1371/journal.pone.0272152

Moher, D., Liberati, A., Tetzlaff, J., Altman, D. G., & PRISMA Group*. (2009). Preferred reporting items for systematic reviews and meta-analyses: The PRISMA statement. *Annals of Internal Medicine, 151*(4), 264–269.

Noël, T., & Dardenne, B. (2022). Relationships between Green Space Attendance, Perceived Crowdedness, Perceived Beauty and Prosocial Behavior in Time of Health Crisis. *International Journal of Environmental Research and Public Health, 19*(11), 6778. https://doi.org/10.3390/ijerph19116778

Rao, L. L., Han, R., Ren, X. P., Bai, X. W., Zheng, R., Liu, H., . . . & Li, S. (2011). Disadvantage and prosocial behavior: The effects of the Wenchuan earthquake. *Evolution and Human Behavior, 32*(1), 63–69.

Reny, T. T., & Barreto, M. A. (2022). Xenophobia in the time of pandemic: Othering, anti-Asian attitudes, and COVID-19. *Politics, Groups, and Identities, 10*(2), 209–232.

Rodríguez, H., & Aguirre, B. E. (2006). Hurricane Katrina and the healthcare infrastructure: A focus on disaster preparedness, response, and resiliency. *Frontiers of Health Services Management, 23*(1), 13–24.

Shillington, K. J., Vanderloo, L. M., Burke, S. M., Ng, V., Tucker, P., & Irwin, J. D. (2022). A cross-sectional examination of Canadian adults' prosocial behavior during the COVID-19 pandemic. *Journal of Rural Mental Health, 46*(3), 174. https://psycnet.apa.org/doi/10.1037/rmh0000201

Tekin, S., Sager, M., Bushey, A., Deng, Y., & Uluğ, Ö. M. (2021). How do people support each other in emergencies? A qualitative exploration of altruistic and prosocial behaviours during the COVID-19 pandemic. *Analyses of Social Issues and Public Policy, 21*(1), 1113–1140. https://doi.org/10.1111/asap.12277

Thu, T. V., Vu, D., Lee, K., Thi Mai, L. N., Minh, N. L., Dinh Bao, P. P., Hoang Thi Diem, N. T., Xuan, L. N., & Tien, N. P. (2021). Prosocial behaviors among the Vietnamese population during the COVID-19 pandemic: Implications for social education programs. *The Open Psychology Journal, 14*(1).

Turner, J. C., Hogg, M. A., Oakes, P. J., Reicher, S. D., & Wetherell, M. S. (1987). *Rediscovering the social group: A self-categorization theory.* basil Blackwell.

Varma, M. M., Chen, D., Lin, X., Aknin, L. B., & Hu, X. (2022). Prosocial behavior promotes positive emotion during the COVID-19 pandemic. *Emotion, 23*(2), 538–553. https://doi.org/10.1037/emo0001077

Vieira, J. B., Jangard, S., Pierzchajlo, S., Marsh, A. A., & Olsson, A. (2021). Acute anxiety during the COVID-19 pandemic was associated with higher levels of everyday altruism. *Scientific Reports, 12*(1), 1–13. https://doi.org/10.1038/s41598-022-23415-2

Zaki, J. (2020). Integrating empathy and interpersonal emotion regulation. *Annual Review of Psychology, 71*, 517–540.

Zhu, P., Chi, X., Ryu, H. B., Ariza-Montes, A., & Han, H. (2022). Traveler prosocial behaviors at heritage tourism sites. *Frontiers in Psychology, 13*. https://doi.org/10.3389/fpsyg.2022.901530

SECTION 2

Coping Strategies

4

EFFECTIVENESS OF COGNITIVE BEHAVIOURAL THERAPY FOR ADULTS WITH DEPRESSION AND ANXIETY DURING COVID-19

A Systematic Review of Randomised Controlled Trials

Garima Joshi, Charu Joshi, Bhawna Tushir and Akancha Srivastava

Introduction

Coronavirus Disease (COVID-19) has posed a severe public health concern worldwide. Recent scientific evidence has indicated that COVID-19 led to an increase in mental health disorders such as anxiety, depression, and corona-phobia, significantly impacting the quality of life of individuals (Tyrer, 2020). The COVID-19 pandemic led to a significant rise in anxiety and fear, with individuals becoming anxious about contracting the virus, acquiring essential medical supplies, and accessing timely medical assistance (Kini et al., 2020). In addition, governments' abrupt discontinuation of social, economic, educational, and recreational activities had further contributed to feelings of insecurity and a perceived lack of access to necessities such as food items (Brooks et al., 2020).

The world grappled with the loss of access to in-person mental healthcare services. The instability of healthcare facilities caused due to COVID-19, along with significant issues with access to mental healthcare facilities in person, also led to an increase in mental health issues in the general population, severely impacting those already under care due to limitations with access to their mental healthcare professionals (Ornell et al., 2021). Anxiety and depression were found to be the most common mental health conditions during COVID-19, and increasing interest and need for innovation had led to the use of telemedicine and Internet-based Cognitive and Behavioural Interventions.

Previous research has indicated that during the early stages of public health emergencies like SARS, individuals may experience anxiety, depression, and psychotic symptoms, which could result in severe consequences such as suicide. Studies have also shown that patients with COVID-19 may suffer from high levels of negative emotions such as anxiety, depression, loneliness, despair, and anger (Liu et al.,

DOI: 10.4324/9781003357209-6

2003; Zhang & Feei, 2020; Tyrer, 2020). According to a meta-analysis (Li et al., 2020), the percentage of patients with COVID-19 experiencing anxiety and depression was significantly higher than the general population and medical staff. Additionally, a few patients had exhibited extreme behaviours, such as blaming and mistreating medical staff and putting frontline workers at a greater risk (Ferreira, 2022; Xiang et al., 2020).

Cognitive Behavioural Therapy is a psychotherapy proven effective through evidence-based research and used globally to prevent and treat psychological and physical issues (Schure et al., 2019; Chan et al., 2018). This therapy involves various methods that assist individuals in identifying their stress levels, modifying their beliefs and behaviours, and receiving social support (Beck, 1979). Cognitive restructuring, behavioural changes, and social support are some techniques used to eliminate or reduce psychological distress symptoms and aid individuals in returning to their everyday daily lives. Numerous studies have indicated that Cognitive Behavioural Therapy can significantly reduce anxiety, improve somatic symptoms and psychological stress, and increase the overall quality of life (Hartley et al., 2016). Moreover, it is the most cost-effective and successful psychotherapy in reducing and relieving psychological distress (Tang & Kreindler, 2017).

The positive effects of cognitive behaviour and the effectiveness of Cognitive Behavioural Therapy (CBT) have been well established in in treating mental health conditions. However, given the pandemic situation, CBT had to be delivered either through the internet or in person under the looming circumstances of COVID-19 to patients. Therefore, conducting a systematic review to understand the effectiveness of CBT and internet-delivered CBT (iCBT) on conditions of depression and anxiety during the pandemic was essential to understand the impetus of the therapy via different modalities and in varying populations.

The COVID-19 pandemic has significantly impacted global mental health, with depression and anxiety being two of the most common conditions reported. While Cognitive Behavioural Therapy (CBT) and internet-delivered CBT (iCBT) have been established as effective treatments for depression and anxiety, there is a lack of research on their effectiveness during the COVID-19 pandemic. This gap in the literature highlights the need for further investigation to determine the efficacy of CBT and iCBT interventions in treating depression and anxiety during the pandemic. Additionally, evidence-based clinical guidelines for these interventions are needed to ensure that mental health professionals access the most effective and appropriate treatment strategies. Identifying this gap in the literature can help justify the need for future studies and provide a rationale for the importance of evidence-based clinical guidelines for CBT and iCBT interventions during the COVID-19 pandemic.

Method and Analysis

Three researchers retrieved the relevant literature on CBT and internet-delivered CBT for patients with anxiety and depression during the COVID-19 pandemic. PubMed and Web of Science, Cochrane Library, and Clinical Trials Registry of

India were searched for literature starting from December 2019. The grey literature and pertinent trials and references of the contained literature were also looked for. The researchers independently gathered data and pertinent information, and the calibre of the literature was also assessed. The scientific paper maintained methodological rigor by adhering to the guidelines set forth by PICOT and PRISMA (Page et al., 2021), ensuring comprehensive adherence to establish standards (Lalu et al., 2021).

Key Questions

The review questions are listed as follows:

1 What is the comparative effectiveness of CBT and iCBT in treating anxiety and depression during COVID-19, as evidenced in the literature?
2 How does the relative efficacy of CBT and iCBT differ between patients and clinicians?

Table 4.1 gives the description of the population, intervention, comparators, outcomes, and settings (PICOTS) for our review.

Criteria of Inclusion/Exclusion of Studies in the Review

The following criteria included and excluded studies from the searched literature.

The review focuses on the evidence provided in original research articles that are available in full-text, are published in English, and involve randomised controlled trials with at least 30 total individuals (15 in each arm of the study with two arms). Studies from December 2019 till the present were included, with a

TABLE 4.1 Population, intervention, comparators, outcomes, and settings (PICOTS)

Domain	Description
Population	Recipients of mental healthcare therapy – Cognitive Behavioural Therapy or Internet-based Cognitive Behavioural Therapy during COVID-19 population – diagnosed with anxiety or depression
Intervention	Specific clinical intervention is as follows: • Cognitive Behavioural Therapy • Internet-Based Cognitive Behavioural Therapy
Comparator	Treatment-as-usual (TAU)
Outcome measures	Any psychological rating scales describing mood, stress, anxiety, and quality of life.
Study Design	Randomised Controlled Trials
Timing	Any length of time for therapeutic intervention
Settings	Clinical or community settings globally: • In-patient and out-patient settings and clinics of all types • Academic healthcare institutions • Organisations, professional clubs, organisational settings

focus on the adult population aged 18 years and older, including the general public and clinical population, which has been diagnosed with or has presented with the symptoms of depression and anxiety and received psychological intervention in the form of Cognitive Behavioural Therapy or Internet-based Cognitive Behavioural Therapy. Studies on children, and incarcerated populations in jails, were excluded. Admissible settings included in-patient and out-patient settings, clinics of all types, academic institutions in healthcare, and community-based and organisation-based settings located globally.

The studies had at least one outcome of interest: a psychological scale measuring symptoms of anxiety, depression, stress, or quality of life. Any parameter did not limit the duration of the intervention.

Searching for Evidence: Literature Search Strategies

The authors systematically searched, reviewed, and synthesised the scientific evidence for the research questions following the PRISMA guideline (Lalu et al., 2020). The steps are listed as follows: (a) the identification of literature and relevant articles for the research questions through focused searches on the comparative effectiveness of CBT and iCBT in anxiety and depression disorders during COVID-19 and (b) the identification of any clinician and patient-specific characteristics which affected the effectiveness of CBT and iCBT during the COVID-19 pandemic. The literature search was carried out using a variety of Medical Subject Headings (MeSH terms), and major headings, free-text, titles, and abstract text-word searches were also carried out. Relevant terms are listed in Table 4.3. Search results were limited according to the inclusion and exclusion criteria as mentioned in Table 4.2. Randomised trials and the following experimental study types were included: comparative, controlled clinical trials, and crossover studies. The scope of this review was limited to studies published in English only.

The search terms listed in Table 4.3, were searched in the Cochrane Library, Cochrane Central Trials Registry for these topics, and the Clinical Trials Registry of India were searched. PubMed and Web of Science databases were also searched for relevant literature. Duplicates were removed from the database using Zotero, yielded data from these searches, and then screened on the basis of title and abstract. Studies investigating other topics, such as reviews, protocols, electrophysiological studies, and other interventions, were excluded on the basis of title and abstract. The selected full-text articles were evaluated on the inclusion criteria and analysed. Further, the reviewers evaluated the finally selected studies on Cochrane's Risk of Bias (RoB) (Higgins et al., 2011).

Authors Dr Garima Joshi, Charu Joshi and Dr Bhawna Tushir independently evaluated the articles at each selection stage, that is identification, screening, eligibility, and inclusion. Any disagreements were resolved by consultation with another author, Dr Akancha Srivastava, through consensus-based discussions.

TABLE 4.2 Study-specific inclusion and exclusion criteria

Category	Criteria for Inclusion	Criteria for Exclusion
Language	English	All non-English literature
Dates of Publications	December 2019 to present	–
Study Design	• Individual randomised controlled trials • Clustered randomised controlled trials • Quasi-experimental trials • Non-randomised trials	• All non-experimental studies • Qualitative research
Study Duration	No limits	
Publications	Complete full-text articles	• Systematic reviews • Meta-analysis • Protocols • Stand-alone abstracts • Studies lacking original/experimental data • Narrative reviews • Editorials, letters to the editors, and similar publications
Populations	Adults (18 years and above) • General public/patients • Clinicians	• Children (<18 years), incarcerated population
Comparators	Treatment as usual (pharmacological)	• Other psychological interventions
Settings	Clinical or community settings globally	• In-patient and out-patient settings and clinics of all types • Academic healthcare institutions • Primary and secondary schools • Prisons and jails • Organisations, professional clubs, organisational settings
Geographical settings	Any country	
Sample size	• N > 30 • No limits on the size of clusters	N < 30
Other	• Access to full-text article	• Inability to retrieve the full-text article

Data Abstraction and Management

Electronic spreadsheets were used to extract and tabulate the data. From each trial, one continuous health anxiety, depression, quality of life, and stress measure was employed. This was often the trial's central finding, typically a self-rated questionnaire. When there was no stated primary outcome, we selected the first health anxiety and depression outcome that had been reported.

TABLE 4.3 Search terms

Interventions	*Search Terms*
Cognitive Behavioural Therapy	"Cognitive Behavioural Therapy/Intervention" AND "COVID-19" OR "2019 Coronavirus Disease" OR "2019-nCoV", cognitive behavioural therapy, CBT, cognitive behavioural treatment
Cognitive Behavioural Therapy	"Internet-based Cognitive Behavioural Therapy/Intervention "OR "telemedicine and cognitive intervention" AND "COVID-19" OR "2019 Coronavirus Disease" OR "2019-nCoV", cognitive behavioural therapy, CBT, cognitive behavioural treatment
Database	Web of Science, PubMed, Cochrane Library, and Clinical Trial Databases

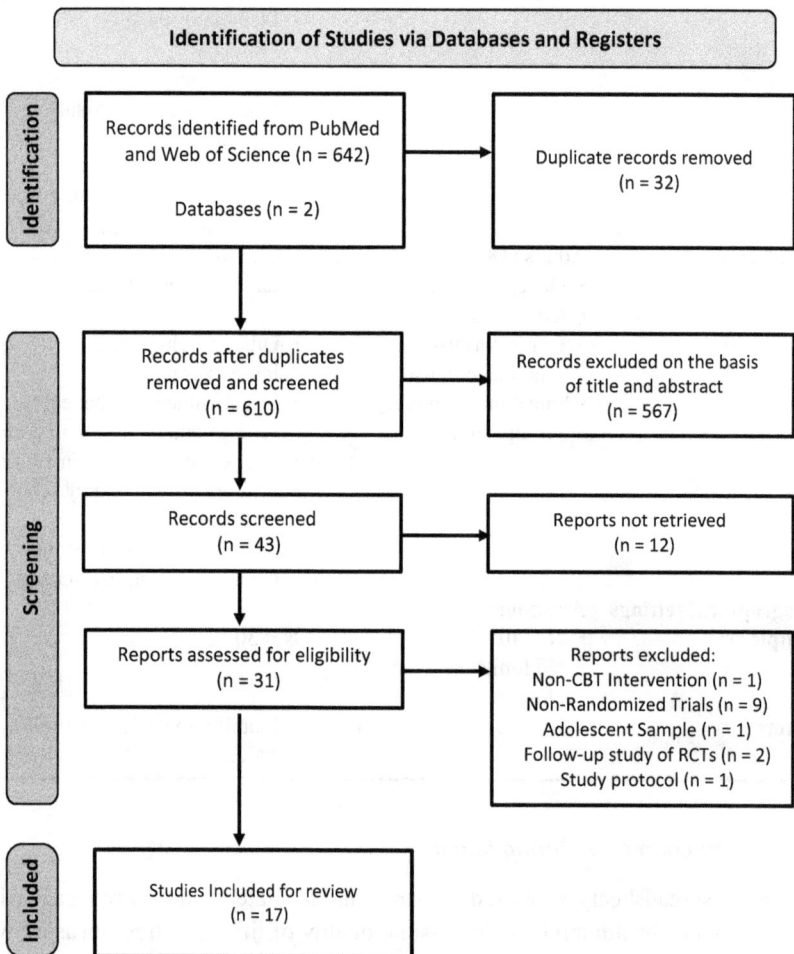

FIGURE 4.1 PRISMA flow diagram describing the selection process for relevant clinical trials used in this systematic review

TABLE 4.4 Data items to extract

Data to Extract	Examples
Study characteristics and methods	• Study design
	• Study objectives
	• Intervention and comparators
	• Settings
	• Duration
	• Outcome measures
	• Sample size
	• Eligibility criteria
	• Sampling technique
	• Statistical analysis
Participant characteristics	• Age group
	• Gender/sex
	• Education
	• Income
	• Health literacy
Outcome characteristics	• Definition of outcome
	• Measures used
	• Source of outcome data
	• Results in intervention and control groups

For studies that met the inclusion criteria, relevant information was further arranged into evidence tables to gather pertinent information from each article based on acharacteristics of studies as mentioned in Table 4.4. Data was then reviewed for completeness and accuracy by three research team members (G.J., B.T., C.J.). Methodological quality was assessed by each of them independently, followed by a discussion.

Assessment of Methodological Quality of Studies

Utilising the Cochrane Risk of Bias Tool (Higgins et al., 2011), the Risk of Bias (RoB) was evaluated to identify the possibility of selection, measurement, confounding, power, and reporting biases. The studies which were determined on a rating of low and medium risks of bias were included. Additionally, two reviewers evaluated each study's risk of bias separately, and team members settled any discrepancies through discussion and agreement.

Results and Discussion

Selection of Studies for Inclusion

A total of 641 articles were obtained from a search in four databases, out of which 610 articles were screened after removing duplicates; the screening was based on the title and abstracts' relevance to the objectives. Forty-three records were further screened, and 31 articles were eligible for full-text search. Out of the remaining 31 articles, an additional 14 were excluded on the basis of the inclusion criteria for the systematic review.

The excluded articles were returned for the following reasons: Weiner et al. (2020) was a study protocol; Samantaray et al. (2022) was a follow-up study to a previously conducted study. Heckendorf et al. (2022) were omitted as the intervention was not CBT, while Wisman et al. (2023) were conducted on adolescents. The other nine studies were excluded because they were not randomised controlled trials (Sharrock et al., 2021; Song et al., 2021; Nesset et al., 2022; Milosevic et al., 2021; Korpilahti-Leino et al., 2022; Mahoney et al., 2021; Puertas-Gonzales et al., 2021; Ying et al., 2022).

All the studies were found to be of low risk regarding selection bias, attrition bias, and reporting bias.

Specifications of the Included Studies

All the studies were randomised controlled trials and were conducted during the COVID-19 period. The smallest and the most significant sample consisted of 24 (Sharma et al., 2022) and 670 elements (Wahlund et al., 2020). Out of the studies conducted, one study was done on patients admitted due to COVID-19 infection (Puertas-Gonzalez, 2020), and one study was done on patients with acute stress disorder (Perri et al., 2021), while one was conducted on inpatients with severe psychological disorder (Sharma et al., 2022). Three studies were done on university students (El Morr et al., 2020; Shabahang et al., 2021; Aminoff et al., 2021). Three of the included studies were done on a population with clinical depression and anxiety (Liu et al., 2021; Zhou et al., 2022; Sockalingam et al., 2022), and one study was done on women with postpartum depression (PPD) (Van Lieshout et al., 2021). Shapira et al. (2021) conducted the study on community-dwelling older adults, while four studies conducted their intervention on community-dwelling adults with symptoms of anxiety and depression (Al-Alawi et al., 2021; Egan et al., 2021; Wahlund et al., 2020; Akin-Sari et al., 2022). One study was conducted on healthcare workers (HCWs) (Amra et al., 2022), and another study was done on pregnant women (Puertas-Gonzalez et al., 2022).

The scales used in the study were PTSD checklist for DSM-V (PCL-5) (Blevins et al., 2015), State-Trait Anxiety Inventory (STAI-Y1) (Spielberger et al., 1983), Beck Depression Inventory-II (BDI-II) (Beck et al., 1996), the Mini International Neuropsychiatric Interview (MINI), version 5.0 (Sheehan et al., 1998), Patient Health Questionnaire (PHQ-9) (Kroenke et al., 2001), Generalised Anxiety Disorder – 7-Item Scale (Spitzer et al., 2006), Emotional Eating Scale (EES) (Arnow et al., 1995), Binge Eating Scale (BES) (Gormally et al., 1982), Hamilton Depression Scale (1960), Hamilton Anxiety Scale (1959), Self-Rating Depression Scale (SDS) (Dunstan & Scott, 2019), the Self-Rating Anxiety Scale (SAS) (Dunstan & Scott, 2020), and the Athens Insomnia Scale (AIS) (Soldatos et al., 2000).

Prevalence of Anxiety and Depression During COVID-19 Pandemic

COVID-19 is one of the most rapidly spreading viruses globally, with severe and debilitating after-effects and lasting physical and psychological burden of the disease (Romagnoli et al., 2020). The most commonly reported symptoms are anxiety (35.7%), depression (32.6%), and insomnia (41.9%) (Nie et al., 2021; Rogers et al., 2020). The uncertainty of the severity and spread has had a significant psychological impact across all strata of society. It poses a severe risk factor for psychiatric conditions (Pfefferbaum & North, 2020), with an increase in reports of stress, insomnia, anxiety, depression, and post-traumatic stress disorder (PTSD) (Chew et al., 2020).

Several studies have reported increased levels of stress and insomnia during the COVID-19 pandemic. In a review, stress levels in China ranged between 8.1% and 29.9% in a survey (Wang et al., 2020), while India experienced a prevalence of 11.6% (Verma & Mishra, 2020).

There has been a reported increase in the prevalence of anxiety disorders during the pandemic, with 76 million new cases between March 2020 and January 2021, indicating a 25% increase in cases (Matthew et al., 2021). The disruption in routine, uncertainty, government-imposed lockdown and isolation, and concerns about health and well-being are the leading causes of anxiety (Santomauro et al., 2021).

In a review, the prevalence of symptoms of depression ranged between 8.3% and 48.3% in China (Huang & Zhao, 2020; Gao et al., 2020), and 25% prevalence in India also accounted for extreme-to-mild depression (Verma & Mishra, 2020) during the pandemic. This made the COVID-19 pandemic not just a respiratory syndrome but also a pandemic of mental and psycho-social issues (World Health Organization n.d.).

Cognitive Behavioural Therapy Intervention During COVID-19 Pandemic

The symptoms of anxiety, depression, stress, and insomnia have been comorbidly reported in varying severity across the literature since 2020. Several studies have reported the efficacy of CBT as a treatment method for the conditions mentioned earlier, and several studies have reported the effects of CBT, disseminated by various modalities, that is in-person and virtual or telephonic, across varying populations – both general and clinical settings. Next, we summarise the findings of our review study characteristics as listed in Table 4.5.

We have stratified the studies based on sample universes into studies conducted on the general population, clinical population, and university students, and into RCTs conducted on women during the pandemic until December 2022.

The analysis found that CBT is a treatment effective in improving the symptoms in the studies done in a clinical set-up. CBT is also found to be effective in studies done on adult populations that included patients admitted for bariatric surgery

TABLE 4.5 Characteristics of selected studies

Authors	Intervention on	Comparator	Settings	Session Details	Outcome Measure	Sample size	Age range	Findings in Intervention and Control Group
Zhou et al., 2022	E-aid cognitive behavioural therapy (eCBT-I)	Control group	Clinical	Once per week for six weeks	Chronic insomnia	118	24 to 44 years	Frontline nurses' sleep quality, anxiety, and depression during COVID-19 prevention and control considerably improved after six weeks of treatment compared to the control group, indicating that eCBTI had a strong therapeutic efficacy.
Sockalingam et. al., 2022	Tele-CBT	Control group	Clinical	Six weekly one-hour sessions	Anxiety and depression	81	18 and above	From pre- to post-intervention, the Tele-CBT group experienced significant reductions in binge eating symptoms (44%), emotional eating (22%), depression (49%), and anxiety (47%), and these reductions persisted over the three-month follow-up.
Liu et al., 2021	Computerised CBT (cCBT)	Baseline control group	Clinical	One week	Depression and anxiety (primary) insomnia (secondary)	252	18–75 years	During the postintervention and follow-up periods, there was a significant reduction in the symptoms of depression ($p = .001$), anxiety ($p = .001$), and sleeplessness ($p = .002$) in the cCBT + TAU group. Improvement in insomnia was not significantly different between the cCBT + TAU group and the TAU group for females ($p = .14$) or those with middle school education ($p = .48$).

| Li et al., 2020 | CBT (in person) | A control group with no intervention and TAU | Clinical (in-patients with COVID-19) | 30 minutes | DASS-21 | 93 | 18 years and above | Significant mean decreases in the depression, anxiety, stress, and total DASS-21 scales occurred in the intervention group (p = 0.001) and the control group (p = 0.001), with participants in the intervention group seeing a more significant mean decline. After the intervention, more people in the intervention group than in the control group showed no symptoms of depression or anxiety. However, there were no statistically significant differences (p > 0.05). Comparing participants with and without chronic disease, those without chronic disease saw a much higher decline in their overall DASS-21 score (coefficient = -4.74, 95% CI: -9.31; -0.17). |
| Sharma et al., 2022 | MindShift CBT app based CBT | Control group (TAU) | Clinical | Ten minutes at least for six days across six sessions | GAD-7 PHQ-9 Kessler Psychological Distress Scale (K10) | 24 | 18-65 years | No patient was admitted primarily for an anxiety illness, and 13/20 patients, or 65% of the included patients, were admitted for a psychotic disease. Twenty days on average (SD = 4.4; range = 321) were spent in the hospital, and 35% (7/20) of the patients were admitted against their will. The intervention group showed significant improvements in all domains assessed. |

(Continued)

TABLE 4.5 (Continued)

Authors	Intervention on	Comparator	Settings	Session Details	Outcome Measure	Sample size	Age range	Findings in Intervention and Control Group
Perri et al., 2021	Trauma-focused CBT	Eye movement desensitisation and reprocessing (EMDR) control group	Clinical	Seven-session therapy: two sessions per week for a total duration of about three weeks	PCL-5 STAI-Y1 BDI-II	38	18 and 65 years	The major conclusions showed that both the brief EMDR and TF-CBT were equally effective and significantly improved the end measures. In particular, following the seven-session therapy, state anxiety fell by about 30%. In comparison, the traumatic and depressed symptoms were decreased by about 55% in line with earlier studies that showed PTSD therapies were also linked to improvements in depressive symptoms.
Egan et al., 2021	CBT	Control group	General	Six hours;self-help	FAD-7 PHQ-9,	225	18–80 years	Results showed modest but substantial decreases in sadness (d = 0.28) and anxiety (d = 0.36) compared to controls on the wait list.
Wahlund et al., 2020	Three-week self-guided online cognitive behavioural intervention targeting dysfunctional COVID-19 worry and associated symptoms	Wait-list	General	Three-week long self-guided CBT	GAD-7	670	18 years and above	The intervention group significantly reduced COVID-19-related worry as compared to the waiting list, according to the main pre-specified intention-to-treat analysis (= 1.14, Z = 9.27, p = 0.001), which corresponds to a medium effect size (bootstrapped d = 0.74 [95% CI: 0.58–0.90]). All secondary variables, including mood, everyday functioning, sleeplessness, and intolerance of uncertainty, all showed improvements. There was excellent participant satisfaction. There were no significant adverse effects noted.

| Al-Alawi et al., 2021 | Participants in the intervention group were allocated to receive one online session per week for six weeks from certified psychotherapists based on CBT and Acceptance and Commitment Therapy | in the Oman control group received an automatic weekly newsletter via email containing self-help information and tips to cope with distress associated with COVID-19 | General | Six sessions; once per week across six weeks | CAD-7 PHQ-9 | 46 | 18–65 years | After accounting for baseline scores, the analysis of covariance revealed a significant decline in GAD-7 scores between the two groups (F(1, 43)=7.307; p = .01). Participants in the intervention group had significantly lower GAD-7 scores than those in the control group (β = 3.27; P = .01). Additionally, individuals in the intervention group showed a higher decline in mean PHQ-9 scores than those in the control group (F(1, 43)=8.298; p = .006) (β = 4.311; p = .006). Although both study groups had a decrease in their feelings of anxiety and sadness, the intervention group experienced a greater decrease (p = .049) than the control group (p = .02). |

(Continued)

TABLE 4.5 (Continued)

Authors	Intervention on	Comparator	Settings	Session Details	Outcome Measure	Sample size	Age range	Findings in Intervention and Control Group
Akin-Sari et al., 2022	App-based CBT	Wait-list, delayed intervention	General	Four minutes a day, for 12 days	OCI-R OBQ-44 DASS-21 IUS-12 CDS	55	18–65	Participants in the immediate-app usage group (iApp; n = 25) began using the app at baseline (T0), 4 minutes per day, for 12 days (T0–T1). The mobile application was made available to participants in the delayed-app group (dApp; n = 20) at T1 (crossover), and they utilised it for the next 12 days (T1–T2). Intention to treat analyses showed that using the app for 12 straight days was linked to significant effect-size decreases in OCD symptoms and dysfunctional thought patterns in the iApp group (from T0 to T1) and dApp group (Cohen's d ranged from 0.87 to 2.73). (from T1 to T2). At the follow-up, these reductions were still there.

| Shapira et al., 2021 | iCBT | Wait-list | Older adults | Seven online sessions over 3.5 weeks | PHQ-9 | 82 | 65–90 years | The changes in depressive symptoms showed a marginally significant main impact of time-by-group interaction (F(1, 79) = 3.82, p = 0.05, 2 = 0.05), indicating a marginally significant difference between the groups post-intervention. Statistically, the main effect of time was insignificant (F(1, 79) = 0.35, p = 0.55, 2 = 0.00). |
| Amra et al., 2022 | CBT | control group with no intervention | HCW | One shot CBTi | Five-minute heart rate variability epochs, Iranian version of the insomnia severity index | 57 | 18 years and above | The difference between the insomnia severity index score before and after the intervention was also statistically significant when comparing the two groups (p = 0.001). The mean insomnia severity index score in the intervention group was lower than the control group after the intervention (6.7, 4.5 vs. 13.6, 6.3, respectively; p = 0.001). |

(Continued)

TABLE 4.5 (Continued)

Authors	Intervention on	Comparator	Settings	Session Details	Outcome Measure	Sample size	Age range	Findings in Intervention and Control Group
Aminoff et al., 2021	ICBT	Control group baseline	University	Seven-week long	BDI-II BBQ, PHQ-9 GAD-7	52	18 years or older	According to the regression model's findings, the group condition on the BDI-II had a significant unstandardised regression coefficient with the following values: b = 5.48, 95% CI [0.43, 10.53], t = 2.130, and p = 0.034. This demonstrates that, on average, the treatment group outperformed the control group by 5.48 points on the BDI-II at the post-treatment measurement. Cohen's d = 0.63 [95% CI: 0.07–1.18] was the between-group effect size, which is a significant effect size. b = 2.86, 95% CI [5.29, 10.94], t = 0.68, p = 0.49; no significant unstandardised regression coefficient for group condition was identified for the BBQ. The Cohen's d value for the between-group effect size was 0.15 [95% CI: 0.39–0.70].

Shabahang et al., 2021	video-based, cognitive–behavioural intervention	Wait-list	University	15–20 minutes; three sessions per week for three weeks	COVID-19 Anxiety Questionnaire SHAI, Anxiety Sensitivity Index-3, Somatosensory Amplification Scale, Experience of Parasocial Interaction Scale Source Credibility Scale.	150	18–40	Between the intervention and control groups, there were significant differences in health anxiety (F = 42.97; p 0.01), anxiety sensitivity (F = 40.47; p 0.01), COVID-19 anxiety (F = 139.22; p 0.01), and somatosensory amplification (F = 38.74; p 0.01). According to Cohen51, the small, medium, and large impact sizes are 0.2, 0.5, and 0.8, respectively. Small to medium effect sizes were discovered for COVID-19 anxiety, health anxiety, anxiety sensitivity, and somatosensory amplification. According to our research, after receiving a video-based cognitive-behavioural intervention, people with high COVID-19 anxiety showed a slight to moderate reduction in their anxiety sensitivity, health anxiety, COVID-19 anxiety, and somatosensory amplification.

(Continued)

TABLE 4.5 (Continued)

Authors	Intervention on	Comparator	Settings	Session Details	Outcome Measure	Sample size	Age range	Findings in Intervention and Control Group
El Morr et al., 2020	Eight-week web-based guided web-based mindfulness	Wait-list	University	20 minutes on the web platform; 24 sessions spanning eight weeks	PHQ9 BAI PSS FFMQ-SF	148	18 years and above	According to the adjusted comparisons, at the postintervention follow-up, there were statistically significant increases in mindfulness (β = 4.84, p = .02) compared to the WLC group, as well as between-group decreases in depression and anxiety scores (β = −2.21, p = .01). When compared to WLC, there were no statistically significant differences between MVC and WLC in terms of subjective stress (β = .64, p = .48).

| Van Lieshout et al., 2021 | interactive online 1-day CBT-based workshop delivered by a registered psychotherapist, psychiatrist, or clinical psychology graduate student, in addition to treatment as usual | Wait-list and TAU | Women with PPD | Seven-hour single session in a workshop mode | PPD (EPDS scores) GAD-7 Social support Social Provisions Scale Postpartum Bonding Questionnaire Infant Behaviour Questionnaire – Revised Very Short Form. | 403 | 18 years and above | Participants had a mean (SD) age of 31.8 (4.4) years, and all identified as females. The workshop resulted in a significant mean (SD) EPDS score decrease (from 16.47 [4.41] to 11.65 [4.83]; B = 4.82; p = .001) and was linked to greater odds of displaying a clinically meaningful EPDS score reduction (odds ratio, 4.15; 95% CI, 2.66–6.46). After the workshop, the mean (SD) GAD-7 scores dropped from 12.41 (5.12) to 7.97 (5.54), and participants were more likely to experience a clinically significant change (odds ratio, 3.09; 95% CI, 1.99–4.81). Mothers reported reductions in infant-focused anxiety (B = 1.64; 95% CI, 2.25–1.00; p = .001), bonding (B = 3.22; 95% CI, 4.72–1.71), and other factors. |

(Continued)

TABLE 4.5 (Continued)

Authors	Intervention on	Comparator	Settings	Session Details	Outcome Measure	Sample size	Age range	Findings in Intervention and Control Group
Puertas-Gonzalez et al., 2022	Online Cognitive Behavioural Therapy	Control group (pregnant women who received online psychological support, pregnant women who received the usual care).	Pregnant women	1.5–2 hours for each session; eight consecutive weekly online sessions	Stress and resilience (primary) Psychopathological symptoms (secondary)	207 pregnant women	18 years and above	Regarding psychopathological symptoms, the interaction between pre-and post-treatment obsession-compulsion (OBS), depressive (DEP), and anxious (ANX) symptom scores was discovered using linear mixed models. According to the findings, the o-CBT group experienced a higher reduction in post-treatment pregnancy-specific stress levels and perceived stress levels than the other groups. Regarding susceptibility to stress, which is the propensity for being affected by perceived stress, there was no evidence of improvement in any of the groups.

Note: GAD-7, Generalised Anxiety Disorder – 7-Item Scale; DASS-21, Depression Anxiety Stress Scale – 21 Item; PHQ-4, Patient Health Questionnaire – 4 Item; SAS, Self-Rating Anxiety Scale; HARS, Hamilton Anxiety Rating Scale; SCL-90, Symptom Checklist – 90 Item; CAS, Coronavirus Anxiety Scale; PROMIS, Patient-Reported Outcomes Measurement Information System; STAI, State-Trait Anxiety Inventory; HADS, Hospital Anxiety and Depression Scale; BDI, Beck's Depression Inventory-II; BAI, Beck's Anxiety Inventory; FFMQ-SF, the Five Facet Mindfulness Questionnaire – Short Form; OCI-R, Obsessive Compulsive Inventory-Revised; OBQ-44, Obsessional Beliefs Questionnaire (OBQ-44); IUS-12, Intolerance of Uncertainty Scale-12; CDS, COVID-19 Distress Scale; PCL5, PTSD Checklist for DSM-5 (PCL-5).

(Sockalingam et al., 2022) with a focus on psychological distress and in-patients with COVID-19 diagnosis (Li et al., 2020) and anxiety and depression symptoms. However, the sample sizes were small, and both studies had short follow-up periods, limiting the knowledge of long-term efficacy in managing the symptoms without active intervention.

Studies done on healthcare workers have indicated that the prevalence of mental health disorder symptoms is higher in healthcare workers than in other professionals (Mattila et al., 2021). In keeping with the literature, Amra et al. (2022) explored the effectiveness of a one-shot CBT session for insomnia (CBTi) on frontline HCWs with acute insomnia. The mean insomnia severity index score in the intervention group was lower than the control group after the intervention (6.7, 4.5 vs. 13.6, 6.3, respectively; p-value 0.001). They indicate that a one-shot CBT session effectively manages acute insomnia symptoms.

Similar findings have been reported by Zhou et al. (2022) in a randomised trial using eCBT-I where the eCBT-I group's GAD-7 and PHQ-9 scores were lower after treatment than they were before (p 0.05). Many studies have confirmed the efficacy of eCBT-I in treating insomnia and improving sleep quality and efficiency (Seyffert et al., 2016; Lopez et al., 2019). eCBT-I also reduces the symptoms of comorbid anxiety and depression (Ye et al., 2015).

Virtually delivered CBT and in-person CBT do not have a considerable difference, indicating a moderate effect of the intervention. The mode of administration does not make a huge difference.

Future Implications and Limitations

Insomnia can increase the risk of developing mental health issues (Baglioni et al., 2011). However, Cognitive Behavioural Therapy (CBT) is an effective treatment for insomnia symptoms as well as symptoms of anxiety, depression, and stress, regardless of the mode of delivery (in-person or virtual) (Cassin et al., 2016; Sockalingam et al., 2019). Studies have shown that virtual care, including Internet-based CBT, is cost-effective, convenient, and increases access to treatment (Murphy et al., 2020; Santiago et al., 2021). Therefore, a hybrid dissemination model, utilising both virtual and traditional methods, is recommended to overcome the limitations of virtual care. These findings suggest that Internet-based CBT will continue to be used in different capacities, alongside traditional CBT, even after the pandemic (Sockalingam et al., 2022). The COVID-19 situation has emphasised the importance of virtual care, including Internet-based CBT, as an effective tool for mental health treatment. As a result, virtual care will likely continue to be a critical component of mental health treatment even after the pandemic.

Through the current review, we aimed to inform current Cognitive Behavioural Therapy (CBT) guidelines in the context of COVID-19. The review identified the most effective modes of delivery of CBT, whether in-person or virtual and identified the populations that would benefit the most from these interventions. The study also provided insights into the most effective techniques and strategies used in

CBT to address the specific mental health challenges faced by individuals during the pandemic.

The findings will inform the existing recommendations for developing CBT guidelines specific to the COVID-19 situation by synthesising the available evidence. These guidelines include best practices for adapting CBT to the virtual environment, such as strategies for addressing technological challenges and maintaining therapeutic relationships remotely. Additionally, the guidelines highlight the importance of addressing the unique challenges of the pandemic, such as anxiety related to health concerns and social isolation.

Limitations

The studies did not, in particular, focus on therapist and patient characteristics and their effects on the effectiveness of treatment. The sample demographics across studies were not homogenous or compared; therefore, the effects of clinician and patient-specific characteristics and their role in CBT and iCBT could not be ascertained with surety.

Most studies also had a very short follow-up period or did not report a follow-up, leaving the question of the long-term efficacy of CBT in managing symptoms of stress, anxiety, and depression unanswered. Most studies focused on anxiety and depression as outcome measures, the most prevalent disorders during the COVID-19 pandemic.

Most studies did not explore the quality of life as a construct and indicator of well-being, and the primary focus was psychopathological symptoms. The functional effectiveness of the treatment, therefore, still needs to be explored.

Method-wise, the studies also used varying sessions, and the duration of CBT intervention differed in each study; the limited homogeneity of intervention also limits our understanding of the recommended CBT treatment. This also paves the way for the necessity to create an evidence-based hybrid strategy that combines in-person and online sessions to maximise each modality's advantages while lowering implementation hurdles (Yeo et al., 2020; Strudwick et al., 2021) through meta-analysis and understanding the individual clinical and client characteristics and the effect of their interaction on the therapeutic outcome.

Conclusion

There is growing evidence that Cognitive Behavioural Therapy (CBT) can be effective in helping individuals at high risk avoid developing psychiatric illnesses such as post-traumatic stress disorder, anxiety, and depression. With the ongoing COVID-19 outbreak, the importance of adequate mental health treatment has become increasingly apparent. This systematic review aimed to evaluate the efficacy of CBT in reducing symptoms of anxiety and depression and enhancing the overall quality of life for patients during the COVID-19 pandemic.

Previous research has demonstrated that individuals who maintain close relationships with their loved ones and receive support from medical professionals experience improved psychological health. This is particularly important during epidemics like SARS and COVID-19, where social distancing measures can lead to feelings of isolation and loneliness. By using CBT techniques to enhance patients' self-esteem and lessen the psychological stress response, mental health professionals can significantly improve their patient's physical and mental well-being.

The findings of this systematic review can inform the existing guidelines for CBT and mental health treatment in the context of the COVID-19 pandemic. By providing evidence-based recommendations for best practices in adapting CBT to the virtual environment, addressing technological challenges, and maintaining therapeutic relationships remotely, mental health professionals can be equipped with the most effective and appropriate interventions to support individuals during these challenging times. Ultimately, this review aims to ensure that individuals receive the necessary care and support to maintain their mental health and well-being during the COVID-19 pandemic.

References

Akin-Sari, B., Inozu, M., Haciomeroglu, A. B., Cekci, B. C., Uzumcu, E., & Doron, G. (2022). Cognitive training via a mobile application to reduce obsessive-compulsive-related distress and cognitions during the COVID-19 outbreaks: A randomised controlled trial using a subclinical cohort. *Behaviour Therapy, 53*(5), 776–792. https://doi.org/10.1016/j.beth.2021.12.008

Al-Alawi, M., McCall, R. K., Sultan, A., Al Balushi, N., Al-Mahrouqi, T., Al Ghailani, A., Al Sabti, H., Al-Maniri, A., Panchatcharam, S. M., & Al Sinawi, H. (2021). Efficacy of a six-weeklong therapist-guided online therapy versus self-help internet-based therapy for COVID-19–induced anxiety and depression: Open-label, pragmatic, randomised controlled trial. *JMIR Mental Health, 8*(2). https://doi.org/10.2196/26683

Aminoff, V., Sellén, M., Sörliden, E., Ludvigsson, M., Berg, M., & Andersson, G. (2021). Internet-based cognitive behavioural therapy for psychological distress associated with the COVID-19 pandemic: A pilot randomised controlled trial. *Frontiers in Psychology, 12.* https://doi.org/10.3389/fpsyg.2021.684540

Amra, B., Ghadiry, F., Vaezei, A., Nematollahy, A., Radfar, N., Haghjoo, S., Penzel, T., & Morin, C. M. (2022). *Effect of the one-shot cognitive behavioural therapy on health care workers' insomnia and heart rate variability during the COVID-19 pandemic: A randomised controlled trial.* https://doi.org/10.21203/rs.3.rs-2067887/v1

Arnow, B., Kenardy, J., & Agras, W. S. (1995). The Emotional Eating Scale: The development of a measure to assess coping with the negative effect of eating. *International Journal of Eating Disorders, 18*(1), 79–90. https://doi.org/10.1002/1098-108X(199507)18:1<79::AID-EAT2260180109>3.0.CO;2-V

Baglioni, C., Battagliese, G., Feige, B., Spiegelhalder, K., Nissen, C., Voderholzer, U., Lombardo, C., & Riemann, D. (2011). Insomnia as a predictor of depression: A meta-analytic evaluation of longitudinal epidemiological studies. *Journal of Affective Disorders, 135,* 10–19. https://doi.org/10.1016/j.jad.2011.01.011

Beck, A. T. (1979). *Cognitive therapy of depression.* Guilford Press.

Beck, A. T., Steer, R. A., Brown, G. K. (1996). *Manual for the beck depression inventory-II.* Psychological Corporation.

Blevins, C. A., Weathers, F. W., Davis, M. T., Witte, T. K., Domino, J. L. (2015). The post-traumatic stress disorder checklist for DSM-5 (PCL-5): Development and initial psychometric evaluation. *Journal of Traumatic Stress, 28*, 489–498. https://doi.org/10.1002/jts.22059

Brooks, S. K., Webster, R. K., Smith, L. E., et al. (2020). The psychological impact of quarantine and how to reduce it: A rapid review of the evidence. *Lancet, 395*(10227), 912–920. https://doi.org/10.1016/S0140-6736(20)30460-8

Cassin, S. E., Sockalingam, S., Du, C., Wnuk, S., Hawa, R., Parikh, S. V. (2016). A pilot randomised controlled trial of telephone-based cognitive behavioural therapy for preoperative bariatric surgery patients. *Behaviour Research and Therapy, 80*, 17–22. https://doi.org/10.1016/j.brat.2016.03.001

Chan, P., Bhar, S., Davison, T. E., Doyle, C., Knight, B. G., Koder, D., et al. (2018). Characteristics of cognitive behavioural therapy for older adults living in residential care: Protocol for a systematic review. *JMIR Research Protocols, 7*(7), e164.

Chew, N. W. S., Lee, G. K. H., Tan, B. Y. Q., Jing, M., Goh, Y., Ngiam, N. J. H., Yeo, L. L. L., Ahmad, A., Ahmed Khan, F., Napolean Shanmugam, G., Sharma, A. K., Komalkumar, R. N., Meenakshi Christ, C., Schouten, M. J., Blankers, M., van Schaik, D. J., Beekman, A. T., Wisman, M. A, et al. (2020). Internet and computer-based cognitive behavioural therapy for anxiety and depression in adolescents and young adults: Systematic review and meta-analysis. *Journal of Medical Internet Research, 22*, e17831. https://doi.org/10.2196/17831

Dunstan, D. A., & Scott, N. (2019). Clarification of the cut-off score for Zung's self-rating depression scale. *BMC Psychiatry, 19*(1), 177. doi: 10.1186/s12888-019-2161-0

Dunstan, D. A., & Scott, N. (2020). Norms for Zung's Self-rating Anxiety Scale. *BMC Psychiatry, 20*(1), 90. https://doi.org/10.1186/s12888-019-2427-6

Dunstan, D. A., & Scott, N. Clarification of the cut-off score for Zung's self-rating depression scale.

Egan, S. J., McEvoy, P., Wade, T. D., Ure, S., Johnson, A. R., Gill, C., Greene, D., Wilker, L., Anderson, R., Mazzucchelli, T. G., Brown, S., & Shafran, R. (2021). Unguided low-intensity cognitive behaviour therapy for anxiety and depression during the COVID-19 pandemic: A randomised trial. *Behaviour Research and Therapy, 144*, 103902. https://doi.org/10.1016/j.brat.2021.103902

El Morr, C., Ritvo, P., Ahmad, F., & Moineddin, R. (2020). Effectiveness of an 8-week web-based Mindfulness Virtual Community Intervention for university students on symptoms of stress, anxiety, and depression: Randomized Controlled Trial. *JMIR Mental Health, 7*(7). https://doi.org/10.2196/18595

Ferreira, T. B. (2022). The impact of Healthcare Workers' mental health during a COVID-19 pandemic. *Journal of Quality in Health Care & Economics, 5*(6), 1–5. https://doi.org/10.23880/jqhe-16000303

Gao, J., Zheng, P., Jia, Y., et al. (2020). Mental health problems and social media exposure during the COVID-19 outbreak. *PLoS One, 15*(4), e0231924.

Gormally, J., Black, S., Daston, S., & Rardin, D. (1982). The assessment of binge eating severity among obese persons. *Addictive Behaviour, 7*(1), 47–55. https://doi.org/10.1016/0306-4603(82)90024-7

Hamilton, M. (1959). The assessment of anxiety states by rating. *British Journal of Medical Psychology, 32*(1), 50–55. https://doi.org/10.1111/j.2044-8341.1959.tb00467.x

Hamilton, M. (1960). A rating scale for depression. *Journal of Neurology, Neurosurgery, and Psychiatry, 23*, 56–62. https://doi.org/10.1136/jnnp.23.1.56

Hartley, S., Dagneaux, S., Londe, V., Liane, M.-T., Aussert, F., des ColasFrancs, C., & Royant-Parola, S. (2016). Self-referral to group cognitive behavioral therapy: Is it effective for treating chronic insomnia? *L'Encéphale, 42*(5), 395–401. https://doi.org/10.1016/j.encep.2016.08.013

Heckendorf, H., Lehr, D., & Boß, L. (2022). Effectiveness of an internet-based self-help intervention versus public mental health advice to reduce worry during the COVID-19 pandemic: A pragmatic, parallel-group, randomized controlled trial. *Psychotherapy and Psychosomatics, 91*(6), 398–410. https://doi.org/10.1159/000521302

Higgins, J. P., Altman, D. G., Gotzsche, P. C., Juni, P., Moher, D., Oxman, A. D., Savovic, J., Schulz, K. F., Weeks, L., & Sterne, J. A. (2011). The Cochrane Collaboration's tool for assessing the risk of bias in randomised trials. *BMJ, 343*, d5928. https://doi.org/10.1136/bmj.d5928

Huang, Y., & Zhao, N. (2020). Generalised anxiety disorder, depressive symptoms and sleep quality during COVID-19 outbreak in China: A web-based cross-sectional survey. *Psychiatry Research, 288*, 112954.

Kajdy, A., Feduniw, S., Ajdacka, U., et al. (2020). Risk factors for anxiety and depression among pregnant women during the COVID-19 pandemic: A web-based cross-sectional survey. *Medicine (Baltimore), 99*, e21279.

Kini, G., Karkal, R., & Bhargava, M. (2020). All's not well with the "worried well": Understanding health anxiety due to COVID-19. *Journal of Preventive Medicine and Hygiene, 61*(3), E321–E323. https://doi.org/10.15167/2421–4248/JPMH2020.61.3.1605

Korpilahti-Leino, T., Luntamo, T., Ristkari, T., Hinkka-Yli-Salomäki, S., Pulkki-Råback, L., Waris, O., Matinolli, H.-M., Sinokki, A., Mori, Y., Fukaya, M., Yamada, Y., & Sourander, A. (2022). Single-session, internet-based cognitive behavioral therapy to improve parenting skills to help children cope with anxiety during the COVID-19 pandemic: Feasibility Study. *Journal of Medical Internet Research, 24*(4). https://doi.org/10.2196/26438

Kroenke, K., Spitzer, R. L., & Williams, J. B. (2001). The PHQ-9: Validity of a brief depression severity measure. *Journal of General Internal Medicine, 16*, 606–613. https://doi.org/10.1046/j.15251497.2001.016009606.x

Lakhan, R., Agrawal, A., & Sharma, M. (2020). Prevalence of depression, anxiety, and stress during COVID-19 pandemic. *Journal of Neurosciences in Rural Practice, 11*(4), 519–525. https://doi.org/10.1055/s0040–1716442

Lalu, M. M., Li, T., Loder, E. W., Mayo-Wilson, E., McDonald, S., McGuinness, L. A., Stewart, L. A., Thomas, J., Tricco, A. C., Welch, V. A., Whiting, P., & Moher, D. (2021). 26th Cochrane Colloquium, Santiago, Chile. Vol. 0. 2021. PRISMA 2020 statement: Updated guidelines for reporting systematic reviews and meta-analyses.

Li, J., Li, X., Jiang, J., Xu, X., Wu, J., Xu, Y., Lin, X., Hall, J., Xu, H., Xu, J., & Xu, X. (2020). The effect of cognitive behavioural therapy on depression, anxiety, and stress in patients with COVID-19: A randomised controlled trial. *Frontiers in Psychiatry, 11*. https://doi.org/10.3389/fpsyt.2020.580827

Liu, T., Chen, X., Miao, G., Qian, M., He, Y., Yu, X., et al. (2003). Recommendations on diagnostic criteria and prevention of SARS-related mental disorders. *Journal of Clinical Psychology in Medical Settings, 13*, 188–191. https://doi.org/10.3969/j.issn.1005–3220.2003.03.043

Liu, Z., Qiao, D., Xu, Y., Zhao, W., Yang, Y., Wen, D., Li, X., Nie, X., Dong, Y., Tang, S., Jiang, Y., Wang, Y., Zhao, J., & Xu, Y. (2021). The efficacy of computerised cognitive behavioural therapy for depressive and anxiety symptoms in patients with COVID-19: Randomised controlled trial. *Journal of Medical Internet Research, 23*(5). https://doi.org/10.2196/26883

Lopez, R., Evangelista, E., Barateau, L., Chenini, S., & Dauvilliers, Y. (2019). French language online cognitive behavioural therapy for insomnia disorder: A randomised controlled trial. *Frontiers in Neurology, 110*, 1273. https://doi.org/10.3389/fneur.2019.01273.

Mahoney, A., Li, I., Haskelberg, H., Millard, M., & Newby, J. M. (2021). The uptake and effectiveness of online cognitive behaviour therapy for symptoms of anxiety and depression during COVID-19. *Journal of Affective Disorders, 292*, 197–203. https://doi.org/10.1016/j.jad.2021.05.116

Matthew, P., Joanne, M., Patrick, B., Isabelle, B., Tammy, H., Cynthia, M., Shamseer, L., Tetzlaff, J. M., Akl, E. A., Brennan, S. E., Chou, R., Glanville, J., Grimshaw, J. M., Hróbjartsson, A., Lalu, M. M., Li, T., Loder, E. W., Mayo-Wilson, E., McDonald, S., McGuinness, L. A., Stewart, L. A., Thomas, J., Tricco, A. C., Welch, V. A., Whiting, P., & Moher, D. (2021). PRISMA 2020 statement: Updated guidelines for reporting systematic reviews and meta analyses. *26th Cochrane Colloquium*, Santiago, Chile.

Mattila, E., Peltokoski, J., Neva, M. H., Kaunonen, M., Helminen, M., & Parkkila, A.-K. (2021). COVID-19: Anxiety among hospital staff and associated factors. *Annals of Medicine, 53*, 237–246. https://doi.org/10.1080/07853890.2020.1862905

Milosevic, I., Cameron, D. H., Milanovic, M., McCabe, R. E., & Rowa, K. (2021). Face-to-face versus video teleconference group cognitive behavioural therapy for anxiety and related disorders: A preliminary comparison. *The Canadian Journal of Psychiatry, 67*(5), 391–402. https://doi.org/10.1177/07067437211027319

Murphy, R., Calugi, S., Cooper, Z., & Dalle Grave, R. (2020). Challenges and opportunities for enhanced cognitive behaviour therapy (CBT-E) in light of COVID-19. *Cognitive Behavioral Therapy, 13*, e14.

Nesset, M. B., Lauvrud, C., Meisingset, A., Nyhus, E., Palmstierna, T., & Lara-Cabrera, M. L. (2022). Development of nurse-led videoconference-delivered cognitive behavioural therapy for domestic violence: Feasibility and acceptability. *Journal of Advanced Nursing, 79*(4), 1503–1512. https://doi.org/10.1111/jan.15347

Nie, X., Wang, Q., Wang, M., Zhao, S., Liu, L., Zhu, Y., & Chen, H. (2020). Anxiety and depression and its correlates in patients with coronavirus disease 2019 in Wuhan. *International Journal of Psychiatry in Clinical Practice*, 1–6.

Ornell, F., Borelli, W. V., Benzano, D., Schuch, J. B., Moura, H. F., Sordi, A. O., Kessler, F. H., Scherer, J. N., & von Diemen, L. (2021). The next pandemic: Impact of covid-19 in mental healthcare assistance in a nationwide epidemiological study. *The Lancet Regional Health – Americas, 4*, 100061. https://doi.org/10.1016/j.lana.2021.100061

P. V., Shah, K., Patel, B., Chan, B. P. L., Sunny, S., Chandra, B., Ong, J. J. Y., Paliwal, P. R., Perri, R., Castelli, P., La Rosa, C., Zucchi, T., & Onofri, A. (2021). COVID-19, isolation, quarantine: The efficacy of internet-based eye movement desensitisation and reprocessing (EMDR) and cognitive-behavioural therapy (CBT) for ongoing trauma. *Brain Sciences, 11*(5), 579. https://doi.org/10.3390/brainsci11050579

Page, M. J., McKenzie, J. E., Bossuyt, P. M., Boutron, I., Hoffmann, T. C., Mulrow, C. D., Shamseer, L., Tetzlaff, J. M., Akl, E. A., Brennan, S. E., Chou, R., Glanville, J., Grimshaw, J. M., Hróbjartsson, A., Lalu, M. M., Li, T., Loder, E. W., Mayo-Wilson, E., McDonald, S., McGuinness, L. A., Stewart, L. A., Thomas, J., Tricco, A. C., Welch, V. A., Whiting, P., & Moher, D. (2021). The PRISMA 2020 statement: An updated guideline for reporting systematic reviews. *BMJ, 372*(71). doi: 10.1136/bmj.n71

Perri, R., Castelli, P., La Rosa, C., Zucchi, T., & Onofri, A. (2021). COVID-19, isolation, quarantine: On the efficacy of internet-based eye movement desensitization and reprocessing (EMDR) and cognitive-behavioral therapy (CBT) for ongoing trauma. *Brain Science, 11*(5), 579. https://doi.org/10.3390/brainsci11050579

Pfefferbaum, B., & North, C. S. (2020). Mental health and the COVID-19 pandemic. *The New England Journal of Medicine*. https://doi.org/10.1056/NEJMp2008017

Puertas-Gonzalez, J. A., Mariño-Narvaez, C., Romero-Gonzalez, B., Sanchez-Perez, G. M., & Peralta-Ramirez, M. I. (2022). Online cognitive behavioural therapy as a psychological vaccine against stress during the covid-19 pandemic in pregnant women: A randomised controlled trial. *Journal of Psychiatric Research, 152*, 397–405. https://doi.org/10.1016/j.jpsychires.2022.07.016

Rajkumar, R. P. (2020). COVID-19 and mental health: A review of the existing literature. *Asian Journal Psychiatry, 52*, 102066.

Rehman, U., Shahnawaz, M. G., Khan, N. H., Kharshiing, K. D., Khursheed, M., Gupta, K., Kashyap, D., & Uniyal, R. (2020). Depression, anxiety and stress among Indians in times of COVID-19 lockdown. *Community Mental Health Journal, 57*, 42–48.

Rogers, J. P., Chesney, E., Oliver, D., Pollak, T. A., McGuire, P., Fusar-Poli, P., Zandi, M. S., Lewis, G., & David, A. S. (2020). Psychiatric and neuropsychiatric presentations associated with severe coronavirus infections: A systematic review and meta-analysis with comparison to the COVID-19 pandemic. *Lancet Psychiatry, 7*(7), 611–627. https://doi.org/10.1016/S22150366(20)30203-0

Romagnoli, S., Peris, A., De Gaudio, A. R., & Geppetti, P. (2020). SARS-CoV-2 and COVID-19: From the bench to the bedside. *Physiology Review, 100*(4), 1455–1466. https://doi.org/10.1152/physrev.00020.2020

Samantaray, N. N., Kar, N., & Mishra, S. R. (2022). A follow-up study on treatment effects of cognitive-behavioral therapy on social anxiety disorder: Impact of covid-19 fear during post-lockdown period. *Psychiatry Research, 310*, 114439. https://doi.org/10.1016/j.psychres.2022.114439

Santiago, V. A., Cassin, S. E., Wnuk, S., et al. (2021). "If you're offered help, take it": A qualitative study examining bariatric patients' experience of telephone-based cognitive behavioural therapy. *Clinical Obesity, 11*(2), e12431.

Santomauro, D. F., Herrera, A. M. M., Shadid, J., Zheng, P., Ashbaugh, C., Pigott, D. M., Abbafati, C., Adolph, C., Amlag, J. O., Aravkin, A. Y., et al. (2021). Global prevalence and burden of depressive and anxiety disorders in 204 countries and territories in 2020 due to the COVID-19 pandemic. *Lancet, 398*, 1700–1712.

Santomauro, D. F., Mantilla Herrera, A. M., Shadid, J., Zheng, P., Ashbaugh, C., Pigott, D. M., . . . Ferrari, A. J. (2020). Global prevalence and burden of depressive and anxiety disorders in 204 countries and territories in 2020 due to the COVID-19 pandemic. *The Lancet*. https://doi.org/10.1016/S0140-6736(21)02143-7

Schure, M. B., Lindow, J. C., Greist, J. H., Nakonezny, P. A., Bailey, S. J., Bryan, W. L., et al. (2019). Use of a fully automated internet-based cognitive behaviour therapy intervention in a community population of adults with depression symptoms: Randomised controlled trial. *Journal of Medical Internet Research, 21*(11), e14754. https://doi.org/10.2196/14754

Seyffert, M., Lagisetty, P., Landgraf, J., Chopra, V., Pfeiffer, P. N., Conte, M. L., & Rogers, M. A. (2016). Internet-delivered cognitive behavioural therapy to treat insomnia: A systematic review and meta-analysis. *PLoS One, 11*(2), e0149139. https://doi.org/10.1371/journal.pone.0149139

Shabahang, R., Aruguete, M. S., & McCutcheon, L. (2021). Video-based cognitive-behavioural intervention for covid-19 anxiety: A randomised controlled trial. *Trends in Psychiatry and Psychotherapy.* https://doi.org/10.47626/2237-6089-2020-0056

Shapira, S., Cohn-Schwartz, E., Yeshua-Katz, D., Aharonson-Daniel, L., Clarfield, A. M., & Sarid, O. (2021). Teaching and practising cognitive-behavioural and mindfulness skills in a web-based platform among older adults through the COVID-19 pandemic: A pilot randomised controlled trial. *International Journal of Environmental Research and Public Health, 18*(20), 10563. https://doi.org/10.3390/ijerph182010563

Sharma, G., Schlosser, L., Jones, B. D., Blumberger, D. M., Gratzer, D., Husain, M. O., Mulsant, B. H., Rappaport, L., Stergiopoulos, V., & Husain, M. I. (2022). Brief app-based cognitive behavioural therapy for anxiety symptoms in psychiatric in-patients: Feasibility randomised controlled trial. *JMIR Formative Research, 6*(11). https://doi.org/10.2196/38460

Sharrock, M. J., Mahoney, A., Haskelberg, H., Millard, M., & Newby, J. (2021). *The uptake and outcomes of internet cognitive behavioural therapy for health anxiety symptoms during the COVID-19 pandemic.* https://doi.org/10.31234/osf.io/6udqp

Sheehan, D. V., Lecrubier, Y., Sheehan, K. H., Amorim, P., Janavs, J., Weiller, E., Hergueta, T., Baker, R., & Dunbar, G. C. (1998). The Mini-International Neuropsychiatric Interview (M.I.N.I.): The development and validation of a structured diagnostic psychiatric interview for DSM-IV and ICD-10. *Journal of Clinical Psychiatry, 59*(Suppl 20), 22–33; quiz 34-57.

Sheehan, D. V., Lecrubier, Y., Sheehan, K. H., Janavs, J., Weiller, E., Keskiner, A., ... Dunbar, G. C. (19987). The validity of the Mini International Neuropsychiatric Interview (MINI) according to the SCID-P and its reliability. *European Psychiatry, 12*, 232–241. https://doi.org/10.1016/S09249338(97)83297-X

Sockalingam, S., Leung, S. E., Hawa, R., et al. (2019). Telephone-based cognitive behavioural therapy for female patients 1-year post-bariatric surgery: A pilot study. *Obesity Research & Clinical Practice, 13*(5), 499–504. https://doi.org/10.1016/j.orcp.2019.07.003

Sockalingam, S., Leung, S. E., Ma, C., Hawa, R., Wnuk, S., Dash, S., Jackson, T., & Cassin, S. E. (2022). The impact of telephone-based cognitive behavioural therapy on mental health distress and disordered eating among bariatric surgery patients during COVID-19: Preliminary results from a multisite randomised controlled trial. *Obesity Surgery, 32*(6), 1884–1894. https://doi.org/10.1007/s11695-022-05981-6

Soldatos, C. R., Dikeos, D. G., & Paparrigopoulos, T. J. (2000). Athens Insomnia Scale: Validation of an instrument based on ICD-10 criteria. *Journal of Psychosomatic Research, 48*(6), 555–560. https://doi.org/10.1016/s0022–3999(00)00095–7

Song, J., Jiang, R., Chen, N., Qu, W., Liu, D., Zhang, M., Fan, H., Zhao, Y., & Tan, S. (2021). Self-help cognitive behavioral therapy application for covid-19-related mental health problems: A longitudinal trial. *Asian Journal of Psychiatry, 60*, 102656. https://doi.org/10.1016/j.ajp.2021.102656

Spielberger, C. D. (1983). *Manual for the State-Trait Anxiety Inventory STAI (Form Y) ("Self-Evaluation Questionnaire").* Consulting Psychologists Press.

Spitzer, R. L., Kroenke, K., Williams, J. B., & Lowe, B. (2006). A brief measure for assessing generalised anxiety disorder: The GAD-7. *Archives of Internal Medicine, 166*, 1092–1097. https://doi.org/10.1001/archinte.166.10.1092

Strudwick, G., Sockalingam, S., Kassam, I., et al. (2021). Digital interventions to support population mental health in Canada during the COVID-19 pandemic: A rapid review. *JMIR Mental Health, 8*(3), e26550.

Tang, W., & Kreindler, D. (2017). Supporting homework compliance in cognitive behavioural therapy: Essential features of mobile apps. *JMIR Mental Health, 4*(2), e5283. https://doi.org/10.2196/mental.5283

Torales, J., O'Higgins, M., Castaldelli-Maia, J. M., et al. (2020). The outbreak of COVID-19 coronavirus and its impact on global mental health. *International Journal of Social Psychiatry, 66,* 317–320.

Tyrer, P. (2020). COVID-19 health anxiety. *World Psychiatry, 19*(3), 307–308. https://doi.org/10.1002/wps.20798

Van Lieshout, R. J., Layton, H., Savoy, C. D., Brown, J. S., Ferro, M. A., Streiner, D. L., Bieling, P. J., Feller, A., & Hanna, S. (2021). Effect of online 1-day cognitive behavioural therapy – based workshops plus usual care vs usual care alone for postpartum depression. *JAMA Psychiatry, 78*(11), 1200. https://doi.org/10.1001/jamapsychiatry.2021.2488

Verma, S., & Mishra, A. (2020). Depression, anxiety, stress and socio-demographic correlates among general Indian public during COVID-19. *International Journal of Social Psychiatry, 66*(8), 756–762.

Wahlund, T., Mataix-Cols, D., Olofsdotter Lauri, K., de Schipper, E., Ljótsson, B., Aspvall, K., & Andersson, E. (2020). Brief online cognitive behavioural intervention for dysfunctional worry related to the covid-19 pandemic: A randomised controlled trial. *Psychotherapy and Psychosomatics, 90*(3), 191–199. https://doi.org/10.1159/000512843

Wang, C., Pan, R., Wan, X., et al. (2020). A longitudinal study on the mental health of the general population during the COVID-19 epidemic in China. *Brain, Behavior, and Immunity, 87,* 40–48.

Weiner, L., Berna, F., Nourry, N., Séverac, F., Vidailhet, P., & Mengin, A. C. (2020). *Efficacy of an online cognitive behavioral therapy program developed for workers during the COVID-19 pandemic: The REduction of STress (REST) study protocol for a randomized controlled trial.* Trials; Springer Science+Business Media. https://doi.org/10.1186/s13063-020-04772-7

Wisman, M. A., Emmelkamp, J., Dekker, J. J. M., & Christ, C. (2023). Internet-based emotion-regulation training added to CBT in adolescents with depressive and anxiety disorders: A pilot randomized controlled trial to examine feasibility, acceptability, and preliminary effectiveness. *Internet Interventions, 31,* 100596. https://doi.org/10.1016/j.invent.2022.100596

Wong, L. Y. H., Sagayanathan, R., Chen, J. T., Ying Ng, A. Y, Teoh, H. L., Tsivgoulis, G., Ho, C. S., Ho, R. C., & Sharma, V. K. (2020). A multinational, multicentre study on the psychological outcomes and associated physical symptoms amongst healthcare workers during COVID-19 outbreak. *Brain, Behavior, and Immunity, 2020,* 1. https://doi.org/10.1016/j.bbi.2020.04.049.

World Health Organization. (n.d.). COVID-19 pandemic triggers 25% increase in the prevalence of anxiety and depression worldwide. *World Health Organization.* Retrieved January 27, 2023, from www.who.int/news/item/02-03-2022-covid-19-pandemic-triggers-25increase-in-prevalence-of-anxiety-and-depression-worldwide

Xiang, Y., Yang, Y., Li, W., Zhang, L., Zhang, Q., Cheng, T., et al. (2020). Timely mental health care for the 2019 novel coronavirus outbreak is urgently needed. *Lancet Psychiatry, 7,* 228–229. https://doi.org/10.1016/S2215-0366(20)30046-8

Ye, Y. Y., Zhang, Y. F., Chen, J., Liu, J., Li, X. J., Liu, Y. Z., Lang, Y., Lin, L., Yang, X. J., & Jiang, X. J. (2015). Internet-based cognitive behavioural therapy for insomnia (ICBT-i)

improves comorbid anxiety and depression-a meta-analysis of randomised controlled trials. *PLoS One, 10*(11), e142258. https://doi.org/10.1371/journal.pone.0142258

Yeo, C., Ahmed, S., Oo, A. M., Koura, A., Sanghvi, K., & Yeo, D. (2020). COVID-19 and obesity-the management of pre- and post-bariatric patients amidst the COVID-19 pandemic. *Obesity Surgery, 30*(9), 3607–3609. https://doi.org/10.1007/s11695-020-04670-6

Ying, Y., Ji, Y., Kong, F., Wang, M., Chen, Q., Wang, L., Hou, Y., Yu, L., Zhu, L., Miao, P., Zhou, J., Zhang, L., Yang, Y., Wang, G., Chen, R., Liu, D., Huang, W., Lv, Y., Lou, Z., & Ruan, L. (2022). Efficacy of an internet-based cognitive behavioral therapy for subthreshold depression among Chinese adults: A randomized controlled trial. *Psychological Medicine, 53*(9), 3932–3942. https://doi.org/10.1017/s0033291722000599

Zhang, Y., & Feei, Z. (2020). Impact of the COVID-19 pandemic on mental health and quality of life among local residents in Liaoning province, China: A cross-sectional study. *International Journal of Environmental Research and Public Health*. https://doi.org/10.3390/ijerph17072381

Zhou, K., Kong, J., Wan, Y., Zhang, X., Liu, X., Qu, B., Wang, B., & Xue, R. (2022). Positive impacts of e-aid cognitive behavioural therapy on the sleep quality and mood of nurses on-site during the covid-19 pandemic. *Sleep and Breathing, 26*(4), 1947–1951. https://doi.org/10.1007/s11325-021-02547-1

5

SPIRITUAL PROCESS AND CARE FOR COVID-19 PATIENTS, CAREGIVERS, AND HEALTH WORKERS

A Narrative Review

Subhash Meena and Vijeyata Chauhan

Introduction

The coronavirus pandemic has turned people's lives upside down, leaving a scarred memory of the disrupted environment people experienced when the virus outbreak was at its peak. The first case was reported in China in 2020, and within two to three months, the reported number of cases escalated so quickly that there was no time to prepare for the fallout from the outbreak. In February 2020, the World Health Organization (WHO) declared a public health emergency of international concern (PHEIC) (World Health Organization, n.d., January 20, 2020). Since then, around 77 million people have been affected by the novel coronavirus worldwide, resulting in 68 lacs losing their lives to the pandemic (WHO). The effects of the virus varied greatly in different people. It usually started with a common cold symptom, which then progressed to a fever and developed into a complex respiratory illness with a sore throat, loss of taste and smell, and fatigue. Because it was a communicable disease, it could easily spread through contact with the infected person. Over time, the virus could produce more dangerous and unpredictable variants, causing panic and uncertainty. Many studies state that unpredictability, uncertainty, and uncontrollability led to the symptoms of depression and anxiety (Karimi et al., 2020; Rahimi et al., 2021).

The unforeseen pandemic and its biological and social impacts also led to mental health problems in people worldwide. Symptoms of post-traumatic stress disorder, anxiety, and depression were positively associated with psychological distress (Brooks et al., 2020). One of the main reasons for this was a large-scale quarantine that left people feeling socially isolated. Most people felt unable to handle stress, which made them anxious and added to their fear of being trapped and losing control (Usher et al., 2020). Fear is a primal reaction that surfaces in times of danger or uncertainty. The pandemic brought both. Many people worldwide continued visiting shrines and consecratory places in distress, believing that doing so would

DOI: 10.4324/9781003357209-7

alleviate the "hard times". However, shrines and religious centres had been closed in the face of quarantine worldwide, making people feel even more alone and disconnected from the world and the sacred (Baunez et al., 2020). Many Muslim countries banned visiting mosques, which was certainly one of the most difficult decisions (Yezli & Khan, 2020).

This global health crisis profoundly impacted how we perceive our world and everyday lives. Yet, in these difficult times, hope and faith were two powerful healers. Recent research suggests that the process of connecting or reconnecting with their faith has helped people get through the stressful time of the pandemic (Algahtani et al., 2022). In the face of illness and suffering, there was a marked change in attitude that made people think more about the meaning and purpose of life (Kowalczyk et al., 2020). Of all other human experiences, death is the most painful and has the most devastating effects on families (Walsh, 2020). Yet, humanity stood united in the fight against the COVID-19 pandemic. The purpose of this chapter is to explore the process of spiritual care that people suffering from corona virus and their family members have gone through. It also seeks to understand how spiritual and religious beliefs have impacted caregivers and healthcare providers during the pandemic. The reason the author chose to do a narrative review was that spirituality as a variable has not been very well explored during the COVID-19 pandemic due to physical health variables. Therefore, through a narrative review, we could understand how spirituality can contribute to holistic care in situations like COVID pandemic.

Methods

Research articles were selected considering the variables and key words such as spirituality, spiritual caregiving, spiritual health, resilience, caregivers, and healthcare workers. The strategy followed was to search the internet for these articles in various databases and journals including Springer, PubMed, NIMH, ResearchGate, and Google Scholar as well as various journals. For the current study, the inclusion criteria were spirituality studies conducted during COVID-19 and inclusion of healthcare as a variable. The studies unrelated to spirituality and COVID-19 were excluded from the review. Studies from the last three years were considered for this review. First, the authors selected 20 articles for review, and nine studies were chosen for final review. A narrative review was conducted on the basis of the above variables and their interrelationship.

As a result, this study helps us understand how spirituality provides support and functions as part of holistic care for people.

Spirituality in the Times of COVID-19

The term spirituality has a complex meaning and encompasses a broad understanding. The meaning also varies by culture and religion around the world (La Cour & Götke, 2012). Spirituality can be perceived as a multidimensional theoretical construct. It can be a generalized and natural phenomenon, where a person seeks to make a connection between themselves and their higher purpose (Joseph et al., 2017). It can also be seen as a constant exploration of something new in life, trying to push the limits of existence and eventually realizing the true meaning of life (Bożek et al., 2020). Feeling connected to a source allows people to experience meaning and purpose in life (Krause, 2003). The way a person evaluates a situation cognitively and affectively influences their individual experience of the situation. In recent decades, research has focused specifically on health and spirituality, establishing the link among spiritual experience, religiosity, and physical/mental health (Damiano et al., 2016). Spirituality has a positive effect on physical and mental health, improves the quality of life, and helps someone recover from mental illness (Mueller et al., 2001). Religious and spiritual beliefs have enabled people to make sense of many of the events in life that occur and cause grief and suffering. In this sense, faith can be understood as a fulcrum that unites overcoming the psychological crisis associated with an illness and adapting to the illness and its effects (Kowalczyk et al., 2020). When a patient's spiritual needs are curbed due to unavoidable circumstances or by society, spiritual suffering results, which can further lead to sadness, loneliness, impaired social relationships, and interactions.

In the past two years, the impact of COVID-19 has caused people to endure much physical and emotional suffering around the world. The pandemic has caused mental stress not only for those who have contracted COVID-19 but also for those who care for them and provide them with health facilities (Anand et al., 2021). It also impacted careers and education, leaving people financially unstable and dealing with a lot of emotional trauma. The outbreak of the virus was sudden, and most people were not mentally prepared for such a big, alarming situation. The widespread fear brought on by the pandemic affected people individually and interpersonally. The COVID-19 pandemic has gradually sparked interest among researchers in understanding the role of spirituality in times of need (Kasapoğlu, 2022). Some people found peace during the COVID-19 pandemic, but others struggled with their religious beliefs during this time while they or their family members were infected with the virus. Many people seemed to struggle with their faith and hope as they saw untimely deaths all around them on a daily basis. The COVID-19 experience caused many of us to reflect on the quality of our lives, well-being, and, most importantly, death, the end of life. Amid the process of physical and psychological ups and downs, a spiritual process was also observed. With the goal of holistic health in terms of managing illness and dealing with death, spiritual care has been seen as an essential part during this pandemic. Not only the patient, but also the patient's family and frontline health workers experienced a drastic change in their livelihoods and routines that affected their mental health (Ferrell et al., 2020). In the time when treatment was almost contactless, it became more difficult to respond to people's emotional and spiritual needs. Because the disease was ubiquitous and invisible, everyone, including the healthcare workers, was constantly thinking what if it was my turn next (Ferrell et al., 2020).

While the media was deluged with footage and images of people dying in intensive care units and hospitals, their dead bodies were not even given to their loved ones for last rites. Various religious leaders offered prayers, chants, and verses for the dead and their families who were far away from the patient. The situation was both heartbreaking and frightening as this generation had never experienced anything like this before. The anger and fear of the uncertainty rose up every day. It's probably hard to even imagine the feeling when someone's loved one was in the hospital for COVID-19 and they were supposed to leave the patient alone, even if they didn't want to. We can only imagine the mental turmoil and extreme terror and desperation these people experienced. During this pandemic, the need for bereavement support has become clear. The thought of dying alone is one of the few things, which makes people question their very existence (Turner & Caswell, 2020), and that is why almost all cultures around the globe have final rituals for a deceased person.

Spiritual care is not a luxury; it is a necessity for any system that claims to care for people – whether they are lying in bed or wrapped in protective clothing (Ferrell et al., 2020). McSherry et al. (2004) view spirituality as a life-enhancing factor that increases hope for a better future. Spiritual care is broadly understood to be the need for meaning and purpose in life and for dignity and respect in trying to deal with the illness (Ferrell et al., 2020).

Burden of Care During the Pandemic

During the pandemic, the healthcare providers who provided their services to people outside their families (doctors and nurses) were already at a higher risk of developing the symptoms of COVID-19, which certainly burdened them with the responsibility of caring and maintaining their mental health (Bergmann & Wagner, 2021). The requirement of social distancing made it difficult for family members to provide basic services to people with chronic health conditions, and those with physical and cognitive impairments, who were more vulnerable to the health problems associated with the pandemic (Beach et al., 2021). A large part of care comes from the family. Close family members, followed by close relatives, come together to address a crisis when it occurs in a family or an individual. The pandemic altered this help, as the additional family members (or caregivers withdrew) their support; some did so due to quarantine rules, others voluntarily for the fear of the consequences of physical contact with the infected person (Bergmann & Wagner, 2021). In their study, Leggett et al. (2022) found that the association between mental health and caregiver-related stress increased, and lower levels of affectivity related to caregiving and caregivers faced emotional difficulties decreased (Beach et al., 2021). In the closest family, the psycho-social aspects of the pandemic could also be observed in the parents, who are the primary caregivers. Undoubtedly, the COVID-19 virus has been fatal to children and older people. The behavioural and emotional issues the parents suffered impacted the way they looked after their children during the pandemic (Russell et al., 2020). Children learn by imitation, and as the pandemic progressed, their parents' coping mechanisms impacted the way children dealt with their situation (Russell et al., 2020). Some studies examining changes in informal caregiving for older adults found that the burden on caregivers increased among those caring for older people during the COVID-19 pandemic (Cohen et al., 2021). Caregivers already suffer from many problems ranging from socio-economic issues to the availability of finances, food, and transportation (Boyd et al., 2022). In addition, the scenario of the pandemic aggravated the situation amid the panic and chaos of the unavailability of food, hospital wards, and medicines, leading to more burnout among caregivers. The lack of hospital facilities made it worse.

For families struggling to bear the cost of COVID-19 treatment, the main concerns were financial and job jeopardy, which at times left them in debt even if they had lost a family member Rahimi et al., 2021). Much changes when a family takes on the role of a caregiver. The relationship with the patient has a new dimension (Longacre et al., n.d.). It was certainly a case during this pandemic where every one's life was at stake due to the spread of the deadly virus, and yet family members had to care for whoever was sick with the virus, leading to compassion fatigue (Gibbons et al., 2014; Rahimi et al., 2021). Still, the kind of spiritual care that should have been provided was lacking, increasing the need to integrate spiritual care into healthcare.

Spiritual Care for Patients and the Healthcare Workers

As the pandemic has brought much chaos, there has been a huge influx of patients with a total disregard for people's psychological and spiritual needs (Galbadage et al., 2020). Not to mention the psychological needs, because of the quarantine restrictions, some families could not even be there for their loved ones during their deaths, nor could they participate in the final rites and rituals (Mayland et al., 2020). As a result, many people did not have time for the closing that was required at the time of death, and family members considered these deaths undignified, as they could not say a respectful goodbye to their loved ones (Leong et al., 2004; Galbadage et al., 2020). Not being able to witness the loss of loved ones, and to unable to grieve properly anywhere hampered the family's ability to make peace with it. Normally, healthcare providers mostly find themselves in a situation where they have to break the bad news to the patient's family at the time of death. They give them the words and the comfort to help the grieving family members. The pandemic had limited this too, leaving no room for supportive therapies for the families who have lost loved ones. On the other hand, the relationship that develops between the doctor and the patient has healing properties, but due to the physical limitations during COVID-19, this relationship did not have time to develop. The impact of this certainly showed up on the patients' mental health in the form of fear of insecurity and fear of death while being alone on the ward (Galbadage et al., 2020).

Spiritual care is thus becoming an essential part of the healthcare system. At the heart of spiritual care is a biopsycho-socio-spiritual model (Beng, 2004) which is viewed as an integrated model, bringing together the biological, psychological, social, and spiritual aspects of care. Quality of life is also very important in the modern healthcare model (Arya et al., 2021). Providing spiritual care to patients requires assessing the patient's spiritual needs in terms of beliefs, philosophy of life, and active listening skills (should be able to treat the patient with complete respect and, if necessary, recommend them to someone who can provide them greater spiritual guidance) (Roman et al., 2020). Religion and spirituality provided healthy coping mechanisms and helped people cultivate hope and faith, the two vital sources of strength during this distressful time, and helped people make peace with negative events, believing that their deity or supreme power had greater plans with them (Sen et al., 2021). Rathakrishnan et al. (2022) conducted a study hypothesizing that spirituality mediates the relationship between fear and mental health. The results of the study confirmed that spirituality does mediate between fear and mental health. Thus, there lies a connection between spirituality, COVID-19, and mental health. As an indication, when the pandemic was causing stress, people with strong spiritual beliefs have been able to use hope and faith to alleviate the symptoms of anxiety associated with the pandemic and have been able to remain balanced and hopeful during these trying times (Polizzi et al., 2020).

Spiritual care advances the coping skills a person uses when trying to cope with an illness. The first instinct when someone hears about a deadly disease is to clasp their hands and pray to God, while sometimes people get angry and question their belief in God. But a spiritual perspective can make it easier for the person and their family to see life from a new perspective. Caregivers turned to the virtual world to provide religious/spiritual support to people with chronic conditions like Alzheimer's, ultimately resulting in an improvement in their overall mood during the trying time of COVID-19 (Britt et al., 2023). Most caregivers suffered from anxiety as part of the caregiving burden, and therefore it was found that spiritual practices should be encouraged to reduce stress among caregivers (Akkuş et al., 2022). At the time of the pandemic, families who had suffered losses were struggling to get help to build their resilience to cope with their loss, grieve, endure uncertainty, maintain their existing vital ties, and face challenges ahead (Walsh, 2020).

Spirituality provides critical support for positive mental health in times of stress, and individuals suffering from the effects of COVID-19 are in dire need of spiritual support (del Castillo, 2020). Spiritual care continued to be provided amid the chaos and panic of COVID-19, when even medical care was becoming increasingly difficult to obtain. Upon interviewing 19 nurses in the intensive care unit, a study reported that nurses were well aware of the religious beliefs of patients and their families and allowed them to practice their spiritual routines. However, they also believed that in emergencies, such as in the case of an ICU situation, spiritual care takes a back seat and serious medical care takes priority (de Diego-Cordero et al., 2022). Some of the participants also believed that the medical care they provided was characterized by empathy, compassion, resilience, patience, solidarity, and camaraderie towards the patient, which ultimately contributed to the spiritual care of the patient. A clear link was established between the spiritual needs of nurses and the performance they provide. In order to be able to offer the patient this holistic support, however, the nursing staff had to be well-equipped (Karaman et al., 2022). The patient's satisfaction and well-being increase when caregivers are sensitive to the patient and provide spiritual care. However, nurses in this field are not well prepared to respond to the patient's needs and provide appropriate spiritual care once they are identified (Hosseini et al., 2021; Karaman et al., 2022). In addition to nursing practice, nurses have demonstrated a vulnerability to symptoms of depression, anxiety, insomnia, anxiety, and stress amid the corona virus pandemic as they regularly witness patient deaths and have to work exhaustingly during hospital shifts. They put themselves at risk of contagion and also avoided meeting their own family members by isolating themselves (Nicola et al., 2020).

Pastoral care contributed to the holistic care of a patient and included various aspects such as emotional, spiritual, and psychological care. Such form of care usually helped alleviate the burden of illness (Timmins et al., 2022), and, during the COVID pandemic, it helped people deal with their existential crisis. People suffering from the virus felt guilty as if they were being punished for their sins. They often asked themselves what they did to get this disease. That they had such a strong belief in God, but it is not there any more. And some of them prayed to God that they could meet their loved ones one more time before they die. People questioned the meaning of their lives. At that moment, the spiritual foundation began to falter, not only for the patient but also for his family members. During this time, the patient needed spiritual support to reach the level of affective acceptance of infection with the deadly virus. Unfortunately, many patients and their families have not been able to receive the supposed spiritual and emotional help due to the lack of resources and lack of knowledge of the healthcare workers about the knowledge of spiritual care (Ferrell et al., 2020).

One of the main reasons for not being able to seek professional help and care was social distancing. People were afraid of getting infected through contact with other people. Spiritual care advisors present at the hospitals would wear their PPE equipment and act as a bridge between the patient's family and the patient to deliver messages of love, hope, and caring. It was disconcerting for them as they now had to call out those soft words of kindness and prayers to the patient as they were difficult to hear from inside a PPE kit. The counsellors felt helpless at this time, as if there was a mighty storm within them; yet, in the midst of this chaos they had to listen gently to the patient and his family (Busfield, 2020). They were often frustrated and angry at not being able to contribute to the spiritual care of the people due to the restrictions imposed during the pandemic. But over time, they too got used to the new normal (Domaradzki, 2020). They attempted to provide that emotional support through online media, and so there has been a significant shift from the physical setup to the online setup during this pandemic. The process of providing spiritual care and support to alleviate patient distress has changed drastically since the pre-pandemic era. It used to be easy for a spiritual advisor to be present at the bedside and help the person grieve, but the pandemic has made the process stressful (Byrne & Nuzum, 2020). At a time when there was no cure, spiritual support was of the utmost importance to keep people from losing hope (Domaradzki, 2020).

It wasn't just the people who were infected, but also the nurses and doctors whose spiritual needs were not being met. Since the beginning of the pandemic, healthcare workers have been on the front lines, risking their lives to attend to the needs of others. This pandemic has left them exhausted and desperate physically, emotionally, psychologically, and spiritually. Sarmiento (2021) calls these health-care workers "the wounded healers" and also calls for a comprehensive spiritual mentoring programme for healthcare workers so they are better able to contribute to the needs of patients and their families. "We are the wounded healers – called to recognize the sufferings of this time in our own hearts and to make this recognition the starting point of our service" (Ferrell et al., 2020).

Every day when these wounded healers came out, separated from their fami-lies to save a number of lives in the hospitals, many of them never returned and gave their lives (Pandey & Sharma, 2020). Their families were in deep mourning and proud of their selfless service to humanity. It has been observed that front-line healthcare workers promoted compassionate care while risking their own lives every day, treating patients in the hospital (Roman et al., 2020). The extreme feel-ing of burnout due to the increased working hours led to fatigue and exhaustion, and the doctors' quality of life and health is directly proportional to the type of services they provide (Amiel & Ulitzur, 2020).

Emerging from the wisdom of the East, some people showed perseverance and paved the way for others to navigate through disturbing thoughts and feelings throughout the day. Accepting one's feelings was paramount, followed by learning the knowledge of what can and cannot be controlled. There were few things you could control and many other things you couldn't control. To dwell and reflect on one's emotions, a reflection space had been created for people to manage their feel-ings, reflect, and offer prayers to loved ones and to themselves, while also observ-ing social distancing (Drummond & Carey, 2020). It helped people find peace away from chaos. The path of knowing and doing as described in the *Bhagavad Gita* is about being very aware of the nature of ourselves and helping us in the process of metacognition by thinking about ourselves in line with thinking about others. It is also about the selfless acts that have helped caregivers continue their efforts to help other people despite the uncertain consequences (Matcheri S. Keshavan, 2020).

Discussion

Catastrophic events change the perception of normality and make everyday life more difficult. Religious and spiritual beliefs and practices can help create a family structure and view negative events in a positive and meaningful way (Sen et al.,

2022). During this pandemic, the world has adopted a new normal where masks have been worn like accessories, and sanitiser has been an essential item in the bag.

Human beings have the ability to turn moments of pain into growth when given perspective – a different lens to look at their circumstances (Frankl, 1992). In reviewing the research cited before, a topic has come to the fore that can complement the health psychology literature. Spiritual health is an important aspect of general health, and more research needs to be done in this area. Indeed, during the pandemic, a bigger picture emerged that highlighted humanity and our instinct to help one another, despite caste, religion, and name. Scores of people came forward to help, donating money, food, and vehicles to people and families in need. It helped people to feel content, and the feeling of contributing to humanity filled them and made them spiritually stronger. It brought them fulfilment and peace during the pandemic.

The sufferings in the outer world and in the inner world create tensions that often lead a person to question his existence (Ferrell et al., 2020), from where some people take the direction of integrating the new reality into their psyches, and others are devastated and seek help to rebuild. During this pandemic, it has been evident among patients, their families, and healthcare workers. This pandemic has shown alarmingly that our healthcare systems need to integrate a spiritual care system alongside medical care, so that the suffering people are going through can be alleviated and people can come to terms with the spiritual aspects. There is a close connection between spirituality and perception of well-being Jafari et al., 2010). Therefore, there is a need to train medical professionals to recognize the spiritual needs of patients with acute and chronic illnesses, who must be able to provide these patients with the necessary supportive care (Balboni et al., 2014). As mental health aspects of people's lives become better understood, targeting spiritual and psycho-social needs would contribute to people's holistic health and focus on individualized treatment options (Coppola et al., 2021). In addition, there is a need for empirical studies on stress and the burden on nursing staff caused by nursing (Beach et al., 2021). Caregivers of people who had contracted COVID-19 faced much greater difficulties than the other caregivers because they did not know the course of the virus and had no experience in managing the symptoms because the symptoms varied and the illness was unpredictable; moreover, the virus was new to everyone and a challenge in itself (Rahimi et al., 2021).

Religion and spirituality are two of the complex variables and can impact different aspects of mental health. Therefore, studying these two variables becomes important in upcoming future research as it can help psychologists and mental health professionals (Sen et al., 2022) in the development of new therapeutic practices that take into account the holistic growth of an individual and lead to their physical, mental, and spiritual well-being. Therefore, it becomes important to examine religion and spirituality in the context of coping and mental health, so that the evidence for this gains importance and therapies based on that it can be implemented (Walsh, 2020).

Because everyone exhibits a different coping mechanism in times of extreme need, examining the psychological resilience of healthcare workers and COVID combatants on the frontlines during the pandemic can in some way ensure a medically healthy clinical workforce (Chang et al., 2021). Spirituality is gaining importance in healthcare as it promotes coping skills, recovery, and resilience and also helps a person deal with burnout (Roman et al., 2020). Mental health professionals need to arm themselves with knowledge of their patients' religious and spiritual beliefs as this can help patients make sense of their own adversities (Sen et al., 2022) and provide a supportive and helpful solution. The therapist or clinician provides a non-judgemental environment. The COVID-19 pandemic has brought to light not only the many deficiencies in our healthcare systems, but also the importance of spiritual care that must be considered in order to provide holistic service to people (Ferrell et al., 2020).

Limitations and Future Directions

The major limitation of the study is that the entire study is based on a review methodology of specific studies. In the future, further quantitative studies could be conducted in order to obtain the best literature for understanding the role of spirituality in the stressful times. Furthermore, through the use of various research methods, the variable spirituality can be understood in a much better way to improve and promote healthy living.

References

Akkuş, Y., Karacan, Y., Ünlü, K., Deniz, M., & Parlak, A. (2022). The effect of anxiety and spiritual well-being on the care burden of caregivers of cancer patients during the COVID-19 pandemic. *Supportive Care in Cancer*, *30*(2), 1863–1872. https://doi.org/10.1007/s00520-021-06611-0

Algahtani, F. D., Alsaif, B., Ahmed, A. A., Almishaal, A. A., Obeidat, S. T., Mohamed, R. F., Kamel, R. M., Gul, I., & Hassan, S. U. N. (2022). Using spiritual connections to cope with stress and anxiety during the COVID-19 pandemic. *Frontiers in Psychology*, *13*, 915290. https://doi.org/10.3389/fpsyg.2022.915290

Amiel, G. E., & Ulitzur, N. (2020). Caring for the caregivers: Mental and spiritual support for healthcare teams during the COVID-19 pandemic and beyond. *Journal of Cancer Education*. https://link.springer.com/article/10.1007/s13187-020-01859-2

Anand, V., Verma, L., Aggarwal, A., Nanjundappa, P., & Rai, H. (2021). COVID-19 and psychological distress: Lessons for India. *PLoS One*, *16*(8), e0255683. https://doi.org/10.1371/journal.pone.0255683

Arya, R., Kumari, S., Pandey, B., Mistry, H., Bihani, S. C., Das, A., Prashar, V., Gupta, G. D., Panicker, L., & Kumar, M. (n.d.). Structural insights into SARS-COV-2 proteins. *Journal of Molecular Biology*. https://pubmed.ncbi.nlm.nih.gov/33245961/

Balboni, M. J., Puchalski, C. M., & Peteet, J. R. (2014). The relationship between medicine, spirituality and religion: Three models for integration. *Journal of Religion and Health*, *53*(5), 1586–1598. https://doi.org/10.1007/s10943-014-9901-8

Baunez, C., Degoulet, M., Luchini, S., Pintus, P. A., & Teschl, M. (2020). An early assessment of curfew and second COVID-19 lock-down on virus propagation in France [Preprint]. *Health Policy*. https://doi.org/10.1101/2020.11.11.20230243

Beach, S. R., Schulz, R., Donovan, H., & Rosland, A.-M. (2021). Family caregiving during the COVID-19 pandemic. *The Gerontologist*, *61*(5), 650–660. https://doi.org/10.1093/geront/gnab049

Beng, K. S. (2004). The last hours and days of life: A biopsychosocial-spiritual model of care. *Asia Pacific Family Medicine*, *4*, 1–13.

Bergmann, M., & Wagner, M. (2021). The impact of COVID-19 on informal caregiving and care receiving across Europe during the first phase of the pandemic. *Frontiers in Public Health*, *9*, 673874. https://doi.org/10.3389/fpubh.2021.673874

Boyd, K., Winslow, V., Borson, S., Lindau, S. T., & Makelarski, J. A. (2022). Caregiving in a pandemic: Health-related socioeconomic vulnerabilities among women caregivers early in the COVID-19 pandemic. *Annals of Family Medicine*. https://www.ncbi.nlm.nih.gov/pmc/articles/PMC9512563/

Bożek, A., Nowak, P. F., & Blukacz, M. (2020). The relationship between spirituality, health-related behavior, and psychological well-being. *Frontiers in Psychology*, *11*, 1997. https://doi.org/10.3389/fpsyg.2020.01997

Britt, K. C., Richards, K. C., Radhakrishnan, K., Vanags-Louredo, A., Park, E., Gooneratne, N. S., & Fry, L. (2023). Religion, spirituality, and coping during the pandemic: Perspectives of dementia caregivers. *Clinical Nursing Research*, *32*(1), 94–104. https://doi.org/10.1177/10547738221115239

Brooks, S. K., Webster, R. K., Smith, L. E., Woodland, L., Wessely, S., Greenberg, N., & Rubin, G. J. (2020). The psychological impact of quarantine and how to reduce it: Rapid review of the evidence. *The Lancet*, *395*(10227), 912–920. https://doi.org/10.1016/S0140-6736(20)30460-8

Busfield, L. (2020). Listening on the outside-screaming on the inside: Reflections from an acute hospital chaplain during the first weeks of COVID-19. *Health and Social Care Chaplaincy*, *8*(2), 218–222. https://doi.org/10.1558/hscc.41807

Byrne, M. J., & Nuzum, D. R. (2020). Pastoral closeness in physical distancing: The use of technology in pastoral ministry during COVID-19. *Health and Social Care Chaplaincy*, *8*(2), 206–217. https://doi.org/10.1558/hscc.41625

Chang, M.-C., Chen, P.-F., Lee, T.-H., Lin, C.-C., Chiang, K.-T., Tsai, M.-F., Kuo, H.-F., & Lung, F.-W. (2021). the effect of religion on psychological resilience in healthcare workers during the coronavirus disease 2019 pandemic. *Frontiers in Psychology*, *12*, 628894. https://doi.org/10.3389/fpsyg.2021.628894

Cohen, S. A., Kunicki, Z. J., Drohan, M. M., & Greaney, M. L. (2021). Exploring changes in caregiver burden and caregiving intensity due to COVID-19. *Gerontology and Geriatric Medicine*, *7*, 233372142199927. https://doi.org/10.1177/2333721421999279

Damiano, R. F., Costa, L. A., Viana, M. T. S. A., Moreira-Almeida, A., Lucchetti, A. L. G., & Lucchetti, G. (2016). Brazilian scientific articles on spirituality, religion and health. *Archives of Clinical Psychiatry*, *43*(1), 11–16. https://doi.org/10.1590/0101-60830000000073

de Diego-Cordero, R., López-Gómez, L., Lucchetti, G., & Badanta, B. (2022). Spiritual care in critically ill patients during COVID-19 pandemic. *Nursing Outlook*. https://www.ncbi.nlm.nih.gov/pmc/articles/PMC8226065/

del Castillo, F. A. (2020). Health, spirituality and COVID-19: Themes and insights. *Journal of Public Health*, *43*(2), e273-e274. https://doi.org/10.1093/pubmed/fdaa185

Domaradzki, J. (2022). "We are also here" – Spiritual care practitioners' experiences of the COVID-19 pandemic: A qualitative study from Poland. *Journal of Religion and Health, 61*(2), 962–992. https://doi.org/10.1007/s10943-021-01492-3

Drummond, D. A., & Carey, L. B. (2020). Chaplaincy and spiritual care response to COVID-19: An Australian case study-The McKellar Centre. *Health and Social Care Chaplaincy, 8*(2), 165–179. https://doi.org/10.1558/hscc.41243

Ferrell, B. R., Handzo, G., Picchi, T., Puchalski, C., & Rosa, W. E. (2020). The urgency of spiritual care: COVID-19 and the critical need for whole-person palliation. *Journal of Pain and Symptom Management, 60*(3), e7–e11. https://doi.org/10.1016/j.jpainsymman.2020.06.034

Frankl, V. E. (1992). *Man's search for meaning: An introduction to logotherapy* (4th ed). Beacon Press.

Galbadage, T., Peterson, B. M., Wang, D. C., Wang, J. S., & Gunasekera, R. S. (2020). Biopsychosocial and spiritual implications of patients with COVID-19 dying in isolation. *Frontiers in Psychology, 11*, 588623. https://doi.org/10.3389/fpsyg.2020.588623

Gibbons, S. W., Ross, A., & Bevans, M. (2014). Liminality as a conceptual frame for understanding the family caregiving rite of passage: An integrative review: Caregivers' rite of passage. *Research in Nursing & Health, 37*(5), 423–436. https://doi.org/10.1002/nur.21622

Hosseini, S., Behzad Khamesloo, M., Marzband, R., Amouzad Mehdirji, H., & Behzad Khamesloo, M. (2021). The spiritual needs of nurses caring for patients with COVID-19 disease. *Journal of Nursing and Midwifery Sciences, 8*(4), 294. https://doi.org/10.4103/jnms.jnms_171_20

Jafari, E., Dehshiri, G. R., Eskandari, H., Najafi, M., Heshmati, R., & Hoseinifar, J. (2010). Spiritual well-being and mental health in university students. *Procedia – Social and Behavioral Sciences, 5*, 1477–1481. https://doi.org/10.1016/j.sbspro.2010.07.311

Joseph, R. P., Ainsworth, B. E., Mathis, L., Hooker, S. P., & Keller, C. (2017). Incorporating religion and spirituality into the design of community-based physical activity programs for African American women: A qualitative inquiry. *BMC Research Notes, 10*(1), 506. https://doi.org/10.1186/s13104-017-2830-3

Karaman, E., Erkin, Ö., & Göl, İ. (2022). The relationship between spiritual care levels of Turkish nurses with the spiritual well-being of their patients: An exploratory study. *Journal of Religion and Health, 61*(3), 1882–1893. https://doi.org/10.1007/s10943-021-01194-w

Karimi, Z., Fereidouni, Z., Behnammoghadam, M., Alimohammadi, N., Mousavizadeh, A., Salehi, T., Mirzaee, M. S., & Mirzaee, S. (2020). The lived experience of nurses caring for patients with COVID-19 in Iran: A phenomenological study. *Risk Management and Healthcare Policy, 13*, 1271–1278. https://doi.org/10.2147/RMHP.S258785

Kasapoğlu, F. (2022). The relationship among spirituality, self-efficacy, COVID-19 anxiety, and hopelessness during the COVID-19 process in Turkey: A path analysis. *Journal of Religion and Health, 61*(1), 767–785. https://doi.org/10.1007/s10943-021-01472-7

Keshavan, M. (2020). Building resilience in the COVID-19 era: Three paths in the Bhagavad Gita. *Indian Journal of Psychiatry, 62*(5), 459. https://doi.org/10.4103/psychiatry.IndianJPsychiatry_829_20

Kowalczyk, O., Roszkowski, K., Montane, X., Pawliszak, W., Tylkowski, B., & Bajek, A. (2020). Religion and faith perception in a pandemic of COVID-19. *Journal of Religion and Health, 59*(6), 2671–2677. https://doi.org/10.1007/s10943-020-01088-3

Krause, N. (2003). Religious meaning and subjective well-being in late life. *The Journals of Gerontology Series B: Psychological Sciences and Social Sciences, 58*(3), S160–S170. https://doi.org/10.1093/geronb/58.3.S160

La Cour, P., & Götke, P. (2012). Understanding of the word "spirituality" by theologians compared to lay people: An empirical study from a secular region. *Journal of Health Care Chaplaincy, 18*(3–4), 97–109. https://doi.org/10.1080/08854726.2012.720543

Leggett, A., Koo, H. J., Park, B., & Choi, H. (2022). The changing tides of caregiving during the COVID-19 pandemic: How decreasing and increasing care provision relates to caregiver well-being. *The Journals of Gerontology: Series B, Psychological Sciences and Social Sciences.* https://www.ncbi.nlm.nih.gov/pmc/articles/PMC9122649/

Leong, I. Y.-O., Lee, A. O.-K., Ng, T. W., Lee, L. B., Koh, N. Y., Yap, E., Guay, S., & Ng, L. M. (n.d.). The challenge of providing holistic care in a viral epidemic: Opportunities for palliative care. *Palliative Medicine.* https://pubmed.ncbi.nlm.nih.gov/14982202/

Longacre, M. L., Fang, C. Y., Handorf, E. A., & Valdamanis, V. G. (n.d.). *Work impact and emotional stress among informal caregivers for older adults. The Journals of Gerontology: Series B, Psychological Sciences and Social Sciences.* https://pubmed.ncbi.nlm.nih.gov/27048567/

Mayland, C. R., Harding, A. J. E., Preston, N., & Payne, S. (2020). Supporting adults bereaved through COVID-19: A rapid review of the impact of previous pandemics on grief and bereavement. *Journal of Pain and Symptom Management, 60*(2), e33–e39. https://doi.org/10.1016/j.jpainsymman.2020.05.012

McSherry, W., Cash, K., & Ross, L. (2004). Meaning of spirituality: Implications for nursing practice. *Journal of Clinical Nursing, 13*(8), 934–941. doi:10.1111/j.1365-2702.2004.01006.x

Mueller, P. S., Plevak, D. J., & Rummans, T. A. (2001). Religious involvement, spirituality, and medicine: Implications for clinical practice. *Mayo Clinic Proceedings, 76*(12), 1225–1235. https://doi.org/10.4065/76.12.1225

Nicola, M., Alsafi, Z., Sohrabi, C., Kerwan, A., Al-Jabir, A., Iosifidis, C., Agha, M., & Agha, R. (n.d.). The socio-economic implications of the coronavirus pandemic (COVID-19): A review. *International Journal of Surgery (London, England).* https://pubmed.ncbi.nlm.nih.gov/32305533/

Pandey, S., & Sharma, V. (2020). A tribute to frontline corona warriors-Doctors who sacrificed their life while saving patients during the ongoing COVID-19 pandemic. *Indian Journal of Ophthalmology, 68*(5), 939. https://doi.org/10.4103/ijo.IJO_754_20

Polizzi, C., Lynn, S. J., & Perry, A. (n.d.). Stress and coping in the time of covid-19: Pathways to resilience and Recovery. *Clinical Neuropsychiatry.* https://pubmed.ncbi.nlm.nih.gov/34908968/

Rahimi, T., Dastyar, N., & Rafati, F. (2021). Experiences of family caregivers of patients with COVID-19. *BMC Family Practice, 22*(1), 137. https://doi.org/10.1186/s12875-021-01489-7

Rathakrishnan, B., Singh, S. S. B., Yahaya, A., Kamaluddin, M. R., & Aziz, S. F. A. (2022). The relationship among spirituality, fear, and mental health on COVID-19 among adults: An exploratory research. *Frontiers in Psychology, 12*, 815332. https://doi.org/10.3389/fpsyg.2021.815332

Roman, N. V., Mthembu, T. G., & Hoosen, M. (2020). Spiritual care – 'A deeper immunity' – A response to COVID-19 pandemic. *African Journal of Primary Health Care & Family Medicine, 12*(1). https://doi.org/10.4102/phcfm.v12i1.2456

Russell, B. S., Hutchison, M., Tambling, R., Tomkunas, A. J., & Horton, A. L. (2020). Initial challenges of caregiving during COVID-19: Caregiver Burden, mental health, and the parent – Child relationship. *Child Psychiatry & Human Development, 51*(5), 671–682. https://doi.org/10.1007/s10578-020-01037-x

Sarmiento, P. J. D. (2021). Wounded healers: A call for spiritual care towards healthcare professionals in time of COVID-19 pandemic. *Journal of Public Health, 43*(2), e273–e274. https://doi.org/10.1093/pubmed/fdaa232

Sen, H. E., Colucci, L., & Browne, D. T. (2022). Keeping the faith: Religion, positive coping, and mental health of caregivers during COVID-19. *Frontiers in Psychology*, *12*, 805019. https://doi.org/10.3389/fpsyg.2021.805019

Timmins, F., Connolly, M., Palmisano, S., Burgos, D., Juárez, L. M., Gusman, A., Soriano, V., Jewdokimow, M., Sadłoń, W., Serrano, A. L., Caballero, D. C., Campagna, S., & García-Peñuela, J. M. V. (2022). Providing spiritual care to in-hospital patients during COVID-19: A preliminary European fact-finding study. *Journal of Religion and Health*, *61*(3), 2212–2232. https://doi.org/10.1007/s10943-022-01553-1

Turner, N., & Caswell, G. (2020). Moral ambiguity in media reports of dying alone. *Mortality*, *25*(3), 266–281. https://doi.org/10.1080/13576275.2019.1657388

Usher, K., Durkin, J., & Bhullar, N. (2020). The COVID-19 pandemic and mental health impacts. *International Journal of Mental Health Nursing*, *29*(3), 315–318. https://doi.org/10.1111/inm.12726

Walsh, F. (2020). Loss and resilience in the time of COVID-19: Meaning making, hope, and transcendence. *Family Process*, *59*(3), 898–911. https://doi.org/10.1111/famp.12588

World Health Organization. (n.d.). *Coronavirus disease (covid-19)*. World Health Organization. https://www.who.int/emergencies/diseases/novel-coronavirus-2019?gclid=CjwKCAjwysipBhBXEiwApJOcu0tuTnqxu1e1Mi11fmsDElYZWX78Lkb6IzLKtblfUX3f-CtoaES3B-RoCE2MQAvD_BwE

Yezli, S., & Khan, A. (2020). COVID-19 social distancing in the Kingdom of Saudi Arabia: Bold measures in the face of political, economic, social and religious challenges. *Travel Medicine and Infectious Disease*, *37*, 101692. https://doi.org/10.1016/j.tmaid.2020.101692

6

ADDRESSING GRIEF AND BEREAVEMENT

A Scoping Review of Psycho-social Interventions During and Post COVID-19

Ritika Chokhani, Mrinalini Mahajan
and Chetna Duggal

Introduction

The COVID-19 pandemic has been recognised as an international public health crisis. So far, over 650 million confirmed cases and approximately 6.6 million deaths have occurred globally directly due to COVID-19 (World Health Organization [WHO], 2022). The pandemic also led to a significant indirect death toll due to financial repercussions, impact on healthcare systems, increased violence, and physical and psychological stress (Ray & Subramanian, 2020).

Deaths caused by COVID-19 and its associated complications led to grief that was inhibited, disenfranchised, complicated, prolonged, or traumatic (Eisma et al., 2020; Ramadas & Vijayakumar, 2021; Yu et al., 2022). There were various reasons for this. Due to the quarantine rules, social distancing, and safety protocols during the pandemic, the dying and mourning process was impacted. For example usual funeral rites could not be carried out. This contributed to a worsening of grief reactions as it limited opportunities for people to bid goodbye to their loved ones (Gonçalves Júnior et al., 2020), access social support (Eisma et al., 2020), and express their grief freely (Ramadas & Vijayakumar, 2021).

Further, deaths due to COVID-19 were often sudden and unexpected, even among healthy and young individuals (Kaul, 2020), which led to more severe and more traumatic grief reactions among bereaved individuals (Kokou-Kpolou et al., 2020). Healthcare professionals, too, were impacted by death during COVID-19, as they were at a greater risk for witnessing loss (Inchausti et al., 2020).

Hence, many healthcare institutions, organisations, and researchers trialled psycho-social interventions to address grief and bereavement during COVID-19 and focused on reducing the adverse consequences of bereavement and promoting positive adaptation after the loss (Yu et al., 2022). However, the pandemic created

DOI: 10.4324/9781003357209-8

unique demands for the provision of such mental health services, namely, adaptation to the shifting nature of the pandemic; navigation of the move towards briefer, remotely delivered sessions; the usage of appropriate methods to identify levels of need; and the consideration of the needs of vulnerable populations (Duan & Zhu, 2020; Inchausti et al., 2020, Moreno et al., 2020; Rosen et al., 2020). Further, increased collaboration between mental health professionals and other professionals was required, sometimes through task-shifting of the delivery of psychological interventions either through digital means or through different professional groups (Békés & Aafjes-van Doorn, 2020).

Research identified mental healthcare needs specific to loss and grief during COVID-19 which would need to be addressed through psycho-social interventions. Examples included making challenging end-of-life decisions (e.g. when patients requiring mechanical support are unable to be extubated), assisting families in using social support networks despite social distancing protocols, addressing anticipatory grief, and acknowledging the different nature of loss during COVID-19 (LeRoy et al., 2021; Stroebe & Schut, 2021). The need for an evidence-based, trauma-informed, resilience-focused, and culturally sensitive response to bereavement was highlighted (Kokou-Kpolou et al., 2020; Stroebe & Schut, 2021), as was the need for a systems' response to mass bereavement, including collective meaning-making practices (Harrop et al., 2020). Specific subgroups identified as needing mental health support included older adults, healthcare workers, and children (Albuquerque & Santos, 2021; Stroebe & Schut, 2021). With respect to the nature of interventions, remotely delivered, proactive interventions aimed at crisis counselling were preferred (Harrop et al., 2020). Key components of grief interventions identified included structured psychoeducation, drawing on existing peer and social support (including group-based support) and formal risk assessment and referral (Laranjeira et al., 2022; Stroebe & Schut, 2021). Innovative approaches such as theatre-based interventions were also proposed (Rushton et al., 2020). Theoretical frameworks suggested to address grief included the Dual-Process Model (DPM; Stroebe & Schut, 2021) and Cognitive Behavioural Therapy (CBT; Harrop et al., 2020). DPM posits that people who are grieving oscillate between confrontation and avoidance of the tasks of grieving, and such oscillation is both normative and healthy (Stroebe & Schut, 2021). Hence, DPM aims to assist and facilitate oscillation between loss and restoration-oriented tasks of grieving. CBT focuses on helping individuals identify and differentiate between thoughts, feelings, and behaviours related to grieving and use this increased awareness to modify thoughts and behaviours (Harrop et al., 2020). However, empirical evidence for the efficacy of these models during COVID-19 was lacking in the current literature.

To highlight two particular reviews previously conducted, Stroebe and Schut (2021) reviewed the literature on existing knowledge about adaptation to grief and bereavement in the pandemic, and Laranjeira et al. (2022) conducted a scoping review of interventions for family bereavement during COVID-19. One limitation identified by both reviews was the lack of studies providing empirical data or including detailed description of interventions, with most articles describing expert commentaries, reviews of studies conducted in previous pandemics, and quick surveys (Stroebe & Schut, 2021). Stroebe and Schut's (2021) review included studies published up to June 2020, approximately three months into the pandemic; hence there is a need to conduct an updated review. Laranjeira et al. (2022) did not include a detailed narrative synthesis of the nature and components of grief and bereavement interventions, which would be important to elucidate to aid in deriving implications for research and practice.

Hence, there is a strong rationale to comprehensively identify and review the nature and components of psycho-social interventions used to address grief and bereavement during the past two years of the COVID-19 pandemic, with specific focus on delivered interventions or interventions described in sufficient detail. Such a review would have implications for future research and practice on interventions used to address grief and bereavement in emergency contexts as well as implications for policy around mental healthcare in emergencies. Due to the nascent nature of literature in this area (Munn et al., 2018), a scoping review methodology was considered appropriate.

Hence, we aimed to conduct a scoping review to review and analyse the current knowledge on interventions to address grief and bereavement during and post COVID-19 pandemic reported in the academic literature. It had two main objectives:

- To identify the interventions employed to address grief and bereavement during and post COVID-19 pandemic in the academic literature and
- To elucidate and critically review the nature and components of these interventions and further derive implications for future research.

Methods

Inclusion and Exclusion Criteria

Target Population

Interventions targeted at all age groups were included. Interventions could be targeted towards bereaved relatives or friends or healthcare workers. The loss need not have occurred as a consequence of acquiring COVID-19 – only that it occurred during the period of the COVID-19 pandemic.

Type of Interventions

Interventions targeted at helping people with grief and bereavement were included. Interventions needed to be aimed, primarily, or at least substantially, at addressing grief and bereavement, if they formed part of another larger intervention. Grief and bereavement were defined as the loss of a loved one and did not include grief re-lated to losses such as the loss of a home, job, educational opportunities, and so on. Individual, group, and family-based interventions using any theoretical framework were included.

Type of Settings

Interventions delivered face-to-face in hospital, clinic, community or home set-tings, or digitally were included.

Type of Studies

Quasi-experimental, observational, or uncontrolled pre-post studies were included. RCT protocols and qualitative studies were also included. Studies were included irrespective of whether they measured outcomes. Theoretical articles, policy docu-ments, and papers that described recommendations for interventions without deliv-ering them were excluded. Studies published in peer-reviewed journals in English between March 2020 and October 2022 were included.

Selection of Sources of Evidence

The following databases were searched: ProQuest, PubMed, Scopus, Web of Sci-ence, and APA PsycNet. Searches were conducted between 17 October 2022 and 23 November 2022. The search strategies were decided on the basis of discussion between two reviewers and preliminary trials (Table 6.1).

Titles and abstracts of all studies were screened for Scopus and PubMed (R.C.) as well as for APA PsycNet, Web of Science, and ProQuest (M.M.). Duplicates were deleted, and relevant full-texts were accessed. Two full-texts could not be accessed for the review. Both reviewers (M.M. and R.C.) independently read each full-text and determined the eligibility of the study. A spreadsheet was used to record decisions, and disagreements between reviewers were resolved through dis-cussion and input from a third reviewer (C.D.).

TABLE 6.1 Example of search strategies

Search Strategies for Scopus
(TITLE-ABS-KEY (covid-19 OR covid OR pandemic OR sars-cov-2 OR coronavirus) AND TITLE-ABS-KEY (grief OR griev* OR mourn* OR bereavement OR bereave*) AND TITLE-ABS-KEY (therap* OR "psycho-social intervention" OR counselling OR counseling OR "psycho-social support" OR psychotherap* OR psychoeducation OR teletherapy OR intervention OR cognitive-behavioural AND therapy OR "psychological intervention" OR "social support" OR "digital health" OR e-health))

Data Extraction

A template consisting of the following categories was designed in Microsoft Excel: study title, author(s), month and year of publication, location, methodology, aims, sample characteristics, intervention details, components of intervention, and any quantitative/qualitative outcomes. Data was extracted by both reviewers independently and then reviewed together to resolve discrepancies.

Data Synthesis

Thematic analysis was used to identify relevant themes about the interventions. First, two reviewers (R.C. and M.M.) independently read through the data extraction spreadsheet line by line and identified preliminary themes from the data. All three reviewers then examined and discussed the preliminary themes, leading to a final list of themes.

Ethical Considerations

Since the review involved using already-published data that is in the public domain, ethical approval was not required.

Results and Discussion

Overview of Study Characteristics

The final list of eligible studies included 16 studies describing 15 interventions. The flow of studies in the review is displayed in Figure 6.1.

Locations of studies included China, Hong Kong, Italy, Spain, France, Portugal, the Netherlands, Mexico and the United States, indicating a fairly global distribution. All selected studies were published in peer-reviewed journals; however, the study by Mallet et al. (2021) was published as a letter to the editor. Three studies were uncontrolled pre-post studies, five were RCT protocols, and three were case studies. The other five studies described interventions carried out in a routine clinical setting; these will be referred to as "real-world" studies hereon (US Food and Drug Administration, 2018). Sample sizes ranged between 1 (for case studies) to 1,500 (Mellins et al., 2020). In the majority of studies (n = 14), the primary aim of the intervention was addressing grief and bereavement, while two studies included grief and bereavement as a significant component of larger interventions (Mellins et al., 2020; Tao et al., 2022). Table 6.2 summarises these details of the interventions included.

The themes have been discussed in two categories: the nature of interventions and the components of interventions. The nature of interventions pertains to how interventions were delivered, and the components of interventions pertain to what

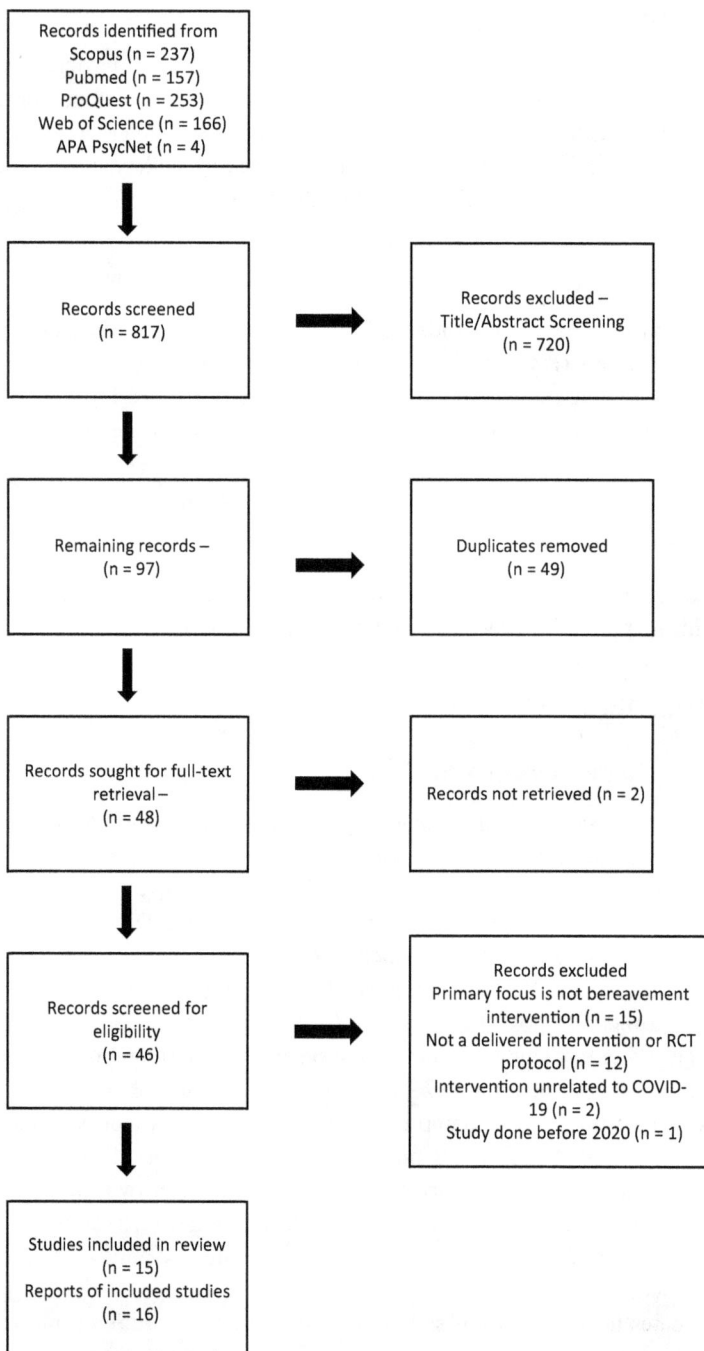

FIGURE 6.1   Flow diagram of study selection

TABLE 6.2 Details of the study included in the review

S. No.	Title	Author/Year	Location	Methodology	Aims	Sample Characteristics
1.	A Phone-Based Early Psychological Intervention for Supporting Bereaved Families in the Time of COVID-19 Phone follow-up to the families of COVID-19 patients who died at the hospital: families' grief reactions and clinical psychologists' roles	Borghi et al., 2021 Menichetti et al., 2021	Milan, Italy	Real-world	The aim was to describe a phone-based primary preventive psychological intervention delivered to bereaved families by the Clinical Psychology unit of an Italian hospital. The aim of the study was to explore the families' experiences and needs and identify the role of the psychologists in this endeavour.	Bereaved family members (n = 246)
2.	End of Life Intervention Program During COVID-19 in Vall d'Hebron University Hospital	Beneria et al., 2021	Barcelona, Spain	Real-world	The aim was to describe an End of Life intervention programme implemented during COVID-19 in the Vall d'Hebron University Hospital (HUVH)	Relatives of end-of-life patients (n = 359)
3.	"Sustaining the unsustainable: Rapid implementation of a Support Intervention for Bereavement during the COVID-19 pandemic"	Mallet et al., 2021	Paris, France	Real-world	The aim was to provide informal peer-support to frontline staff using a rapid implementation of a Support Intervention for Bereavement (SIB) in a large academic hospital.	Bereaved relatives (n = 15)
4.	Psycho-social Intervention on the Dual-Process Model for a Group of COVID-19 Bereaved Individuals in Wuhan: A Pilot Study	Yu et al., 2022	Wuhan, China	Uncontrolled pre-post study	The objective of the paper was to review and analyse how the "Be Together Program", a public welfare programme for grief intervention, worked and to discuss its results	Bereaved family members (n = 45)

(Continued)

TABLE 6.2 (Continued)

S. No.	Title	Author/Year	Location	Methodology	Aims	Sample Characteristics
5.	The Story Listening Project: Feasibility and Acceptability of a Remotely Delivered Intervention to Alleviate Grief during the COVID-19 Pandemic	Reblin et al., 2022	Vermont, the United States	Uncontrolled pre-post study	The aim was to determine the feasibility and acceptability of a brief, remotely delivered Story Listening storytelling intervention for individuals experiencing grief during the COVID pandemic	Bereaved family members or clinicians (n = 62; 48 relatives, 16 clinicians)
6.	Death Cafés for Prevention of Burnout in Intensive Care Unit Employees: Study Protocol for a Randomised Controlled Trial (STOPTHEBURN)	Bateman et al., 2020	New Orleans, the United States	RCT Protocol	The aim of the study was to assess whether the participation in regular debriefing can prevent burnout in intensive care unit (ICU) clinicians	Healthcare workers (n = 200 ICU staff; 100 physicians and 100 non-physicians)
7.	A Self-Applied Multi-Component Psychological Online Intervention Based on UX, for the Prevention of Complicated Grief Disorder in the Mexican Population During the COVID-19 Outbreak: Protocol of a Randomised Clinical Trial	Dominguez-Rodriguez et al., 2021	Mexico	RCT Protocol	The aim of the study was to design and implement a self-applied intervention composed of 12 modules focusing on decreasing the risk of developing Complicated Grief Disorder and increasing the life quality; with the secondary objective of reducing anxiety, depression, and increasing sleep quality.	Bereaved relatives with symptoms of depression, anxiety, or Acute Stress Disorder; within six months of death (n = 49)

#	Title	Author, Year	Location	Type	Objectives	Sample
8.	Grief Reactions and Grief Counseling among Bereaved Chinese Individuals during COVID-19 Pandemic: Study Protocol for a Randomised Controlled Trial Combined with a Longitudinal Study	Tang et al., 2021	Hong Kong, China	RCT Protocol	The objectives were to investigate demographic and related factors associated with prolonged grief symptoms among Chinese individuals bereaved due to COVID-19 (including grief reaction, trauma response, depression, anxiety, and suicide risk), develop training and evaluation programmes for Chinese professional grief counsellors to develop and examine their competence and provide grief counselling for the bereaved during the pandemic; and assess the effect of the intervention.	Bereaved adults Phase 1: n=300 Phase 2: n=500 Phase 3: n=160
9.	Online Treatment of Persistent Complex Bereavement Disorder, Posttraumatic Stress Disorder, and Depression Symptoms in People Who Lost Loved Ones during the COVID-19 Pandemic: Study Protocol for a Randomised Controlled Trial and a Controlled Trial	Reitsma et al., 2021	The Netherlands	RCT Protocol	The aim was to evaluate the short-term and long-term effectiveness of grief-specific online CBT in reducing PCBD, PTSD, and depression symptom-levels for adults who lost a loved one during the COVID-19 pandemic.	Bereaved relatives (died at least three months earlier; have symptoms of PCBD, PTSD, or depression) Phase 1: n = 62 Phase 2: n = 102

(Continued)

TABLE 6.2 (Continued)

S. No.	Title	Author/Year	Location	Methodology	Aims	Sample Characteristics
10.	Supporting People Who Have Lost a Close Person by Bereavement or Separation: Protocol of a Randomised Controlled Trial Comparing Two French-Language Internet-Based Interventions	Debrot et al., 2022	Switzerland but French-speaking people throughout the world will be recruited	RCT Protocol	The aim of the intervention was to use the web-based application to increase the well-being and decrease the distress of the participants. It was also compared to the previous application and improved on the same.	Bereaved adults or those experiencing separation (n = 234)
11.	EMDR Therapy Treatment of Grief and Mourning in Times of COVID-19	Solomon & Hensley, 2020	The United States	Case Study	The aim was to present a framework for treatment of grief and mourning with eye movement desensitisation and reprocessing (EMDR) therapy.	Individual client who had lost his father (n = 1)
12.	Case Report: Parental Loss and Childhood Grief During COVID-19 Pandemic	Santos et al., 2021	Portugal	Case Study	The aim was to describe the intervention for loss of a parent during the COVID-19 pandemic	Individual client who had lost her father (n = 1)
13.	Mourning from COVID-19 and Post-Traumatic Stress Disorder: New Therapeutic Tools in the Treatment of Pathological Bereavement	Spurio, 2021	Rome, Italy	Case Study	The aim was to describe the intervention for loss of spouse during the COVID-19 pandemic	Thirty-five-year-old woman, bereaved by death of husband (n = 1)

No.	Title	Author	Location	Study type	Aim	Sample
14.	Supporting the Well-Being of Healthcare Providers during the COVID-19 Pandemic: The CopeColumbia Response	Mellins et al., 2020	New York City, the United States	Real-world	The aim was to describe CopeColumbia, a peer support programme developed by faculty in a large urban medical centre's Department of Psychiatry to support emotional well-being and enhance the professional resilience of healthcare workers.	Healthcare workers Groups: n = 186 (participants ranging from 1 to 30) Workshops = 43 Individual calls = 141 Total = 1,500
15.	The Effectiveness of the Moving to Emptiness Technique on Clients Who Need Help during the COVID-19 Pandemic: A Real-World Study	Tao et al., 2022	Mainland China	Uncontrolled pre-post study	The aim of the study was to introduce and understand the effectiveness of a new technique called moving to emptiness technique (MET), which combined Western structural progress and core factors of Chinese culture	General adult population who might have trauma symptoms because of the pandemic (n = 107)

was delivered within the interventions. Both of these are described in Tables 6.2 and 6.3, which display the interventions included in the review.

Nature of Interventions

Tables 6.2 and 6.3 provide data on the nature of all included interventions.

Aim of Interventions

Interventions could be categorised into Level 1 (preventive and supportive interventions) or Level 2 responses (treatment for mental health disorders) as per Rosen et al. (2020). Most delivered interventions (n = 8) were supportive interventions for bereaved individuals and contained no formal assessment of symptoms of complicated, prolonged, or traumatic grief. These interventions can be categorised as Level 1 interventions. On the other hand, most RCT protocols (n = 4) formulated interventions including the assessment of symptoms of depression, anxiety, stress, trauma, or grief with explicit aims of preventing or reducing pathological grief. These interventions can be categorised as Level 2 interventions.

Target Population of Interventions

Interventions were mostly targeted towards bereaved relatives (n = 11). However, Tao et al. (2022) focused on individuals who experienced psychological difficulties during the pandemic – a subset of whom was also bereaved. Other studies focused on interventions for healthcare workers (Bateman et al., 2020; Mellins et al., 2020), who had seen an unprecedented increase in witnessing death of patients. Thus, interventions were primarily directed towards those most likely to be exposed to loss during the pandemic.

Delivery of Interventions

While mental health professionals delivered a majority of the interventions (psychiatrists, clinical psychologists, counsellors; n = 7), three interventions were delivered in concert by psychologists and healthcare social workers, one by nurses (Mallet et al., 2021), and one by trained doulas (Reblin et al., 2022). Other studies (n = 3) used self-guided web-based applications to deliver interventions. Two of these were completely unguided interventions, whereas one study proposed to compare an unguided version of the intervention with a therapist-guided (through email contact only) version of the same treatment (Reitsma et al., 2021). Overall, there was a trend towards (a) using diverse professionals to deliver interventions, rather than only highly qualified mental healthcare professionals (b) using self-guided interventions, both of which may be attempts to increase the scalability and accessibility of the interventions.

TABLE 6.3 Interventions described in the identified studies

S. No.	Author/Year	Intervention Details	Components of Intervention	Outcomes
1.	Borghi et al., 2021 Menichetti et al., 2021	*Delivery professionals:* clinical psychologists *Modality:* telephone *No. of sessions:* 1 *Type of intervention:* supportive	The intervention consisted of active listening and emotional validation, assessment of psycho-social needs and resources, information-sharing, psycho-education about stages of grief, brief therapeutic actions like relaxation pills, and assessment of early risk and protective factors and referrals for further psychological support	*Quantitative outcomes:* not measured *Qualitative outcomes:* notes of the psychologists reflected the gratitude of the relatives
2.	Beneria et al., 2021	*Delivery professionals:* healthcare social workers and clinical psychologists *Modality:* face-to-face and telephone *No. of sessions:* unclear **Type of intervention:** supportive	The intervention consisted of social assessment by social workers and psychological assessment by clinical psychologists. It comprised of bad news communication, allowing face to face farewell to the patient, psychological support for bereavement, assessment of risk and protective factors and provision of information and referral	**Quantitative outcomes:** not measured **Qualitative outcomes:** intervention allowed the bereaved to say goodbyes. The emotional impact on practitioners was identified and addressed
3.	Mallet et al., 2021	*Delivery professionals:* nurse *Modality:* telephone *No. of sessions:* 1–4 calls *Type of intervention:* supportive	Hospital staff referred patients for intervention. Nurses called patients on hotlines. The first line intervention used consisted of empathic statements, written psychoeducation, referrals, medical information, and providing contact details of religious representatives. The second line intervention focused on facilitating the acceptance of loss and restoring a sense of possibility of future happiness	*Quantitative outcomes:* not measured *Qualitative outcomes:* not measured

(Continued)

TABLE 6.3 (Continued)

S. No.	Author/Year	Intervention Details	Components of Intervention	Outcomes
4.	Yu et al., 2022	*Delivery professionals*: social workers supervised by professional mental health specialists *Modality*: WeChat *No. of sessions*: variable (participants can choose) *Type of intervention*: DPM-based grief intervention	The intervention included Chinese cultural elements: memory ceremony; components on health anxiety, mindfulness, Yoga, dancing therapy, heart-healing reading, letter-writing on a festival day, and loss-oriented and restoration-oriented psychoeducation	*Quantitative outcomes*: these were measured using the Inventory of Complicated Grief (ICG-19) (Prigerson et al., 1995) *Qualitative outcomes*: not measured
5.	Reblin et al., 2022	*Delivery professionals*: doulas *Modality*: video conferencing *No. of sessions*: 1 *Type of intervention*: supportive	The intervention focused on inviting stories of loss and listening to experiences of the bereaved, identifying key themes and reflection, expressing gratitude for sharing, journaling and identifying and referring participants who needed greater intervention	*Quantitative outcomes*: rates of enrolment, retention, and completion of assessments were used to understand the feasibility of the intervention. *Qualitative outcomes*: thematic analysis of interviews post-intervention

| 6. | Bateman et al., 2020 | *Delivery professionals:* psychotherapists
Modality: video conferencing
No. of sessions: 4
Type of intervention: supportive (debriefing) | Group-based sessions ("Death Cafes") focusing on informal discussions related to themes of death, loss, grief, and illness. The participants will be encouraged to reflect together about stressful events and be offered a space for community and collaboration for the employees which is not in the workspace | **Quantitative outcomes:** Primary outcome will be clinician burnout (measured by the Maslach Burnout Inventory; MBI). Secondary outcomes included depression (as measured by Patient Health Questionnaire-8, PHQ-8) and anxiety (measured by the Generalised Anxiety Disorder 7-item scale, GAD-7). These will be administered prior to the intervention, and then at one month, three months, and six months of post enrolment
Qualitative outcomes: no clarity on how these will be measured, but it will be done |
| 7. | Dominguez-Rodriguez et al., 2021 | *Delivery professionals:* unguided digital course
Modality: A web-based platform on desktop or mobile
No. of sessions: 12 "modules"
Type of intervention: CBT, mindfulness, and positive psychology | Different modules would include psychoeducation about grief phases, managing the pain of loss, and understanding the experience of loss during COVID-19, for example deprived of rights; saying goodbye through parting strategies, adapting to loss through self-care, restoring daily activities and integrating with supportive networks, and repositioning deceased person in lives and preventing relapse | *Quantitative outcomes:* grief symptoms would be assessed
Qualitative outcomes: not measured |

(Continued)

TABLE 6.3 (Continued)

S. No.	Author/Year	Intervention Details	Components of Intervention	Outcomes
8.	Tang et al., 2021	*Delivery professionals*: Psychologist, social worker, or occupational psychological counsellor *Modality*: online *No. of sessions*: 8–10 sessions *Type of intervention*: Prolonged Grief Disorder Therapy (Columbia University), adapted to the context of Chinese psychotherapy; based on DPM	Sessions focused on understanding and accepting grief reactions, managing painful emotions, learning to care of the self, increasing contact with others, coping with difficult days, and adapting to a new life	*Quantitative outcomes*: primary outcomes to be assessed by the Prolonged Grief Questionnaire (PG-13), the 20-item PTSD Checklist for DSM-5 (PCL-5), the Depression Anxiety and Stress Scale (DASS-21), and the Posttraumatic Growth Inventory (PTGI) *Qualitative outcomes*: not measured
9.	Reitsma et al., 2021	*Delivery professionals*: Part 1 – unguided digital course Part 2 – guided by therapists through email contact *Modality*: online, through secure website *No. of sessions*: 8 sessions *Type of intervention*: CBT	Sessions focused on psychoeducation about emotional reactions to bereavement, exposure to loss through structured writing, cognitive restructuring assignments, and behavioural experiments and behavioural activation assignments	*Quantitative outcomes*: measured using Traumatic Grief Inventory – Clinician Administered; PTSD Checklist for DSM-5; Patient Health Questionnaire (PHQ-9); COVID-19 Stressful Events self-report questionnaire *Qualitative outcomes*: not measured
10.	Debrot et al., 2022	*Delivery professionals*: unguided digital course *Modality*: online *No. of sessions*: ten sessions: one introductory, one closing, and the rest eight are based on four modules *Type of intervention*: psychoeducational model grounded in DPM	Current intervention included sessions on introduction (focusing on psychoeducation), cognition-focused loss and restoration-oriented sessions, emotion-focused loss and restoration-oriented sessions, behaviour-focused loss and restoration-oriented sessions, identity-focused loss and restoration-oriented sessions and conclusion (focusing on assessing the experience of intervention and preventing relapse)	*Quantitative outcomes*: primary outcomes to be measured are grief symptoms, depressive symptoms, and eudemonic well-being, while secondary outcomes included anxiety symptoms, coping strategies, aspects related to self-identity reorganisation, and programme satisfaction *Qualitative outcomes*: not measured

11.	Solomon & Hensley, 2020	*Delivery professionals*: EMDR-trained therapist *Modality*: video conferencing *No. of sessions*: eight phases of EMDR completed; but the number of sessions was unspecified *Type of intervention*: EMDR, attachment theory, DPM	History, preparation, assessment, desensitisation, installation, and body scan, closure, and re-evaluation	*Quantitative outcomes*: not measured *Qualitative outcomes*: more engagement with family was seen. The patient was able to adapt to the new schedule and focus on work also increased
12.	Santos et al., 2021	*Delivery professionals*: authors were the therapists for the child *Modality*: fortnightly telephone calls; monthly face-to-face appointments *No. of sessions*: unspecified *Type of intervention*: art-based and talk-based therapy	Dealing with the loss of a parent and sharing adaptive ways to think about them by choosing a linking object as memento, recalling positive experiences with them, and creating a memory book including family stories, photographs, drawings, etc.	*Quantitative outcomes*: not measured *Qualitative outcomes*: not measured
13.	Spurio, 2021	*Delivery professionals*: psychotherapist *Modality*: face-to-face *No. of sessions*: unspecified *Type of intervention*: psychotherapy + nature-based intervention	Narrative questions, forest bathing, and walks in the forest with the therapist	*Quantitative outcomes*: not measured *Qualitative outcomes*: not measured

(Continued)

TABLE 6.3 (Continued)

S. No.	Author/Year	Intervention Details	Components of Intervention	Outcomes
14.	Mellins et al., 2020	*Delivery professionals*: psychiatrists and psychologists *Modality*: video conferencing *No. of sessions*: 186 groups and 43 workshops *Type of intervention*: positive psychology, CBT, ACT	Peer-support groups for identifying unique stressors and their influence on healthcare workers' well-being and resilience; one-to-one peer support sessions for personalised discussion and to facilitate referrals; town halls (virtual talks) on relevant topics like stress management, anxiety, trauma, loss and grief, self-care; 24/7 access to resources through CopeColumbia website	*Quantitative outcomes*: measured using rating scales for perceived helpfulness of the group (consistently high) and emotional distress (decreased over time) and willingness to recommend the group (high). *Qualitative outcomes*: not measured
15.	Tao et al., 2022	*Delivery professionals*: therapists *Modality*: face-to-face *No. of sessions*: two or three sessions for most participants; highest sessions: nine *Type of intervention*: Moving to Emptiness Technique	Three-step intervention: the trio relaxation exercise; visualising and locating target symptom; and visualising symbolic container.	*Quantitative outcomes*: measured using influence rating (1–10) which decreased significantly post the intervention *Qualitative outcomes*: word cloud analysis was done for target symptom and location

Modality of Interventions

A majority of interventions (n = 11) were delivered completely through digital means. Modalities included telephone (n = 4), videoconferencing (n = 3), and web-based applications (n = 3). Two studies did not specify the exact delivery modalities (Tang et al., 2021; Yu et al., 2022).

Two interventions were blended. This included a case report wherein the sessions had started before the pandemic and were shifted to telephonic mode due to lockdown (Santos et al., 2021) and an end-of-life intervention at a hospital where relatives were given opportunities to connect through video calls to the patients in ICUs (Beneria et al., 2021).

Face-to-face interventions were reported in two studies: a single-session body-based intervention from China (Tao et al., 2022) and a case report about nature-based therapy (Spurio, 2021). Hence, remote methods served as the primary modality to deliver interventions under specific COVID-19 protocols whereas the nature of the therapy or setting specifications (end-of-life hospital setting, in the above instance) necessitated the use of face-to-face modalities.

Duration and Frequency of Interventions

A majority of interventions were brief (fewer than six sessions; n = 5), with two interventions including only one session for all participants (Borghi et al., 2021; Reblin et al., 2022). Mallet et al. (2021) did one to four sessions for all participants, based on perceived need. Self-guided interventions included 8–12 modules accessed by mobile apps. The total number of sessions was not specified for some studies (n = 4). Overall, a trend towards briefer interventions was seen.

Format of Interventions

Most interventions (n = 12) were delivered in individual formats. Studies by Mellins et al. (2020) and Yu et al. (2022) had provisions for individual and group interventions, with Mellins et al. (2020) and Bateman et al. (2020) running groups for healthcare workers. One-on-one interventions were used to support at-risk individuals (e.g. those recently bereaved) as well as provide more intensive services, while group interventions were used to draw on community resources to cope with a calamity (COVID-19) that was affecting people at a community level as well – not only individual level.

Components of Interventions

Table 6.3 outlines the components of all included interventions.

Theoretical Frameworks on Grief and Bereavement

Dual Process Model (DPM)

Four interventions used the DPM, which posits that grieving involves two kinds of stressors: loss and restoration-oriented stressors. Adaptive coping involves an oscillation between confrontation and avoidance of these two different tasks of grieving (Schut, 1999). Tang et al. (2021) used Complicated Grief Therapy, based on DPM, developed at Columbia (Shear et al., 2005), and Solomon and Hensley (2020) incorporated DPM principles into their EMDR-based therapy. DPM interventions had a mix of techniques aimed at both loss (e.g. confronting the avoidance of emotions) and restoration (e.g. focusing on positive life aspects), oscillating between one loss session and one restoration-oriented session, aiming to parallel the model's process of grief oscillation (Debrot et al., 2022; Yu et al., 2022).

Therapeutic Approaches and Interventions

Counselling Micro Skills

In several studies (n = 5), interventions were emphasised using micro skills such as validation, summarising, reflection of feeling, and content during the sessions. For example Reblin et al. (2022) trained doulas to invite stories of loss, identify their key themes, and reflect them to participants. Other studies did not explicitly refer to micro skills but presumably used them as part of their larger intervention. Self-guided interventions, by their very nature, did not have opportunities for their use. Overall, counselling micro skills were considered a vital component of primarily supportive interventions.

Cognitive Behavioural Therapy (CBT)

Interventions using CBT (n = 3) focused on differentiating emotions, thoughts, and behaviours as well as linking these three aspects to each other. Two interventions integrated CBT with other approaches. A common theme in CBT interventions was reducing avoidance, both to negative emotions and to desired behaviours, through exposure exercises and behavioural activation.

Positive Psychology

Two studies included elements from positive psychology (Dominguez-Rodriguez et al., 2021; Mellins et al., 2020). Mellins et al. (2020) described peer-support groups that focused on identifying ways to cultivate resilience by discussing coping strategies, valuing one's contribution, and encouraging participants to reflect on what went well and express gratitude. Resilience was also reconceptualised as not "snapping back" to how one was before but rather integrating difficult experiences into one's identity and growing from the process.

Mindfulness

Two studies reported using mindfulness (Dominguez-Rodriguez et al., 2021; Mellins et al., 2020). Dominguez-Rodriguez et al. (2021) presented a mindfulness exercise at the beginning and end of every session to situate the participant in the present moment along with containing mindfulness-based experiential exercises, such as identifying needs, difficulties, preoccupations, and emotions in three modules. Mellins et al. (2020) shared weblinks to mindfulness-based meditation and exercises on their CopeColumbia website.

Body-Based Techniques

Many studies (n = 4) used body-based techniques such as relaxation (Borghi et al., 2021), Yoga and dance therapy (Yu et al., 2022), and body scan (Solomon & Hensley, 2020). A culturally derived body-based technique called "moving to emptiness" technique was used by Tao et al. (2022). It involved asking participants to identify and locate a target symptom in a body part ("symbolic object"), visualising a symbolic container having their internal resources, and moving the symbolic object into the container. The relationship between grief and its bodily manifestation was acknowledged and addressed in these studies.

Eye-Movement Desensitisation and Retraining (EMDR)

Solomon and Hensley (2020) demonstrated the use of EMDR in the context of grief, trauma, and the pandemic in their case report. Eight phases of EMDR were described: (a) history taking and building therapeutic rapport; (b) preparation, (psychoeducation, stabilisation, and coping strategies); (c) assessment; (d) desensitisation; (e) installation; (f) body scan; (g) closure; and (h) re-evaluation of the therapeutic process.

Core Content of Interventions

Addressing Basic Needs and Sharing Information

Several studies (n = 6) helped participants with practical and logistical difficulties and shared information regarding the same (e.g. helping family members to organise the funeral, contacts for religious representatives). Hence, addressing physical and social needs was seen as important in supportive interventions.

Screening and Assessment for Referral

Many studies (n = 5) included screening and assessment components (assessing risk factors, protective factors, and psycho-social resources) and, accordingly, referred individuals needing more specialist support. This showed that the briefer, supportive interventions acted as quick screenings, rather than intensive interventions.

Psychoeducation

Psychoeducation about the expected process, stages, and emotions related to grief were a part of many interventions (n = 6). Debrot et al. (2022) specifically described their intervention as a psychoeducational model, including components on cognitions, emotions, behaviours, and identity. Hence, psychoeducation was aimed at normalising the experience of grief and reducing the uncertainty of participants' grieving experiences.

Facing Towards (Rather Than Turning Away From) the Emotional Pain of Grief

Studies used a number of techniques to help participants access their emotional pain, such as identifying and naming felt emotions (Dominguez-Rodriguez et al., 2021) and telling the story of the loss (Reblin et al., 2022). Some studies used expressive writing to facilitate emotional processing, for example, journaling (Reblin et al., 2022) and structured writing prompts (Reitsma et al., 2021). Thus, processing, rather than avoiding, painful emotions related to grief became an important target of interventions.

Making Memories of the Deceased and Readapting to Life Without Them

Some studies reported unique ways of commemorating loved ones such as a memory ceremony, heart-healing reading, letter-writing, cultivating a linking object to the deceased, and creating memory books (Santos et al., 2021; Yu et al., 2022). Another study included a module on alternative parting rituals for those who were unable to say goodbye in a traditional manner (Dominguez-Rodriguez et al., 2021). These studies highlighted how creative methods to honour the memories of the deceased became important, especially when the usual grieving process was interrupted. Further, some studies (n = 3) included components on helping bereaved persons reposition the role of the deceased person in their lives, adapt to a new life without them, and restore a sense of future possibilities.

Self-Care

Interventions targeted at bereaved relatives as well as healthcare workers (n = 3) encouraged participants to gradually return to activities of daily living and promoted self-care in various domains: physical, emotional, cognitive, and spiritual. According to Mellins et al. (2020), self-care was framed as essential, not selfish, using the metaphor of oxygen masks on an aeroplane. Thus, it is seen that interventions kept the costs of caring in mind and tried to destigmatise self-care.

Drawing on Community Resources and Social Connections

Studies by Bateman et al. (2020) and Mellins et al. (2020) targeted healthcare workers and drew on community as the basis of the intervention (e.g. Death Cafes aim to help staff reflect on distressing events related to patient care while focusing on the development of a sense of community for themselves). Some studies (n = 3) also encouraged participants to connect with their social support networks. In fact, in Reitsma et al.'s (2021) intervention, participants were encouraged to invite someone close to them to be a part of the programme. Thus, social support and community were seen as important resources, especially in the context of social distancing protocols.

Finding Meaning

Two studies encouraged participants to consciously make meaning and identify values (Mellins et al., 2020; Tang et al., 2021). For example, Mellins et al. (2020) encouraged healthcare professionals to identify their professional values and reasons for joining the medical profession and to reconnect to the same to find meaning in one's work during the pandemic.

Outcomes of Interventions

Quantitative Outcomes

Majority of the studies (n = 9) measured or proposed to measure the outcomes of the interventions through quantitative means. RCT protocols usually proposed to study the outcomes through structured questionnaires whereas other studies involved rating scales to assess the outcomes. This may be because RCT protocols targeted symptoms of disorders such as PTSD and Complicated Grief Disorder, while other interventions focused more on general well-being and preventive aspects.

Qualitative Outcomes

Some studies (n = 6) measured the qualitative outcomes of their intervention. Some of the outcomes were related to the symptoms of the participants (Tao et al., 2022), while others used qualitative measures to understand how the participants felt post the intervention (n = 4). One of the interventions (Bateman et al., 2020) did not mention which qualitative outcomes would be measured.

Unique Adaptations to the Pandemic

Interventions were adapted to the specific context of COVID-19 in the ways given in the subsequent sections.

Meeting Specific Needs

Interventions attempted to address the specific nature of grieving during the pandemic. For example some case studies showed the challenges of working with unexpected losses: a child who lost her father (Santos et al., 2021) and a wife who had lost her husband (Spurio, 2021). Dominguez-Rodriguez et al. (2021) included a module on rights-deprived grief, which highlighted alternative ways of bidding goodbye when the usual processes of mourning were not possible.

Creative Approaches

Some studies incorporated elements from different approaches such as arts-based intervention (Santos et al., 2021) and nature-based interventions to address grief (Spurio, 2021). Further, self-guided interventions as well as a component of Yu et al.'s (2022) intervention called the "supermarket mode" (which gave participants a choice of attending any module) provided increased agency and flexibility to participants.

Acknowledging the Cultural Context

All studies based in China (n = 3) acknowledged and especially incorporated cultural context in their intervention. This included incorporating culturally relevant activities such as a memory ceremony on the Zhongyuan festival (Yu et al., 2022), adapting an existing model to the researchers' cultural context (Tang et al., 2021), and using a technique based on the Chinese cultural concept of "emptiness" (Tao et al., 2022).

Addressing the Needs of Vulnerable Populations

Specific subgroups such as older adults, healthcare workers, and children have been identified as being at-risk by a previous literature review (Stroebe & Schut, 2021). Out of the studies selected in the current review, only one study reporting on a child's therapy (Santos et al., 2021) was found. Yu et al. (2022) included components on how adults could cope with losing their children due to COVID-19. Two studies focused on healthcare workers' needs (Bateman et al., 2020; Mellins et al., 2020).

Critical Review and Future Directions

The pandemic necessitated quick responses to its specific needs. Many interventions aimed to address the unprecedented grief during the pandemic through the immediate deployment of clinical resources. On the other hand, RCT protocols elaborated more detailed interventions to further evidence-based research on grief. Next, we discuss gaps in the literature, methodological limitations of the studies, and limitations in intervention content.

Gaps in the Literature

Although there was a fairly global distribution of studies, the absence of published studies from South-East Asia, South America, Africa, and Australia was notable. While there were some interventions focusing on special populations such as healthcare workers and children, overall, most interventions did not specifically target vulnerable populations, which were disproportionately affected due to the pandemic (Stroebe & Schut, 2021). Family-focused interventions were also missing. This is an important lacuna as bereavement generally affects entire families (Lebow, 2020).

Methodological Limitations of Studies

Most studies that reported delivered interventions did not measure outcomes, and the few studies that did measure outcomes did not have control groups, precluding conclusions about the effectiveness of interventions. All studies did not report detailed information on interventions. In fact, the number of sessions in the interventions, theoretical frameworks of the interventions as well as the components of the interventions were unclear in several studies.

Limitations in Intervention Content

Some missing themes in the content of interventions were addressing anger towards sociopolitical systems, the impact of media, and components on spirituality and faith in grief and bereavement. Although trauma was mentioned in some studies, no study elaborated on how trauma-informed approaches were incorporated in their intervention. No intervention incorporated intersectionality or systems lens with qualitative studies giving voice to the lived experience of people being notably missing. Overall, there was a gap between the theoretical and policy recommendations in the research literature (Harrop et al., 2020) and reported interventions. Further, studies did not explore the possibility that those delivering these interventions may have experienced bereavement, thus, their training and supervision needs were not addressed.

Implications for Future Research and Practice

Overall, it was seen that experiences of grief and bereavement during this pandemic were distinctive and necessitated flexible and dynamic psycho-social interventions.

While these interventions had a positive impact on the participants, certain limitations were also present. Hence, we would recommend that future research can focus on (a) describing lived experiences; (b) interventions for children, older adults, vulnerable populations, and families; (c) methodological robustness with detailed documentation; (d) incorporating themes such as anger, impact of media, and spirituality and faith; (e) trauma-informed, systemic, and intersectionality-based approaches; and (f) addressing specific training and supervision needs for those delivering interventions. Future reviews could incorporate broader definitions of grief including grief for intangible losses. One limitation of our review was that we restricted ourselves to academic literature; future reviews could also include interventions conducted by non-governmental organisations (NGOs), governments, and commercial and public healthcare sectors. Future research must also take a resilience-focused perspective to examining people's responses to grief and bereavement.

Conclusion

Our aim was to conduct a scoping review of the grief and bereavement interventions reported in the research literature during and after COVID-19. We found 16 studies (real-world, pre-post, and RCT protocol studies) reporting on 15 interventions.

The interventions were preventive or early interventions, targeted towards bereaved family members and healthcare workers, and delivered by diverse healthcare professionals and through self-guided modes, mostly through remote means, with a brief number of sessions, in individual as well as group formats.

Further, interventions used DPM as a primary theoretical approach as well as adapted approaches such as CBT to grief. Core components included screening and assessment for referral, addressing basic needs and sharing information, psychoeducation, facing towards (rather than turning away from) the emotional pain of grief, making memories of the deceased and readapting to life without them, encouraging community and social connection, promoting self-care, and finding meaning.

Although interventions attempted to adapt to the unique context of the pandemic by addressing specific needs, using innovative approaches, acknowledging the cultural context, and addressing the needs of special populations, certain limitations were also present. Interventions lacked well-defined theoretical underpinnings and did not take a trauma-informed, systemic, or intersectionality lens. Future research, including intervention design and evaluation, may take these factors into consideration.

References

Albuquerque, S., & Santos, A. R. (2021). "In the same storm, but not on the same boat": Children grief during the COVID-19 pandemic. *Frontiers in Psychiatry*, *12*(January), 10–13. https://doi.org/10.3389/fpsyt.2021.638866

Bateman, M. E., Hammer, R., Byrne, A., Ravindran, N., Chiurco, J., Lasky, S., . . . Denson, J. L. (2020). Death Cafés for prevention of burnout in intensive care unit employees: Study protocol for a randomized controlled trial (STOPTHEBURN). *Trials*, *21*(1), 1–9. https://doi.org/10.1186/s13063-020-04929-4

Békés, V., & Aafjes-van Doorn, K. (2020). Psychotherapists' attitudes toward online therapy during the COVID-19 pandemic. *Journal of Psychotherapy Integration*, *30*(2), 238–247. https://doi.org/10.3389/fpsyg.2021.705699

Beneria, A., Castell-Panisello, E., Sorribes-Puertas, M., Forner-Puntonet, M., Serrat, L., García-González, S., . . . Ramos-Quiroga, J. A. (2021). End of life intervention program during COVID-19 in Vall d'Hebron University Hospital. *Frontiers in Psychiatry*, 583–592. https://doi.org/10.3389/fpsyt.2021.608973

Borghi, L., Menichetti, J., Vegni, E., & Early Bereavement Psychological Intervention Working Group. (2021). A phone-based early psychological intervention for supporting bereaved families in the time of COVID-19. *Frontiers in Public Health*, *9*, 625–691. https://doi.org/10.3389/fpubh.2021.625691

Debrot, A., Kheyar, M., Efinger, L., Berthoud, L., & Pomini, V. (2022). Supporting people who have lost a close person by bereavement or separation: Protocol of a randomized controlled trial comparing two French-language internet-based interventions. *JMIR Research Protocols*, *11*(6), e39026. https://doi.org/10.2196/39026

Dominguez-Rodriguez, A., Martínez-Luna, S. C., Hernández Jiménez, M. J., De La Rosa-Gómez, A., Arenas-Landgrave, P., Esquivel Santovena, E. E., . . . Vargas, R. O. C. (2021). A self-applied multi-component psychological online intervention based on UX, for the prevention of complicated grief disorder in the Mexican population during the COVID-19 outbreak: Protocol of a randomized clinical trial. *Frontiers in Psychology*, *12*, 644–782. https://doi.org/10.3389/fpsyg.2021.644782

Duan, L., & Zhu, G. (2020). Psychological interventions for people affected by the COVID-19 epidemic. *Lancet Psychiatry*, *7*, 300–302. https://doi.org/10.1016/S2215-0366(20)30073-0

Eisma, M. C., Boelen, P. A., & Lenferink, L. I. M. (2020). Prolonged grief disorder following the Coronavirus (COVID-19) pandemic. *Psychiatry Research*, *288*, 113–31. https://doi.org/10.1016/j.psychres.2020.113031

Gonçalves Júnior, J., Moreira, M. M., & Rolim Neto, M. L. (2020). Silent cries, intensify the pain of the life that is ending: The COVID-19 is robbing families of the chance to say a final goodbye. *Frontiers in Psychiatry*, *11*, 570773. https://doi.org/10.3389/fpsyt.2020.570773

Harrop, E., Mann, M., Semedo, L., Chao, D., Selman, L. E., & Byrne, A. (2020). What elements of a systems' approach to bereavement are most effective in times of mass bereavement? A narrative systematic review with lessons for COVID-19. *Palliative Medicine*, *34*(9), 1165–1181. https://doi.org/10.1177/0269216320946273

Inchausti, F., MacBeth, A., Hasson-Ohayon, I., & Dimaggio, G. (2020). Telepsychotherapy in the age of COVID-19: A commentary. *Journal of Psychotherapy Integration*, *30*(2), 394–405. https://doi.org/10.1037/int0000222

Kaul, R. (2020, December 19). 88% of COVID-19 fatalities, 40% of cases in 45+ age group: Govt data. *Hindustan Times*. Retrieved from www.hindustantimes.com/india-news/88-of-covid-fatalities-40-of-cases-in-45-age-group-govt-data/story-0RvZ2kT1CXM-RonZjl6pGlL.html

Kokou-Kpolou, C., Fernández-Alcántara, M., & Cénat, J. (2020). Prolonged grief related to COVID-19 deaths: Do we have to fear a steep rise in traumatic and disenfranchised griefs? *Psychological Trauma: Theory, Research, Practice, and Policy*, *12*(S1), S94–S95. https://doi.org/10.1037/tra0000798

Laranjeira, C., Moura, D., Salci, M. A., Carreira, L., Covre, E., Jaques, A., Cuman, R. N., Marcon, S., & Querido, A. (2022). A scoping review of interventions for family bereavement care during the COVID-19 pandemic. *Behavioral Sciences*, *12*(5). https://doi.org/10.3390/bs12050155

Lebow, J. L. (2020). Family in the age of COVID-19. *Family Process*, *59*(2), 309–312. https://doi.org/10.1111/famp.12543

Mallet, J., Le Strat, Y., Colle, M., Cardot, H., & Dubertret, C. (2021). Sustaining the unsustainable: Rapid implementation of a support intervention for bereavement during the COVID-19 pandemic. *General Hospital Psychiatry*, *68*, 102–103. https://doi.org/10.1016/j.genhosppsych.2020.11.015

Mellins, C. A., Mayer, L. E., Glasofer, D. R., Devlin, M. J., Albano, A. M., Nash, S. S., . . . Baptista-Neto, L. (2020). Supporting the well-being of health care providers during the COVID-19 pandemic: The CopeColumbia response. *General Hospital Psychiatry*, *67*, 62–69. https://doi.org/10.1016/j.genhosppsych.2020.08.013

Menichetti, J., Borghi, L., Cao di San Marco, E., Fossati, I., & Vegni, E. (2021). Phone follow up to families of COVID-19 patients who died at the hospital: Families' grief reactions and clinical psychologists' roles. *International Journal of Psychology*, *56*(4), 498–511. https://doi.org/0.1002/ijop.12742

Moreno, C., Wykes, T., Galderisi, S., Nordentoft, M., Crossley, N., Jones, N., Cannon, M., Correll, C. U., Byrne, L., Carr, S., Chen, E. Y. H., Gorwood, P., Johnson, S., Kärkkäinen, H., Krystal, J. H., Lee, J., Lieberman, J., López-Jaramillo, C., Männikkö, M., . . . Arango, C. (2020). How mental health care should change as a consequence of the COVID-19 pandemic. *The Lancet Psychiatry*, *7*(9), 813–824. https://doi.org/10.1016/S2215-0366(20)30307-2

Munn, Z., Peters, M. D. J., Stern, C., Tufanaru, C., McArthur, A., & Aromataris, E. (2018). Systematic review or scoping review? Guidance for authors when choosing between a systematic or scoping review approach. *BMC Medical Research Methodology*, *18*(1), 1–7. https://doi.org/10.1186/s12874-018-0611-x

Prigerson, H. G., Maciejewski, P. K., Reynolds III, C. F., Bierhals, A. J., Newsom, J. T., Fasiczka, A., . . . & Miller, M. (1995). Inventory of complicated grief: A scale to measure maladaptive symptoms of loss. *Psychiatry Research*, *59*(1–2), 65–79. https://doi.org/10.1016/0165-1781(95)02757-2

Ramadas, S., & Vijayakumar, S. (2021). Disenfranchised grief and COVID-19: How do we make it less painful? *Indian Journal of Medical Ethics*, *VI*(2), 1–4. https://doi.org/10.20529/IJME.2020.123

Ray, D., & Subramanian, S. (2020). India's lockdown: An interim report. *NBER Working Paper Series* (No. 27282). https://doi.org/10.3386/w27282

Reblin, M., Wong, A., Arnoldy, F., Pratt, S., Dewoolkar, A., Gramling, R., & Rizzo, D. M. (2022). The StoryListening project: Feasibility and acceptability of a remotely delivered intervention to alleviate grief during the COVID-19 pandemic. *Journal of Palliative Medicine*. https://doi.org/10.1089/jpm.2022.0261

Reitsma, L., Boelen, P. A., de Keijser, J., & Lenferink, L. I. M. (2021). Online treatment of persistent complex bereavement disorder, posttraumatic stress disorder, and depression symptoms in people who lost loved ones during the COVID-19 pandemic: Study protocol for a randomized controlled trial and a controlled trial. *European Journal of Psychotraumatology*, *12*(1), 1987687. https://doi.org/10.1080/20008198.2021.1987687

Rosen, C. S., Glassman, L. H., & Morland, L. A. (2020). Telepsychotherapy during a pandemic: A traumatic stress perspective. *Journal of Psychotherapy Integration, 30*(2), 174–187. https://doi.org/10.1037/int0000221

Rushton, C. H., Doerries, B., Greene, J., & Geller, G. (2020). Dramatic interventions in the tragedy of the COVID-19 pandemic. *The Lancet, 396*(10247), 305–306. https://doi.org/10.1016/S0140-6736(20)31641-X

Santos, S., Sá, T., Aguiar, I., Cardoso, I., Correia, Z., & Correia, T. (2021). Case report: Parental loss and childhood grief during COVID-19 pandemic. *Frontiers in Psychiatry, 12*, 626–631. https://doi.org/10.3389%2Ffpsyt.2021.626940

Schut, M. (1999). The dual process model of coping with bereavement: Rationale and description. *Death Studies, 23*(3), 197–224. https://doi.org/10.1080/074811899201046

Shear, K., Frank, E., Houck, P. R., & Reynolds, C. F. (2005). Treatment of complicated grief: A randomized controlled trial. *JAMA, 293*(21), 2601–2608. https://doi.org/10.1001/jama.293.21.2601

Solomon, R. M., & Hensley, B. J. (2020). EMDR therapy treatment of grief and mourning in times of COVID-19 (coronavirus). *Journal of EMDR Practice and Research, 14*(3), 163–176. https://psycnet.apa.org/doi/10.1891/EMDR-D-20-00031

Spurio, M. G. (2021). Mourning from COVID-19 and post traumatic stress disorder: New therapeutic tools in the treatment of pathological bereavement. *Psychiatria Danubina, 33*, 102–107.

Stroebe, M., & Schut, H. (2021). Bereavement in times of COVID-19: A review and theoretical framework. *Omega, 82*(3), 500–522. https://doi.org/10.1177/0030222820966928

Tang, R., Xie, T., Jiao, K., Xu, X., Zou, X., Qian, W., & Wang, J. (2021). Grief reactions and grief counseling among bereaved Chinese individuals during COVID-19 pandemic: Study protocol for a randomized controlled trial combined with a longitudinal study. *International Journal of Environmental Research and Public Health, 18*(17), 9061. https://doi.org/10.3390/ijerph18179061

Tao, Y., Chen, Y., Zhou, W., Lai, L., & Liu, T. (2022). The effectiveness of the moving to emptiness technique on clients who need help during the COVID-19 pandemic: A real-world study. *Frontiers in Public Health, 10*–18. https://doi.org/10.3389/fpubh.2022.890960

US Food and Drug Administration (FDA). (2018). *Framework for FDA's Real World evidence program.* Retrieved from www.fda.gov/downloads/ScienceResearch/SpecialTopics/RealWorldEvidence/UCM 627769.pdf

World Health Organization. (2022, December 22). *WHO coronavirus disease (COVID-19) dashboard.* Retrieved from https://covid19.who.int

Yu, Z., Liang, J., Guo, L., Jiang, L., Wang, J. Y., Ke, S., . . . Liu, X. (2022). Psychosocial intervention on the dual-process model for a group of COVID-19 bereaved individuals in Wuhan: A pilot study. *Omega.* https://doi.org/10.1177%2F00302228221083067

7

EXPLORING POSITIVE ADAPTATION TO COVID-19

The Indian Context

Shikha Soni and Amrita Deb

The past few years have witnessed the world getting severely impacted by the Corona Virus Disease of 2019 (COVID-19). COVID-19 belongs to a family of coronavirus which also includes the Severe Acute Respiratory Syndrome (SARS)-CoV and the Middle East Respiratory Syndrome (MERS)-CoV (Nikolich-Zugich et al., 2020). On March 11, 2020, the World Health Organization (WHO) declared COVID-19 outbreak a pandemic (WHO, 2020), a situation in which a new and highly pathogenic viral subtype, one to which no one in the human population has immunological resistance, rapidly starts increasing (WHO, 2011). As COVID-19 emerged with an unmatched severity, human lives were threatened, and survival became challenging. Many countries have adopted multiple steps to decrease the virus' transmission and save lives, such as imposing lockdown and social distancing (Anderson et al., 2020; McCloskey & Heymann, 2020). These steps, though necessary, impacted the general population psychologically by increasing stress and anxiety among them, as evidenced by Bao et al. (2020). Dong et al. (2020) confirm a mental health crisis, especially in countries with high COVID-19 caseloads. Therefore, in addressing this major concern, it is imperative to explore the various psychological factors that assist people in overcoming adversities caused by COVID-19.

Positive Psychology: Shift From Deficits to Strengths

Seligman and Csikszentmihalyi (2000) presented positive psychology as a new orientation to social sciences which, along with repairing damages and understanding negative human behaviour, also concentrated on developing positive qualities and upholding what is right in individuals. Positive psychology aims to treat mental health issues by making individuals aware of and acknowledging their strengths.

DOI: 10.4324/9781003357209-9

As opposed to a deficit-based approach which is determined to fix what is broken (Seligman & Csikszentmihalyi, 2000), positive psychology shifted the perspective towards building on the positive characteristics of an individual, such as optimism, gratitude, happiness, and the like.

Positive Adaptation After Adversity

As such events often leave individuals with overwhelming emotions and long-term scars, strong resources are required to recover from them. Various resources, such as positive emotions, self-esteem, and self-efficacy that are either inherent or built over time, aid in successful adaptation (Seligman, 2004). With the growing zeal to study post-traumatic growth and well-being, researchers started emphasising facilitating personal growth and positive change (Tedeschi & Calhoun, 2004). In this context, Zoellner and Maercker (2006) elaborate that the adversity of various forms can foster the development of different adaptation processes and abilities. For example Bonanno (2004) observes that being aware of one's actions, having a purpose, and having a strong belief system contribute towards resilience during stressful situations. Hence, adaptation strategies are expected to vary from case to case.

Impact of Adversities: Sensitisation Versus Strengthening

Adversities are generally believed to render an individual vulnerable. But there are reports of people implementing skills gained from previous adversities to cope better with future challenges. Updegraff and Taylor (2000) summarise that previous exposure to trauma can either reduce or enhance adaptation to any future stress. Additionally, Rutter's (2012) concept of steeling effect supports that an exposure to adversity may either increase vulnerabilities through a sensitisation effect or decrease vulnerabilities through the steeling effect.

The steeling effect was documented in studies where individuals with a history of some lifetime adversity reported better mental and physical health, fewer post-traumatic stress symptoms, well-being, and higher life satisfaction over time (Seery et al., 2010a, 2010b). For example Elder's (1974) classic study on children of the Great Depression found that those exposed to the stress of socio-economic hardships in early life tended to exhibit better emotional and psychological functioning as adults. These studies confirm that individuals with prior exposure to adversity can experience increased resistance to later adversities through steeling or strengthening effect.,

However, studies also show that past adversities can contribute towards increased vulnerabilities to subsequent stressors. Pre-existing mental or physical health conditions such as adults with childhood difficulties (McLaughlin et al., 2010), homelessness (Tsai & Wilson, 2020), and mental illness (Yao et al., 2020) may act as risk factors for future adversities. Therefore, exploring the possibility of vulnerability and strengthening effects in the aftermath of challenges such as the ongoing pandemic is important.

Aftermath of COVID-19: Challenges and Vulnerabilities

The pandemic may be considered a situation of collective adversity and loss. Apart from physical suffering caused due to COVID symptoms, psychological consequences of the pandemic during the subsequent lockdown were observed. Some of these are detailed in the subsequent sections.

Increase in Negative Emotions

A review by Dubey et al. (2020) reports a negative impact on overall psychological functioning and mental health. Studies from the United States, China, and Europe showed that the COVID-19 pandemic increased negative emotions and decreased positive emotions (Brooks et al., 2020; Li et al., 2020; Morales-Vives et al., 2020). Findings reported in the aftermath of previous pandemic outbreaks show that the psychological impact of the quarantine process can vary from irritability, fear of contracting the virus, loneliness, frustration, anxiety, and depression to extreme consequences such as suicide (Brooks et al., 2020; Jeong et al., 2016).

Earlier, Bonanno et al.'s (2007) investigation of the aftermath of a disaster has shown that fear can arise from the presence of others, contact with contaminated surfaces, and withdrawal from everyday activities, leading to decreased opportunities for essential contact with others. These responses are concerning – fear-driven behaviours such as panic buying can accelerate the spread of disease and ignite fear and pain, among others, as observed by Shultz et al. (2016) during the Ebola virus disease outbreak. Based on COVID-19 studies and other disease outbreaks, it can be concluded that such outbreaks negatively affect emotions.

Social Isolation

Social isolation or quarantine to contain the virus was one of the immediate reactions to COVID-19. While it helps to control the spread of the disease, social isolation was observed to have adverse psychological effects (Day et al., 2006) such as escalating the risk of confusion and anger because of increased aloofness due to lockdown (Brooks et al., 2020). Additionally, forced proximity with immediate family members creates the risk of aggression (Greenaway et al., 2015). Previous SARS epidemic studies have demonstrated that a lack of social interaction and quarantine over a long period affect mental health leading to anxiety, depression, fatigue, irritability, and drug dependency (Brooks et al., 2020). These findings are confirmed by a comprehensive review of 24 studies conducted by Brooks et al. (2020), where individuals quarantined for durations ranging from several days to several weeks showed negative psychological effects.

Adaptation to the COVID-19 Pandemic

Recent studies on the COVID-19 impact indicate that tough times build opportunities to resolve difficulties. For example, Plomecka et al. (2020) and Petersen et al. (2021) report that individuals engaged in active social interaction and daily exercise at home displayed fewer psychological symptoms. By focusing on strengths and using adaptive strategies, people can overcome these challenging times and emerge stronger than before (Polizzi et al., 2020; Petersen et al., 2021). It is important to note that Petersen et al. (2021) are among the few researchers using a qualitative approach to study post-pandemic adaptation. In this study, they focused exclusively on physical activity and sedentary behaviour. Furthermore, adaptive strategies have been exhibited by individuals in the aftermath of the 9/11 terrorist attack, as depicted by Bonanno et al. (2006) and Eakman et al. (2016), and other mass traumas such as earthquakes and floods, as affirmed by Polizzi et al. (2020), respectively. Another study conducted in Spain with adults (18~80 years) found that through COVID-19, resilient individuals displayed higher subjective happiness and satisfaction (Morales-Vives et al., 2020). The authors also reported that participants adapted and maintained a better positive attitude and behaviour.

Studies on the Indian population include Dsouza et al.'s (2020) investigation on increased incidences of suicide due to the fear of COVID-19 infection and Singhai et al.'s (2020) study on adaptive difficulties in people with diabetes mellitus during the pandemic. While these findings are crucial to understanding the negative impact of the pandemic, the deficit-based approach only gives us a partial picture of the overall situation. Using a strength-based approach to explore adaptation to adversity is thus important. This chapter studies the process of positive adaptation to COVID-19 by exploring individuals' subjective experiences towards adaptation. As discussed earlier, individuals often navigate through adversities rather than succumb to stress. Accordingly, the broad research question for this research was framed as: what are the subjective experiences of adaptation to COVID-19 among adults with a past history of adversity?

Methodology

Sample Description

This study (N = 10) is part of an ongoing study (N = 27) on positive adaptation after transitional experiences. The qualitative data for the larger study was collected by contacting organisations such as support and storytelling groups. Organisers of events and groups that promote discussions on topics such as life experiences, mental health, and well-being were contacted with the anticipation of finding participants who would be interested in this work. Out of 27 participants, some were approached again if they were interested in sharing their experience of COVID-19. The respondents who were keen and willing to share their adaptation experiences

TABLE 7.1 Demographic data and past adversity as reported by participants

S. No	Age	Gender	Relationship Status	Occupation	Significant Adversity in the Past
1	29	M	Married	Business	Lost one leg in an accident
2	33	F	Widowed	Information technology	Lower-body paralysis in an accident
3	22	M	Single	Freelancing	Diagnosed with bipolar disorder
4	28	M	Single	Information technology	Absence of father since childhood, loss of mother in adulthood due to cancer
5	26	M	Single	Business	Loss of romantic relationship and loss of father
6	26	F	Single	Student	Right-side paralysis due to cerebral stroke
7	23	M	Single	Information technology	Multiple failures in academics and relationship issues with parents
8	28	F	Married	Information technology	Sexual abuse multiple times in childhood
9	27	F	Married	Student	Brother in a coma after an accident leading to several changes in life
10	42	M	Single	Medicine	Sexual abuse in childhood at the age of 11

during COVID-19 were selected. Approval from the Institutional Ethics Committee and consent from all participants were obtained after providing information about the objective of the study. Anonymity and confidentiality were maintained throughout the process.

Table 7.1 represents the participants' details. The final sample comprised ten participants, five males and five females, with a mean age of 27 years.

Sampling

Participants were selected using purposive sampling, which, according to Patton (1990), helps provide richly textured information relevant to the phenomenon under investigation. This approach was suitable for this study as the objective was to uncover unique adaptation experiences among those who have experienced repeated adversities.

Data Collection

Participants from the larger investigation were randomly contacted, and those interested in sharing their adaptation experiences to the COVID situation were called to participate in this study. All interviews were conducted during the lockdown period; hence, all interactions were conducted virtually.

Semi-structured interviews were conducted to obtain data about adaptation to changes brought about by the pandemic. The interview guide covered general views about the situation of COVID-19 and its related outcomes, such as lockdown and social distancing, changes experienced in the present scenario and their consequences, and strategies to overcome these challenges. The interviews were largely participant-driven, with probing questions whenever required. The interviews were planned, executed, and analysed keeping in mind Legard et al.'s (2003) proposition that exploring datasets not as a whole but as individual reports aids in understanding participants' perspectives. This approach suited the objective of the study focusing on subjective experiences.

The interviews lasting between 25 and 45 minutes were audio-taped and transcribed. Data saturation was achieved after ten interviews, revealing in-depth information. At this point, no new information was being reported as per Laimputtong's (2013) criteria of data saturation. This may be understood in the light of Morse's (2000) observation that fewer participants are required when the information collected from each person is insightful.

Data Analysis

Interview transcripts were analysed using Braun and Clarke's (2006) guidelines on thematic analysis. This method minimally organises and describes the data set in rich detail and aids in identifying, analysing, and reporting patterns or themes within the data (Braun & Clarke, 2006). The authors add that this technique is useful for generating themes that may show patterned responses or meaning within the data set. Moreover, it is a flexible approach that may help describe, summarise, and interpret the participants' experiences (Braun et al., 2019). The analysis was primarily data-driven, so inductive thematic analysis was used wherein the themes were strongly linked to the data. The present research is exploratory in nature, and the qualitative query into participants' subjective experiences led to the accumulation of rich information. Hence, this technique was suitable for analysing such data considering this work's objective.

Results and Discussion

Several themes and subthemes were identified from the process of thematic analysis. The four major themes that emerged were *negative emotions, lifestyle change, support of significant others, and increased self-awareness*. A discussion of the major themes is presented in the next subsections.

Negative Emotions

Negative emotions were the most commonly reported theme in the data. All participants reported fear and anxiety prevalent at that time and future circumstances. Participant 3 compares the pre-COVID situation with the present "I used to love to go out on drives, and I really like the late-night moon. But now when I go outside, I feel fearful . . . and I don't enjoy it anymore". This displays anxiety about *leaving the safety of one's home*. Participant 2 also confirms this fear of moving outside freely due to the worry of getting infected, while Participant 10 recounts experiencing breakdowns every 15 minutes or so due to stress. Additionally, participants reported feeling anxious about vulnerable family members, such as the elderly. Clark et al.'s (2020) study on global, regional, and national estimates reports that older individuals with no conditions or comorbid conditions, such as chronic kidney disease, cardiovascular disease, chronic respiratory disease, and diabetes, are at high risk of contracting COVID-19. In view of this, Participant 7 hopes that "my mom and dad should not get the virus, they are old. So, my brother goes out to buy stuff for them . . . and follows all precautions".

Additionally, the uncertainty created by the pandemic led to worry about the future. Participant 9 compares the present with the anticipated future, "I am worried about the future after corona, now we are used to working from home . . . less pollution . . . more (visibility of) stars in the sky . . . I don't know how will I take it . . ." *(life after lockdown)*. Furthermore, Participant 10 outlines several future uncertainties, including the postponement of examinations which is expected to hinder job prospects and career decisions. Wright et al. (2016) suggest that due to such ambiguities, individuals may become intolerant of future uncertainties, which could impact mental health.

Another major reason for experiencing negative emotions was related to employment, particularly the worry of losing one's job. This is reflected in Participant 2's statement, "Even though my organisation is doing well, and nothing of that sort would probably happen, there is always a fear". Similarly, Participant 1 specifies that "layoffs in future and no increment in salary" are the cause of his worry. These accounts are confirmed by Dev and Sengupta's (2020) prediction that the COVID-19 pandemic may lead to significant job losses in India's formal and informal sectors. Furthermore, this agrees with Fernandes' (2020) observation that as the economy gets impacted by COVID-19, millions of people are losing employment globally. Worse still, economic uncertainty followed by mass layoffs and cut-downs may lead to emotional exhaustion and psychological strain, as Newman et al. (2018) and Yousaf et al. (2019) anticipated.

The sense of anxiety is prominently displayed to the extent that Participant 3 claims "no validation is needed" to demonstrate the presence of it. In summary, these findings are in agreement with Bao et al.'s (2020) report that the widespread outbreak of infectious diseases, such as COVID-19, is associated with psychological distress.

Lifestyle Change

Lifestyle changes ranging from mild to radical were reported due to the country's lockdown. This will be discussed under two minor themes reported under this category:

Revaluation of Earlier Lifestyle: Individuals reevaluated their earlier lifestyle and realised the importance of maintaining these measures in future. Considering that the present situation is a health crisis, several changes were reported in this area. For instance, Participant 2 stated, "There is some learning for everyone . . . sanitisation . . . health and cleanliness". Participant 1 reports an increase in precautionary measures to maintain good health in order to avoid other health ailments.

Finance was reported to be another area where a change of perspective was experienced. While Participant 2 mentioned, "We are now saving money from travel and other spending, our expenditures are reduced", Participant 1 shared that "Financial matters are taken more seriously now . . . saving is important . . . and we are controlling our expenses too". Understanding the value of essential goods and avoiding the wastage of food were emphasised by some participants, such as Participant 2, who compared her earlier lifestyle with the COVID-19 situation one and concluded that they were

[S]o much dependent on maids, cooks, online shopping, clothes, and hotels. Now I feel those were a luxury. . . . The difference between luxury and necessity is appreciated now; earlier, we didn't want to put effort. . . . Now we are bringing in those changes. We also realised that wastage of food must be strictly avoided because getting essential items and groceries is a challenge now

Additionally, the decision to use sustainable products leading to minimal wastage was reported by Participant 10. Such reappraisal may eventually lead to better choices. Additionally, the revaluation of the meaning of a stressful situation helps regulate emotions and increases positive emotion (Denny & Ochsner, 2014; Goldin et al., 2014), thereby leading to emotional well-being (Gross & Thompson, 2007).

Using Positive Adaptation Strategies: Even though difficult, adapting to a new way of life has led to several interesting strategies. Individuals reported engaging in different activities at home to cope with the stressors. Participant 4, pursuing virtual courses, revealed that this "online marathon . . . is really good". Some respondents described participating in activities initiated by their organisations, such as those aimed at overcoming stress. For example Participant 2 mentions attending online Yoga classes arranged by her organisation. A recent study reports that during this period, individuals paid more attention to their mental health and spent time resting, relaxing, and exercising (Zhang & Ma, 2020). Evidence shows that web interventions on social media help promote the mental health of large groups of individuals. These studies by Chang et al. (2014) and Ploeg et al. (2017) employed paradigms such as positive psychology, mindfulness, and exercise to address mental health issues.

Time management was also cited as an important adaptive strategy, as observed in Participant 7's comment, "I am managing my time by breaking the day up into . . . intervals". The respondent explains that setting targets every two hours helps him accomplish bigger tasks while keeping up with the activities of the work team. Participant 1, while recognising the importance of time management, admits that he needs to develop better skills to accomplish his tasks. He explains that working from home can be challenging as it involves multitasking between professional demands, such as meeting work deadlines and connecting virtually with colleagues while completing household chores, such as purchasing groceries.

Acceptance, which serves as a protective factor against stressors (Hwei & Abdullah, 2017), was reported by several participants. According to Participant 6, "I have accepted the situation, as there is no other way out". Likewise, Participant 1 says, "I have accepted the challenges now; we . . . manage". This is confirmed by Thompson et al.'s (2011) claim that acceptance is positively associated with psychological adjustment during traumatic events.

Another strategy to counter the situation was reframing negative thoughts, which contributed to positive reappraisal, as reflected in Participant 10's words. She states that before the pandemic, her friends were a strong source of emotional support; however, they were unable to meet like earlier because of the lockdown. Due to this, she blamed her friends for ignoring her. Subsequently, such negative feelings led to the development of a victim mindset. However, she was able to reframe these negative thoughts and eventually accepted the situation. She now acknowledges that this is a commonly experienced feeling and that she is not the only one suffering in the present scenario. She finally realised that one must be kind to others during such adversities. Likewise, Participant 8 reappraised the current situation on the basis of her past experience of adversities and concluded that any situation goes bad before it gets better. This provided her with much-needed reassurance to face the situation. These descriptions of reappraisals are consistent with Veer et al.'s (2020) claim that positive appraisal during the COVID-19 pandemic can lead to greater resilience and psychological well-being. Also, adaptive mindsets help to provide a greater appreciation of life and enhance relationships (English et al., 2012; Tedeschi & Calhoun, 2004), increase positive emotion, reduce negative symptoms, and boost physiological functioning (Crum et al., 2017; Cludius et al., 2020) *when* under stress. This is supported by Hébert et al.'s (2022) recent study, which found that resilient individuals showed the highest probability of a positive adaptation.

Considering several individuals have lost employment, Participant 7 felt lucky to have retained his job despite being hit with a pay cut. The tendency of such individuals to draw parallels with those who lost employment can be explained through downward social comparison. Frieswijk et al. (2004) elaborate that comparing oneself with those who are worse off may help redefine the situation positively, increasing life satisfaction.

Hence, using positive adaptation strategies may help individuals diverge from adversity and engage in positive emotions, thereby facilitating the ability to bounce back from negative experiences.

Support of Significant Others

Along with the adaptation strategies mentioned earlier, participants also shared that positive experiences with significant others helped them to survive the pandemic. Participant 9 expressed that the lockdown has given her time to pursue painting and to spend with her husband. They enjoy cooking together and spending time with their pet. Additionally, significant others, including family, friends, and colleagues, appear to act as supporting factors in this difficult situation. Participant 2 mentions that she is fortunate to have a supportive family and colleagues from whom she learns several things. Additionally, she emphasises the importance of social well-being by stating that "it's important to interact with good people as we get . . . positive vibes" from them. Similarly, Participant 1 is delighted with the opportunity of spending more time with his family, a luxury that he did not have earlier. Thus, it is evident that significant others, such as family and friends, served as an external protective factor facilitating positive adaptation. This agrees with Pandey et al.'s (2022) findings from the Indian population that social support effectively dealt with negative emotions during COVID-19. Furthermore, such interpersonal relationships are reported as crucial criteria for minimising mental health difficulties in specific stressful situations (Sehmi et al., 2019; Sharma & Subramanyam, 2020).

Increased Self-Awareness

Spending long periods in isolation at home, with minimal distractions, helped find more time for oneself in an otherwise busy life. Participant 2 says, "We were all so busy in our day-to-day lives and . . . so much into work, we almost became machine-like. So now it is time for us to take a break . . . take time for ourselves". The positive outcome of focusing on oneself is noted in Participant 9's words,

> I feel a lot at peace with myself; there are no high tides, no stress associated with the office. Even if I am having a bad day and I have a call, I have my space while still making the call and being present at work. Staying at home gives leverage to be present at home. It gives more mental peace.

Spending more time at home also gives access to hobbies and interests, as elaborated by Participant 4, who claims that for several years, he had only been busy with work and had no time to focus on himself. The lockdown period has allowed him to pursue his interests, such as online storytelling classes referred by a friend. This is consistent with Johnston and Scholler-Jaquish's (2007) finding that individuals often find hidden opportunities, new directions, liberation, and deeper meaning following adversity.

Some participants displayed an awareness that optimism can provide hope for recovery. Participant 2, paralysed after an accident and using a wheelchair, expresses that the lockdown has been a transformational experience. This time has allowed her to reflect on the past, wherein she realised that she is not the only one suffering. This motivated her to break the vicious circle of self-pity. Likewise, Participant 3 narrated,

> I have always had a very negative attitude. . . . But now I have realised that bad happens, but there are always good people everywhere and all the time, it's just that we don't see it . . . good in terms of coming forward and helping people.

These observations show that by noticing the positives during this crisis, participants have been able to adapt to it, enhancing their self-awareness. Increased awareness was also found in another study by Singh et al. (2022), wherein participants displayed increased awareness by taking responsibility for their health.

Summary of Themes

Past adversity for participants in this study was perceived to have provided an increased capacity to adapt to the COVID-19 pandemic. Rutter (2012) suggests that past negative experiences may have a steeling effect on the response to later adversity. The powerful remarks of some participants confirm this. For instance, Participant 8 states,

> Because of facing adversity at an early age, you . . . tend to think that this is also . . . adversity and you will get through it. I don't get that feeling of oh! It is too much of a problem.

She also adds that those who have experienced past trauma free themselves from restrictions and demons in their mind and achieve solitude. Participant 8 notes that those who have prior experiences of adversity tend to compare the COVID-19 led adversity to the earlier one and find the strength to overcome them rather than being overwhelmed. While Participant 1 mentions, "I am facing this adversity as any other adversity I have faced in the past", Participant 2 cites, "I have some . . . relatability to the coronavirus situation. It is like . . . bipolar disorder. We cannot cure it, but we can only manage it, so to make myself better, I think like that". Participants repeatedly brought up their experiences with past trauma in recounting how they handled the present crisis. These findings are supported by studies on how steeling effect stemming from lifetime adversity (Seery et al., 2013) and perceived stress (Hagan et al., 2014) impact adaptation to future situations. This may also be explained through the contrast effect (Elder, 1974), which showed that children of the Great Depression who faced hardships in childhood showed greater success and reported greater contentment and happiness later in life.

The aforementioned themes point to the fact that despite expressing a crisis of such great magnitude and the negative emotions stemming from it, individuals were able to display positive adaptation. Additionally, it is important to note that none of the participants or anyone in their close circle was afflicted by COVID-19 during the interview, which may have also contributed to their adaptation.

Limitations of the Study and Future Directions

Although this chapter is limited to ten participants, the qualitative approach has helped gather rich information that can be utilised in future research planning. However, as all participants were highly educated and financially middle class, further research is required to understand the adaptation experiences of those who have low levels of education and poor financial status, such as daily-wage workers and migrant labourers. Furthermore, the study was not focused specifically on sociocultural factors as contributors to adaptation. This aspect was also not intentionally explored as the interviews were largely participant-guided, focusing on participants' experiences of adapting to COVID-19. Future studies can consider emphasising sociocultural factors contributing to adaptation during such adversities.

Further investigations with a larger number of participants and longitudinal designs may help track the adaptation process. Also, researchers may consider employing a strength-based approach and interview methods as they can help to capture subjective experiences of participants' adaptation, which are otherwise challenging to identify through large-scale quantitative surveys. Information from such methods may be useful in developing interventions in the area.

Implications

There is abundant literature on the suffering caused due to COVID-19; comparatively, there is less emphasis on strength-based work. Besides investigations by Mathias et al. (2020) and Sharma and Subramanyam (2020), the present study is one of the few attempts at using a qualitative approach to study adaptation in India in the aftermath of COVID-19. While the former study employed participants from Uttarakhand, the latter was an online mixed method investigation. This methodology has helped highlight several subjective factors that future researchers may consider in developing quantitative measures and suitable interventions for those in similar circumstances. Mental health professionals can implement these findings to help individuals who have faced adversities and are currently adapting to COVID-19. Additionally, the strength-based approach of the interview led participants to think about how they have adapted to this situation rather than focus on their vulnerability and suffering. This provided them with an opportunity for self-reflection. Self-reflection is important in appreciating positive outcomes and in developing awareness about health conditions pertaining to the situation. Awareness of these preventive steps can be developed via self-reflection and deliberation initiated by psychology practitioners. While some organisations have launched mental health support services, these resources are not sufficient for the population of the country. Organisations, practitioners, and policymakers may consider addressing this demand using a preventative approach and cure.

Personal Reflections

This research served as a medium for participants to share their experiences and perspectives, with some reporting that it helped them unburden their feelings. Similarly, while living through the same uncertainties posed by the COVID-19 pandemic, the researchers could also relate to the participants' experiences as they belonged to a similar socio-economic and cultural background. They were able to appreciate the various perspectives shared by participants about COVID-19, which helped them cope with the situation better. It also inculcated a sense of gratitude in them for the resources they were fortunate to have access to during these difficult times.

Conclusion

The COVID-19 pandemic has brought many new challenges in various domains, including that of mental health. Despite several unexpected stressors in the scenario, participants have largely shown positive adaptation. The concept of the steeling effect is well depicted by participants of this study, with several narrations that point directly to how past adversity prepared them for the COVID-19. This, along with the adaptation strategies implemented by the participants, is the major finding of this chapter. These creative strategies developed for survival indicate how human beings can adapt to almost anything. Negative emotions, frequently reported by all participants, were an expected outcome as such reactions are natural in an unprecedented crisis. Nevertheless, it is promising to note that individuals have used available resources and developed useful strategies that led to changes in their perspectives and lifestyles in the process of adaptation to the ongoing crisis.

Acknowledgement

The authors thank all the participants for sharing their experiences and Rishi Kumar for providing valuable inputs.

Declaration of Interest

The authors declare no conflict of interest.

Funding

This work is a part of the first author Shikha Soni doctoral research funded by the Ministry of Education, India.

References

Anderson, R. M., Heesterbeek, H., Klinkenberg, D., & Hollingsworth, T. D. (2020). How will country-based mitigation measures influence the course of the COVID-19 epidemic? *The Lancet, 395*(10228), 931–934. https://doi.org/10.1016/S0140-6736(20)30567-5

Bao, Y., Sun, Y., Meng, S., Shi, J., & Lu, L. (2020). 2019-nCoV epidemic: Address mental health care to empower society. *The Lancet, 395*(10224), e37–e38. https://doi.org/10.1016/S0140-6736(20)30309-3

Bonanno, G. A. (2004). Loss, trauma, and human resilience: Have we underestimated the human capacity to thrive after extremely aversive events?. *American Psychologist, 59*(1), 20–28. https://doi.org/10.1037/0003-066X.59.1.20

Bonanno, G. A., Galea, S., Bucciarelli, A., & Vlahov, D. (2006). Psychological resilience after disaster: New York City in the aftermath of the September 11th terrorist attack. *Psychological Science, 17*(3), 181–186. https://doi.org/10.1111/j.1467-9280.2006.01682.x

Bonanno, G. A., Galea, S., Bucciarelli, A., & Vlahov, D. (2007). What predicts psychological resilience after disaster? The role of demographics, resources, and life stress. *Journal of Consulting and Clinical Psychology, 75*(5), 671–682. https://doi.org/10.1037/0022-006X.75.5.671

Braun, V., & Clarke, V. (2006). Using thematic analysis in psychology. *Qualitative Research in Psychology, 3*(2), 77–101. https://doi.org/10.1191/1478088706qp063oa

Braun, V., Clarke, V., Hayfield, N., & Terry, G. (2019). Thematic analysis. In P. Liamputtong (Ed.), *Handbook of research methods in health social sciences* (pp 843–860). Springer. https://doi.org/10.1007/978-981-10-5251-4_103

Brooks, S. K., Webster, R. K., Smith, L. E., Woodland, L., Wessely, S., Greenberg, N., & Rubin, G. J. (2020). The psychological impact of quarantine and how to reduce it: Rapid review of the evidence. *The Lancet, 395*(10227), 912–920. https://doi.org/10.1016/S0140-6736(20)30460-8

Chang, S.-M., Lin, Y.-H., Lin, C.-W., Chang, H.-K., & Chong, P. P. (2014). Promoting positive psychology using social networking sites: A study of new college entrants on Facebook. *International Journal of Environmental Research and Public Health, 11*(5), 4652–4663. https://doi.org/10.3390/ijerph110504652

Clark, A., Jit, M., Warren-Gash, C., Guthrie, B., Wang, H. H. X., Mercer, S. W., Sanderson, C., McKee, M., Troeger, C., Ong, K. L., Checchi, F., Perel, P., Joseph, S., Gibbs, H. P., Banerjee, A., Eggo, R. M., Nightingale, E. S., O'Reilly, K., Jombart, T., . . . Jarvis, C. I. (2020). Global, regional, and national estimates of the population at increased risk of severe COVID-19 due to underlying health conditions in 2020: A modelling study. *The Lancet Global Health, 8*(8), e1003–e1017. https://doi.org/10.1016/S2214-109X(20)30264-3

Cludius, B., Mennin, D., & Ehring, T. (2020). Emotion regulation as a transdiagnostic process. *Emotion, 20*(1), 37–42. https://doi.org/10.1037/emo0000646

Crum, A. J., Akinola, M., Martin, A., & Fath, S. (2017). The role of stress mindset in shaping cognitive, emotional, and physiological responses to challenging and threatening stress. *Anxiety, Stress, and Coping, 30*(4), 379–395. https://doi.org/10.1080/10615806.2016.1275585

Day, T., Park, A., Madras, N., Gumel, A., & Wu, J. (2006). When is quarantine a useful control strategy for emerging infectious diseases? *American Journal of Epidemiology, 163*(5), 479–485. https://doi.org/10.1093/aje/kwj056

Denny, B. T., & Ochsner, K. N. (2014). Behavioral effects of longitudinal training in cognitive reappraisal. *Emotion, 14*(2), 425–433. https://doi.org/10.1037/a0035276

Dev, S. M., & Sengupta, R. (2020). *COVID-19: Impact on the Indian economy*. [Manuscript in preparation]. Indira Gandhi Institute of Development Research.

Dong, L., Bouey, J., & Bouey, J. (2020). Public mental health crisis during COVID-19 pandemic, China. *Emerging Infectious Diseases, 26*(7) 1616–1618. https://doi.org/10.3201/eid2607.200407

Dsouza, D. D., Quadros, S., Hyderabadwala, Z. J., & Mamun, M. A. (2020). Aggregated COVID-19 suicide incidences in India: Fear of COVID-19 infection is the prominent causative factor. *Psychiatry Research, 290*, 113145. https://doi.org/10.1016/j.psychres.2020.113145

Dubey, S., Biswas, P., Ghosh, R., Chatterjee, S., Dubey, M. J., Chatterjee, S., Lahiri, D., & Lavie, C. J. (2020). Psychosocial impact of COVID-19. *Diabetes & Metabolic Syndrome: Clinical Research & Reviews, 14*(5), 779–788. https://doi.org/10.1016/j.dsx.2020.05.035

Eakman, A. M., Schelly, C., & Henry, K. L. (2016). Protective and vulnerability factors contributing to resilience in post-9/11 veterans with service-related injuries in postsecondary education. *American Journal of Occupational Therapy, 70*(1), 7001260010p1–7001260010p10. https://doi.org/10.5014/ajot.2016.016519

Elder, G. H. (1974). *Children of the great depression: Social change in life experience* (1st ed.). University of Chicago Press.

English, T., John, O. P., Srivastava, S., & Gross, J. J. (2012). Emotion regulation and peer-rated social functioning: A 4-year longitudinal study. *Journal of Research in Personality, 46*(6), 780–784. https://doi.org/10.1016/j.jrp.2012.09.006

Fernandes, N. (2020). *Economic effects of coronavirus outbreak (COVID-19) on the world economy*. Retrieved from https://mediaroom.iese.edu/wp-content/uploads/2020/03/Fernandes-Nuno_20200322-Global-Recession-is-inevitable.pdf

Frieswijk, N., Buunk, B. P., Steverink, N., & Slaets, J. P. J. (2004). The effect of social comparison information on the life satisfaction of frail older persons. *Psychology and Aging, 19*(1), 183–190. https://doi.org/10.1037/0882-7974.19.1.183

Goldin, P. R., Jazaieri, H., & Gross, J. J. (2014). Emotion regulation in social anxiety disorder. In S. G. Hofmann & P. M. DiBartolo (Eds.), *Social anxiety* (3rd ed., pp. 511–529). Academic Press. https://doi.org/10.1016/B978-0-12-394427-6.00017-0

Greenaway, K. H., Jetten, J., Ellemers, N., & van Bunderen, L. (2015). The dark side of inclusion: Undesired acceptance increases aggression. *Group Processes & Intergroup Relations, 18*(2), 173–189. https://doi.org/10.1177/1368430214536063

Gross, J. J., & Thompson, R. A. (2007). Emotion regulation: Conceptual foundations. In J. J. Gross (Ed.), *Handbook of emotion regulation* (pp. 3–24). The Guilford Press.

Hagan, M. J., Roubinov, D. S., Marreiro, C. L. P., & Luecken, L. J. (2014). Childhood interparental conflict and HPA axis activity in young adulthood: Examining nonlinear relations. *Developmental Psychobiology, 56*(4), 871–880. https://doi.org/10.1002/dev.21157

Hébert, M., Tremblay-Perreault, A., Jean-Thorn, A., & Demers, H. (2022). Disentangling the diversity of profiles of adaptation in youth during COVID-19. *Journal of Affective Disorders Reports, 7*, 100308. https://doi.org/10.1016/j.jadr.2022.100308

Hwei, L. K., & Abdullah, H. S. L. B. (2017). Acceptance, forgiveness, and gratitude: Predictors of resilience among university students. *Malaysia Online Journal of Psychology & Counselling, 1*(1), 1–23. https://mojc.um.edu.my/article/view/5563

Jeong, H., Yim, H. W., Song, Y. J., Ki, M., Min, J. A., Cho, J., & Chae, J. H. (2016). Mental health status of people isolated due to Middle East Respiratory Syndrome. *Epidemiology and Health, 38*, e2016048. https://doi.org/10.4178/epih.e2016048

Johnston, N., & Scholler-Jaquish, A. (2007). *Meaning in suffering: Caring practices in the health professions*. University of Wisconsin Press. https://doi.org/10.1177%2F0969733008090527

Legard, R., Keegan, J. and Ward, K. (2003) In-depth Interviews. In J. Richie & J. Lewis (Eds.), *Qualitative research practice* (pp. 139–168). Sage.

Li, S., Wang, Y., Xue, J., Zhao, N., & Zhu, T. (2020). The impact of COVID-19 epidemic declaration on psychological consequences: A study on active web users. *International Journal of Environmental Research and Public Health, 17*(6), 2032–2041. https://doi.org/10.3390/ijerph17062032

Liamputtong, P. (2013). *Qualitative research methods* (4th ed.). Oxford University Press.

Mathias, K., Rawat, M., & Philip, S. (2020). "We've got through hard times before": Acute mental distress and coping among disadvantaged groups during COVID-19 lockdown in North India-a qualitative study. *International Journal for Equity in Health, 19*(224). https://doi.org/10.1186/s12939-020-01345-7

McCloskey, B., & Heymann, D. L. (2020). SARS to novel coronavirus – Old lessons and new lessons. *Epidemiology & Infection, 148*, e22. https://doi.org/10.1017/S0950268820000254

McLaughlin, K. A., Kubzansky, L. D., Dunn, E. C., Waldinger, R., Vaillant, G., & Koenen, K. C. (2010). Childhood social environment, emotional reactivity to stress, and mood and anxiety disorders across the life course. *Depression and Anxiety, 27*(12), 1087–1094. https://doi.org/10.1002/da.20762

Morales-Vives, F., Dueñas, J. M., Vigil-Colet, A., & Camarero-Figuerola, M. (2020). Psychological variables related to adaptation to the COVID-19 lockdown in Spain. *Frontiers in Psychology, 11*, 565634. https://doi.org/10.3389/fpsyg.2020.565634

Morse, J. M. (2000). Determining sample size. *Qualitative Health Research, 10*(1), 3–5. https://https://doi.org/10.1177/104973200129118183

Newman, A., Nielsen, I., Smyth, R., & Hirst, G. (2018). Mediating role of psychological capital in the relationship between social support and wellbeing of refugees. *International Migration, 56*(2), 117–132. https://doi.org/10.1111/imig.12415

Nikolich-Zugich, J., Knox, K. S., Rios, C. T., Natt, B., Bhattacharya, D., & Fain, M. J. (2020). SARS-CoV-2 and COVID-19 in older adults: What we may expect regarding pathogenesis, immune responses, and outcomes. *Geroscience, 42*, 505–514. https://doi.org/10.1007/s11357-020-00193-1

Pandey, V., Talan, A., Mahendru, M., & Shahzad, U. (2022). Studying the psychology of coping negative emotions during COVID-19: A quantitative analysis from India. *Environmental Science and Pollution Research, 29*, 11142–11159. https://doi.org/10.1007/s11356-021-16002-x

Patton, M. Q. (1990). *Qualitative evaluation and research methods* (2nd ed.). Sage Publications. https://doi.org/10.1002/nur.4770140111

Petersen, J. A., Naish, C., Ghoneim, D., Cabaj, J. L., Doyle-Baker, P. K., & McCormack, G. R. (2021). Impact of the COVID-19 pandemic on physical activity and sedentary behaviour: A qualitative study in a Canadian city. *International Journal of Environmental Research and Public Health, 18*(9), 4441. https://doi.org/10.3390/ijerph18094441

Ploeg, J., Markle-Reid, M., Valaitis, R., McAiney, C., Duggleby, W., Bartholomew, A., & Sherifali, D. (2017). Web-based interventions to improve mental health, general caregiving outcomes, and general health for informal caregivers of adults with chronic conditions living in the community: Rapid evidence review. *Journal of Medical Internet Research, 19*(7), e263. https://doi.org/10.2196/jmir.7564

Plomecka, M. B., Gobbi, S., Neckels, R., Radziński, P., Skórko, B., Lazerri, S., Almazidou, K., Dedić, A., Bakalović, A., Hrustić, L., Ashraf, Z., Haghi, S. E., Rodríguez-Pino, L., Waller, V., Jabeen, H., Alp, A. B., Behnam, M. A., Shibli, D., Turska, Z. B., . . . Jawaid, A.

(2020). Mental health impact of COVID-19: A global study of risk and resilience factors. *MedRxiv*. https://doi.org/10.1101/2020.05.05.20092023

Polizzi, C., Lynn, S. J., & Perry, A. (2020). Stress and coping in the time of COVID-19: Pathways to resilience and recovery. *Clinical Neuropsychiatry: Journal of Treatment Evaluation*, *17*(2), 59–62. https://doi.org/10.36131/CN20200204

Rutter, M. (2012). Resilience as a dynamic concept. *Development and Psychopathology*, *24*(2), 335–344. https://doi.org/10.1017/S0954579412000028

Seery, M. D., Holman, E. A., & Silver, R. C. (2010a). Whatever does not kill us: Cumulative lifetime adversity, vulnerability, and resilience. *Journal of Personality and Social Psychology*, *99*(6), 1025–1041. https://doi.org/10.1037/a0021344

Seery, M. D., Leo, R. J., Holman, E. A., & Cohen Silver, R. (2010b). Lifetime exposure to adversity predicts functional impairment and healthcare utilization among individuals with chronic back pain. *Pain*, *150*(3), 507–515. https://doi.org/10.1016/j.pain.2010.06.007

Seery, M. D., Leo, R. J., Lupien, S. P., Kondrak, C. L., & Almonte, J. L. (2013). An upside to adversity?: Moderate cumulative lifetime adversity is associated with resilient responses in the face of controlled stressors. *Psychological Science*, *24*(7), 1181–1189. https://doi.org/10.1177/0956797612469210

Sehmi, R., Maughan, B., Matthews, T., & Arseneault, L. (2019). No man is an island: Social resources, stress and mental health at mid-life. *The British Journal of Psychiatry*, 1–7. https://doi.org/10.1192/bjp.2019.25

Seligman, M. E. P. (2004). *Authentic happiness: Using the new positive psychology to realize your potential for lasting fulfillment*. Simon and Schuster.

Seligman, M. E. P., & Csikszentmihalyi, M. (2000). Positive psychology: An introduction. *American Psychologist*, *55*(1), 5–14. https://doi.org/10.1037/0003-066X.55.1.5

Sharma, A. J., & Subramanyam, M. A. (2020). A cross-sectional study of psychological wellbeing of Indian adults during the COVID-19 lockdown: Different strokes for different folks. *PLoS One*, *15*(9), e0238761. https://doi.org/10.1371/journal.pone.0238761

Shultz, J. M., Cooper, J. L., Baingana, F., Oquendo, M. A., Espinel, Z., Althouse, B. M., Marcelin, L. H., Towers, S., Espinola, M., McCoy, C. B., Mazurik, L., Wainberg, M. L., Neria, Y., & Rechkemmer, A. (2016). The role of fear-related behaviors in the 2013–2016 West Africa Ebola virus disease outbreak. *Current Psychiatry Reports*, *18*(11), 104. https://doi.org/10.1007/s11920-016-0741-y

Singh, T., Mittal, S., Sharad, S., Bhanot, D., Das, S., Varma, R., Kaur, H., Merwal, U., Arya, Y. K., Verma, S. K., Jaiswal, A., & Bharti, B. K. (2022). The silver lining behind the dark cloud: Exploring the psycho-social factors impacting successful adaptation during the COVID-19 pandemic. *Journal of Pacific Rim Psychology*, *16*. https://doi.org/10.1177/18344909221102207

Singhai, K., Swami, M. K., Nebhinani, N., Rastogi, A., & Jude, E. (2020). Psychological adaptive difficulties and their management during COVID-19 pandemic in people with diabetes mellitus. *Diabetes & Metabolic Syndrome: Clinical Research & Reviews*, *14*(6), 1603–1605. https://doi.org/10.1016/j.dsx.2020.08.025

Tedeschi, R. G., & Calhoun, L. G. (2004). Posttraumatic growth: Conceptual foundations and empirical evidence. *Psychological Inquiry*, *15*(1), 1–18. https://doi.org/10.1207/s15327965pli1501_01

Thompson, R. W., Arnkoff, D. B., & Glass, C. R. (2011). Conceptualizing mindfulness and acceptance as components of psychological resilience to trauma. *Trauma, Violence, & Abuse*, *12*(4), 220–235. https://doi.org/10.1177/1524838011416375

Tsai, J., & Wilson, M. (2020). COVID-19: A potential public health problem for homeless populations. *The Lancet: Public Health*, *5*(4), e186–e187. https://doi.org/10.1016/S2468-2667(20)30053-0

Updegraff, J. A., & Taylor, S. E. (2000). From vulnerability to growth: Positive and negative effects of stressful life events. In J. H. Harvey & E. D. Miller (Eds.), *Loss and trauma: General and close relationship perspectives* (pp. 3–28). Brunner-Routledge.

Veer, I. M., Riepenhausen, A., Zerban, M., Wackerhagen, C., Engen, H., Puhlmann, L., Kö-ber, G., Bögemann, S., Weermeijer, J. D., Merlijn, Uściłko, A., Mor, N., Barsuola, G., Cardone, P., Deza-Araujo, Y. I., Farkas, K., Feller, C., Hajduk, M., Ilen, L., Kasanova, Z., . . . Kalisch, R. (2020). Mental resilience in the Corona lockdown: First empirical insights from Europe. *PsyArXiv*. https://doi.org/10.31234/osf.io/4z62t

World Health Organization. (2011). The classical definition of a pandemic is not elusive. *Bulletin World Health Organization, 89*(7), 540–541. https://doi.org/10.2471/blt.11.088815

World Health Organization (2020). *Coronavirus disease (COVID-19) outbreak*. Retrieved from www.who.int/emergencies/diseases/novel-coronavirus-2019

Wright, K. D., Lebell, M. A. N. A., & Carleton, R. N. (2016). Intolerance of uncertainty, anxiety sensitivity, health anxiety, and anxiety disorder symptoms in youth. *Journal of Anxiety Disorders, 41*, 35–42. https://doi.org/10.1016/j.janxdis.2016.04.011

Yao, H., Chen, J. H., & Xu, Y. F. (2020). Patients with mental health disorders in the COVID-19 epidemic. *The Lancet Psychiatry, 7*(4), e21.

Yousaf, S., Rasheed, M. I., Hameed, Z., & Luqman, A. (2019). Occupational stress and its outcomes: The role of work-social support in the hospitality industry. *Personnel Review, 49*(3), 755–773. https://doi.org/10.1108/PR-11-2018-0478

Zhang, Y., & Ma, Z. F. (2020). Impact of the COVID-19 pandemic on mental health and quality of life among local residents in Liaoning Province, China: A cross-sectional study. *International Journal of Environmental Research and Public Health, 17*(7), 2381. https://doi.org/10.3390/ijerph17072381

Zoellner, T., & Maercker, A. (2006). Posttraumatic growth in clinical psychology: A critical review and introduction of a two component model. *Clinical Psychology Review, 26*(5), 626–653. https://doi.org/10.1016/j.cpr.2006.01.008

SECTION 3

Insights for the Future

8

THE EFFECT OF DEMOGRAPHIC AND PSYCHOLOGICAL FACTORS ON VACCINE RELUCTANCE IN COVID-19

A Systematic Review

Divya Bhatia, Deepak Pandiaraj and Sadananda Reddy

Introduction

According to World Health Organization (WHO) in December 2019, the novel coronavirus disease (COVID-19) first came to light in Wuhan, China, and was announced as an emergency on 30 January 2020. Within the next few days, many countries had reported confirmed infections of COVID-19. By December 2022, over 640 million COVID-19 contaminations and over 6.6 million fatalities related to COVID-19 were reported worldwide (WHO, 2022). Considering significant global health threats, vaccine research skyrocketed, and several potential vaccines were developed quickly. In December 2020, Pfizer/BioNTech vaccine received the first emergency approval, followed by several others in the next few months (WHO, 2020). Over two years, 13 vaccines received the WHO emergency use listing for COVID-19, and 13 billion vaccine doses had been administered worldwide as of 12 December 2022, resulting in the most extensive vaccination campaign in history (WHO, 2022). Despite these mass vaccination efforts globally, a substantial percentage of the population has shown hesitancy/reluctance towards the vaccine. Vaccine hesitancy has been defined as a delay in acceptance or refusal of vaccines despite the availability of vaccination services by WHO.

The vaccine acceptance rate, defined as the "degree to which individuals accept, question, or refuse vaccination" for COVID-19, varied in various nations (Thomson et al., 2016). For instance an extensive survey on the Arab population, including participants from 23 Arab communities and 122 other nations, suggested the vaccine hesitancy to be 83% and 81% in Arabs in and outside the Arab region, respectively (Qunaibi et al., 2021). Another global survey depicting data from 17 countries showed more than 90% vaccine acceptance in countries like Australia, China, and Norway. In contrast, high vaccine hesitancy was

DOI: 10.4324/9781003357209-11

reported in nations like Japan, the United States, and Iran (Wong et al., 2021). Another multi-country study from South Asia showed that 66%, 65%, 74%, and 72% of respondents agreeing to receive vaccination against COVID-19 were for India, Bangladesh, Nepal, and Pakistan, respectively (Hawlader et al., 2022). The widely cited reasons for this hesitancy were the concern about the possible side effects of vaccines, the perceived destructive impact of COVID-19, belief regarding vaccine potency, mistrust in health policies, and expedited production of vaccines. Several demographic factors also played a significant role, like age, gender, marital status, comorbidities, physical health status, health insurance, education, and socio-economic status. Psychological factors, such as risk perception, played a critical role in defining vaccine acceptance or reluctance against COVID-19. Several studies have reported that the risk perception/disease severity is dependent on an individual's intention to protect themselves by following preventive behaviours such as personal hygiene, direct contact with people, avoiding crowded places, vaccination, quarantine, and travel restrictions (Group, 2006; Weinstein, 1988; Sjo¨berg, 2000; World Health Organization Writing Group et al., 2006). Moreover, anxiety is another critical factor characterised as a perception of risk. Such factors contribute to the understanding of risk, which leads to a state of psychological distress and affects mental health and subsequent decision-making (Sheeran et al., 2014; Harada et al., 2015; Orita et al., 2013; Takeda et al., 2016). Thus, several variables are found to be associated with the cognitive (risk perception, prosociality), emotional (COVID-19 fear), experiential (direct experience of COVID-19, precautionary behaviours adapted, misinformation), and sociocultural (faith in science, government, and medical personnel) aspects of the COVID-19 and are correlated with vaccine reluctance (Santirocchi et al., 2022; Dryhurst et al., 2020).

One of the most efficacious public health interventions for limiting the scope of the pandemic and minimising contamination risk, disease extremity, and death is vaccination. Hence, it is critical to understand people's willingness to receive vaccination and the factors determining vaccine acceptance and hesitancy. Considering the global data on vaccine hesitancy, reviewing the demographic and psychological determinants contributing to vaccine hesitancy during COVID-19 worldwide becomes pertinent. Therefore, the current chapter, following a systematic review approach, is focused on three essential questions: (a) the vaccine acceptance rate for COVID-19 for the general population globally, (b) demographic factors that determine the vaccine reluctance/hesitancy for COVID-19 in the general population, and (c) psychological factors that determine the vaccine reluctance/hesitancy for COVID-19 in the general population. The current chapter paves the way for public health and government officials to design adequate policies and interventions at the societal level to assist vaccine hesitancy for current and future emergencies by disseminating collective information about the role of different factors in promoting vaccine hesitancy.

Materials and Methods

The current review followed the PRISMA guidelines. An electronic database search was conducted on 15 November 2022 in the PubMed and Scopus databases for published articles in peer-reviewed journals. Studies published from December 2020 to October 2022, published in the English language, were included in the review. All studies within this time range that met the norms for inclusion were examined in the review.

The inclusion criteria were: (a) studies that recruited only the general population of age 18 years and above, (b) evaluation for vaccine acceptance/reluctancy/hesitancy, (c) evaluation for demographic or psychological or both factors for vaccine reluctancy/hesitancy, (d) English as the publication language and (e) peer-reviewed published journal articles.

The exclusion criteria were: (a) no evaluation of vaccine acceptance/reluctancy/hesitancy; (b) no evaluation of demographic or psychological factors for vaccine reluctancy/hesitancy; (c) the study included only specific, focused subgroups and not the general population; (d) unpublished articles, conference proceedings, reports, and case studies.

A search was conducted using the following keywords: combination of coronavirus terms (coronavirus OR corona-virus OR COVID OR COVID-19 OR COVID-2019 OR severe acute respiratory syndrome coronavirus OR 2019-nCoV OR SARS-CoV-2 OR 2019nCoV) and vaccine acceptance/reluctancy terms (vaccine acceptance OR vaccine reluctancy OR vaccine hesitancy) and terms related to demographic factors and psychological factors. See Table 8.1 for further details.

One thousand two hundred and one records were identified and imported into Covidence for further screening. After removing duplicates (n = 65), 1,136 articles were screened for titles and abstracts by two independent reviewers (D.P. and S.R.). In case of discrepancies, a third reviewer (D.B.) was contacted. Therefore, 827 articles were found irrelevant to the current review and were rejected, and 309 articles were eligible for full-text screening. Ninety-four articles were screened by D.P., 127 by S.R. and 88 by D.B.; any discrepancies were resolved by meeting among three reviewers. Out of 309 articles assessed for full-text eligibility, 255 were rejected for critical reasons such as failing to meet eligibility criteria, not including nationally represented data, and data collected before the vaccination campaign started in the country. Fifty-four research articles were considered in the review for final analysis. Data were extracted for various items such as sample size, the timeline of data collection, target population, country of the target population, sampling strategy and type of study, vaccine acceptance rate/hesitancy rate/reluctance rate, response recorded as vaccine acceptance, demographic factors linked with vaccine acceptance/reluctance/hesitancy, and psychological factors linked with vaccine acceptance/reluctance/hesitancy (see Figure 8.1 for review and selection of articles). Data items were extracted by three independent reviewers: 18 by D.P., 19 by S.R., and 17 by D.B.

TABLE 8.1 Search strategy used

Search Strategy	Database	Number of Articles
((Covid*[Title/Abstract] OR Corona*[Title/Abstract] OR severe acute respiratory syndrome coronavirus[Title/Abstract] OR 2019-nCoV[Title/Abstract] OR SARS-CoV-2[Title/Abstract] OR 2019nCoV[Title/Abstract]) AND (Vaccin* hesitancy[Title/Abstract] OR Vaccin* reluctance[Title/Abstract] OR Vaccin* acceptance[Title/Abstract] OR intention to vaccin*[Title/Abstract]) AND (demographic factors[Title/Abstract] OR contextual factors[Title/Abstract] OR psychological factors[Title/Abstract]))	PubMed	68
((Covid*[Title/Abstract] OR Corona*[Title/Abstract] OR severe acute respiratory syndrome coronavirus[Title/Abstract] OR 2019-nCoV[Title/Abstract] OR SARS-CoV-2[Title/Abstract] OR 2019nCoV[Title/Abstract]) AND (Vaccin* hesitancy[Title/Abstract] OR Vaccin* reluctance[Title/Abstract] OR Vaccin* acceptance[Title/Abstract] OR intention to vaccin*[Title/Abstract]) AND (age[Title/Abstract] OR gender[Title/Abstract] OR income[Title/Abstract] OR socioeconomic status[Title/Abstract] OR location[Title/Abstract] OR marital status[Title/Abstract] OR rural[Title/Abstract] OR urban[Title/Abstract] OR race[Title/Abstract] OR ethnicity[Title/Abstract] OR fear[Title/Abstract] OR anxiety[Title/Abstract] OR risk-perception[Title/Abstract] OR perception of risk[Title/Abstract] OR personality[Title/Abstract] OR attitude[Title/Abstract] OR trust in preventive measures[Title/Abstract] OR awareness of the preventive guidelines[Title/Abstract] OR awareness of the preventive measures[Title/Abstract] OR stress[Title/Abstract]))	PubMed	1,106
TITLE-ABS-KEY((Covid* OR Corona* OR severe acute respiratory syndrome coronavirus OR 2019-nCoV OR SARS-CoV-2 OR 2019nCoV) AND (Vaccin* hesitancy OR Vaccin* reluctance OR Vaccin* acceptance OR intention to vaccin*) AND (demographic factors OR contextual factors OR psychological factors))	Scopus	27
TITLE-ABS-KEY((Covid* OR Corona* OR severe acute respiratory syndrome coronavirus OR 2019-nCoV OR SARS-CoV-2 OR 2019nCoV) AND (Vaccin* hesitancy OR Vaccin* reluctance OR Vaccin* acceptance OR intention to vaccin*) AND (age OR gender OR income OR socioeconomic status OR location OR marital status OR rural OR urban OR race OR ethnicity OR fear OR anxiety OR risk-perception OR perception of risk OR personality OR attitude OR trust in preventive measures OR awareness of the preventive guidelines OR awareness of the preventive measures OR stress))	Scopus	0

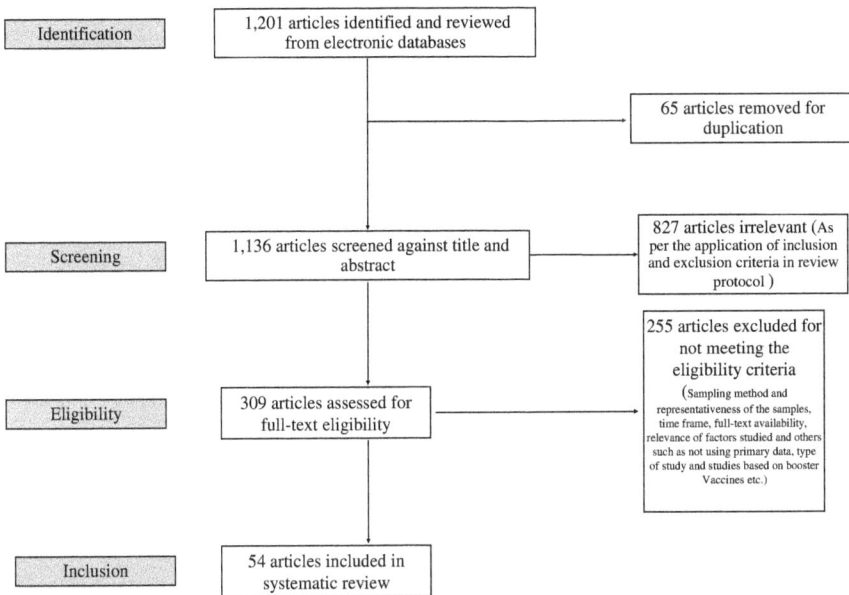

FIGURE 8.1   Review and selection of articles

Three reviewers (D.B., D.P., and S.R.) independently managed the quality assessment of the finally included studies, and discrepancies were resolved by meeting between the reviewers. The Joanna Briggs Institute (JBI) checklist was used to
assess the quality of studies (Porritt et al., 2014). The overall quality of the studies
was "yes" to include in the review. Still, a few items were not applicable in this review, such as identifying confounding factors and strategies to deal with them since
most of the studies were conducted online/web-based, and it would be challenging
to handle confounding factors remotely. Most of the studies used valid and reliable
measures, but a few could have used better-quality tools/interview schedules/semi-
structured questionnaires to assess the COVID-19 vaccine acceptance and hesitancy. To best represent the current level of evidence and quality of research in the
area, studies were not rejected on the basis of quality assessment, and, therefore, all
54 studies were finally considered in the review.

Results

Literature Review Summary

The systematic review includes 54 studies (see Table 8.2). Twenty studies (37.03%)
were published in the year 2021, and 34 studies (62.96%) were recently published
in 2022. Based on the World Bank's country classifications by income for 2021–
2022, each of the 54 studies that were finally included was assigned to one of

TABLE 8.2 Literature review summary

Sr. No.	Authors/Publication Year	Country/Population Studied	Sample Size (N)	Data Collection Timeline	Vaccine Acceptance	Non-vaccine Acceptance	Demographic Factors	Psychological Factors
1	Adzrago et al., 2022	The United States	5,404	13 May 2021 to 9 January 2022	67.34	32.66	9	6
2	Beca-Martinez et al., 2022	Spain	1,001	24 May to 3 June 2021	84.5	15.1	2	8
3	Bagasra et al., 2021	The United States	2080	1 March to 1 April 2021	NA	NA	2	2
4	Ahiakpa et al., 2022	16 African countries	365	December 2020 to March 2021	59	41	1	1
5	King et al., 2021	The United States	5,25,644	6 January to 31 May 2021	NA	16.6	13	2
6	Enders et al., 2022	The United States	2,065	17 July–5 August 2021	72	28	3	6
7	Kumari et al., 2021	India	1,294	13 March 2021, and 25 March 2021	83.6	5.65	2	NA
8	Ahamed et al., 2021	The United Arab Emirates	1003	NA	NA	NA	3	1
9	Morales et al., 2022	The United States	50,359	Between 17 February 2021 and 1 March 2021	79	21	6	NA
10	Paul et al., 2021	Bangladesh	4,175	24 January to 6 February 2021	60.5	39.5	3	1
11	Nguyen et al., 2021	The United States	77,104	6 Jan to 29 March 2021	84.4	7.6	6	1

12	Oyekale, 2022	Nigeria	1,700	Feb 202	85.29	14.71	3	3
13	Burger et al., 2022	South Africa	11,491	2 February and 11 May 2021	74	24	3	2
14	Kadoya et al., 2021	Japan	4,253	Feb-2021	46.62	53.37	6	2
15	Ohlsen et al., 2022	The United States	5,77,110	22 April 2021–29 January 2022	76.9	23.1	1	NA
16	Levin & Bradshaw, 2022	The United States	1,222	27 January to 21 March 2021	NA for overall sample[1]	NA	1	NA
17	Sekizawa et al., 2022	Japan	11,846	23 April till 6 May 2021	59.8	38.4	4	4
18	Touré et al., 2022	Guinea	3,663	23 March 2021 to 25 August 2021	NA[2]	NA	3	5
19	Wafula et al., 2022	Uganda	1,053	Mar-2021	57.8	NA	6	3
20	Burch et al., 2022	The United States	946	Dec-2020	50.00	NA	10	4
21	Piltch-Loeb et al., 2022	The United States	2,013	7 to 22 April 2021	10.5	30.60	14	2
22	Upenieks et al., 2021	The United States	1,247	27 January to 21 March 2021	NA	NA	4	2

(Continued)

TABLE 8.2 (Continued)

Sr. No.	Authors/ Publication Year	Country/ Population Studied	Sample Size (N)	Data Collection Timeline	Vaccine Acceptance	Non-vaccine Acceptance	Demographic Factors	Psychological Factors
23	Wong et al., 2021	17 countries	19,714	4 January and 5 March2021	Australia – 96.4 Bangladesh – 92.2 China – 95.3 India – 95.1 Iran – 72.2 Japan – 65.5 Malaysia – 77.5	Australia – 3.6 Bangladesh – 7.8 China – 4.9 India – 4.9 Iran – 27.9 Japan – 34.6 Malaysia – 10.5	5	3
24	Zarbo et al., 2022	Italy	2,015	3 March to 2 April 2021 and 7 to 20 May 2021	64.6	35.3	9	10
25	Shareef et al., 2022	Iraq	1,221	20 December 2020, through May 2021	56	NA	5	5
26	Frankenthal et al., 2022	Israel	17,99	December 2020 to May 2021	72	16.3	7	6
27	Borga et al., 2022	France, Germany, Italy, Luxembourg, Spain, and Sweden	4,862	Jun-2021	NA	13	14	1
28	Tlale et al., 2022	Botswana	5,300	1 to 28 February 2021	73	31	7	1
29	Adu et al., 2022	Canada	4,515	8 March 2021 and 6 December 2021	56	43	4	1
30	Rogers et al., 2022	The United States	2007	21 December 2020 to 22 January, 2021	97.5	8	14	6

31	Qunaibi et al., 2021	Arab countries and territories	36,220	14 January 2021 to January 29 2021	16.6	83	5	7
32	Szilagyi et al., 2021	The United States	7,832	23 December 2020 to 19 January 2021	57.4	NA	7	6
33	Yahia et al., 2021	Saudi Arabia	531	January and March 2021	62	38	2	1
34	Stead et al., 2021	Great Britain	4,978	January to February 2021	83	NA	6	3
35	Wisniak et al., 2021	Switzerland	4,067	17 March and 1 April 2021	58.5	NA	12	5
36	Dambadarjaa et al., 2021	Mongolia	2,875	16 February 2021 and 25 March 2021	NA	NA	5	6
37	Shah et al., 2022	Singapore	1,009	15 January 2021 to 3 February 2021	NA	NA	6	6
		Australia	1,118	15 January 2021 to 3 February2021	NA	NA		
		Hong Kong	1,006	15 January 2021 to 3 February 2021	NA	NA		
38	Goodwin et al., 2022	Israel, Japan, and Hungary	1,011 (Israel), 997 (Japan), 1,130 (Hungary)	January 2021 (Israel), February 2021 (Japan), April 2021 (Hungary)	Israel (74.1), Japan (51.1), Hungary (31)	NA	2	7
39	Raffetti et al., 2022	Sweden and Italy	2,144 (Sweden), 2,010 (Italy)	13 August 2021 to 23 August 2021	NA	NA	3	1

(Continued)

TABLE 8.2 (Continued)

Sr. No.	Authors/ Publication Year	Country/ Population Studied	Sample Size (N)	Data Collection Timeline	Vaccine Acceptance	Non-vaccine Acceptance	Demographic Factors	Psychological Factors
40	Ebrahimi et al., 2021	Norway	4,571	23 January 2021 to 2 February 2021	NA	10.46	3	6
41	Moore et al., 2021	Brazil	1,73,178	22 January 2021 to 29 January 2021	89.5	10.5	6	7
42	Kollamparambil et al., 2021	South Africa	5,629	February and March 2021	55	45	5	2
43	Okamoto et al., 2022	Japan	5,000	July 2021	33.1[3]	30.4	8	3
44	Ng et al., 2022	Malaysia	804	11 June 2021 to 20 June 2021	82.09	17.92	2	4
45	Hawlader et al., 2022	Bangladesh, India, Pakistan, and Nepal	18,201	17 January 2021 to 2 February 2021	(65) Bangladesh, (65.7) India, (71.5) Pakistan, (74) Nepal	(35) Bangladesh, (34.3) India, (28.5) Pakistan, (26) Nepal	9	9
46	Pérez-Bermejo et al., 2022	Spain	2,462	December 2021	NA	NA	6	NA
47	Seddig et al., 2022	Germany	5,044	9 April 2021 to 28 April 2021	NA	NA	3	5
48	Eshel et al., 2022	Israel	600	February 2022	NA	NA	NA	1
49	Schmidtke et al., 2022	Great Britain	1,201	6 April 2021 to 13 April 2021	NA	79 Low hesitancy, 16 medium, 5 high	2	3

50	Tram et al., 2021	The United States	45,9235	6 January 2021 to 29 March 2021	17.5[4]	18.4	8	6
51	Chen et al., 2022	Hong Kong, Japan, South Korea, Singapore, the United Kingdom, and the United States	6764	5 June to 30 June 2021	NA[5]	No percentage provided[6]	7	4
52	Karabela et al., 2021	Turkey	1,216	1 February 2021 to 28 February 2021	54	46	NA	6
53	Wu et al., 2021	China	29,925	6 August 2021 to 9 August 2021	91.6	8.39	9	2
54	Gerretsen et al., 2021	The United States	7,678	May and July 2020, March 2021	74.9	25.2	7	4

Note: NA for vaccine acceptance and non-vaccine acceptance columns shows that the same was not identified or studied in the corresponding study. NA in the demographic and psychological factors columns shows that the corresponding study either did not identify/report the same factor or wasn't found to be significant at the level of $p < 0.05$.

the three income categories: high-income countries (HICs), upper-middle-income countries (UMICs), or lower-middle-income countries (LMICs) (World Bank, 2022). Thirty-eight studies (70.37%) represented data from HICs such as the United States, Canada, UAE, Japan, Spain, Italy, France, Germany, Luxembourg, Sweden, Iraq, the United Kingdom, Switzerland, Great Britain, Singapore, Israel, Hungary, Norway, Kingdom of Saudi Arabia, Hong Kong, and South Korea. Seven publications (12.96%) contained data from UMICs, including Brazil, South Africa, Botswana, Malaysia, Turkey, and China. Eight studies (14.81%) were representative of the data from the LMICs, such as African countries, India, Bangladesh, Nigeria, Guinea, Uganda, Mongolia, Pakistan, and Nepal. One study (1.85%) reported data from 17 countries, including Australia, Bangladesh, China, India, Iran, Japan, and Malaysia, reporting data from HICs, UMICs, and LMICs. The data collection timeline varied across studies from December 2020 to February 2022, where data collection for most of the studies took place across 2021 when COVID-19 vaccines were licensed for public use in most countries. Thirty-eight studies (70.37%) reported data on the vaccine acceptance rate, whereas 13 (24.07%) did not report data on the vaccine acceptance rate. One study (1.85%) reported data on vaccine hesitancy rate in the subgroup population but not for the overall sample. Two studies (3.70%) reported only the vaccine update data (i.e. individuals in the sample who had already got COVID-19 vaccination). Thirty-five studies (64.81%) reported data on vaccine hesitancy rate, whereas 18 studies (33.33%) did not report hesitancy rate data. One study (1.85%) reported the vaccine hesitancy data in terms of the mean of the vaccine hesitancy scale (on a Likert scale of 1 to 7). Fifty-two studies (96.29%) identified at least one demographic factor, and 49 studies (90.74%) identified at least one psychological factor substantially correlated to COVID-19 vaccine acceptance/rejection.

Vaccine Acceptance and Hesitancy Rates Worldwide

The average rate for acceptance of COVID-19 vaccine for HICs was revealed to be 69.48% (SD = 22.10%), for UMICs 80.89% (SD = 15.36%), and for LMICs 81.13% (SD = 13.58%). The average vaccine hesitancy rate for COVID-19 for HICs was revealed to be 24.36% (SD = 21.51%), for UMICs 19.80% (SD = 15.82%), and for LMICs 16.50% (SD = 11.41%). Within HICs, Arab countries were found to have the lowest vaccine acceptance rate (16.6%) and highest vaccine hesitancy rate (83%). The United States witnessed the highest rate of vaccination acceptance (97.5%), whereas the lowest vaccine hesitancy was reported in Australia (3.6%). Within UMICs, China was reported to have the highest vaccine acceptance rate (95.3%) and the lowest hesitancy rate (4.9%). Turkey was reported to have the lowest vaccine acceptance rate (54%) and highest hesitancy rate (46%). Within LMICs, India was reported to have the highest vaccine acceptance rate (95.1%) and lowest hesitancy rate (4.9%). African nations were found to have the lowest vaccination acceptance rates (59%) and the highest vaccination hesitancy rates (41%). Figure 8.2 shows a graphic representation of the global vaccination acceptance and hesitancy rate.

Vaccine Acceptance

Vaccine Hesitancy

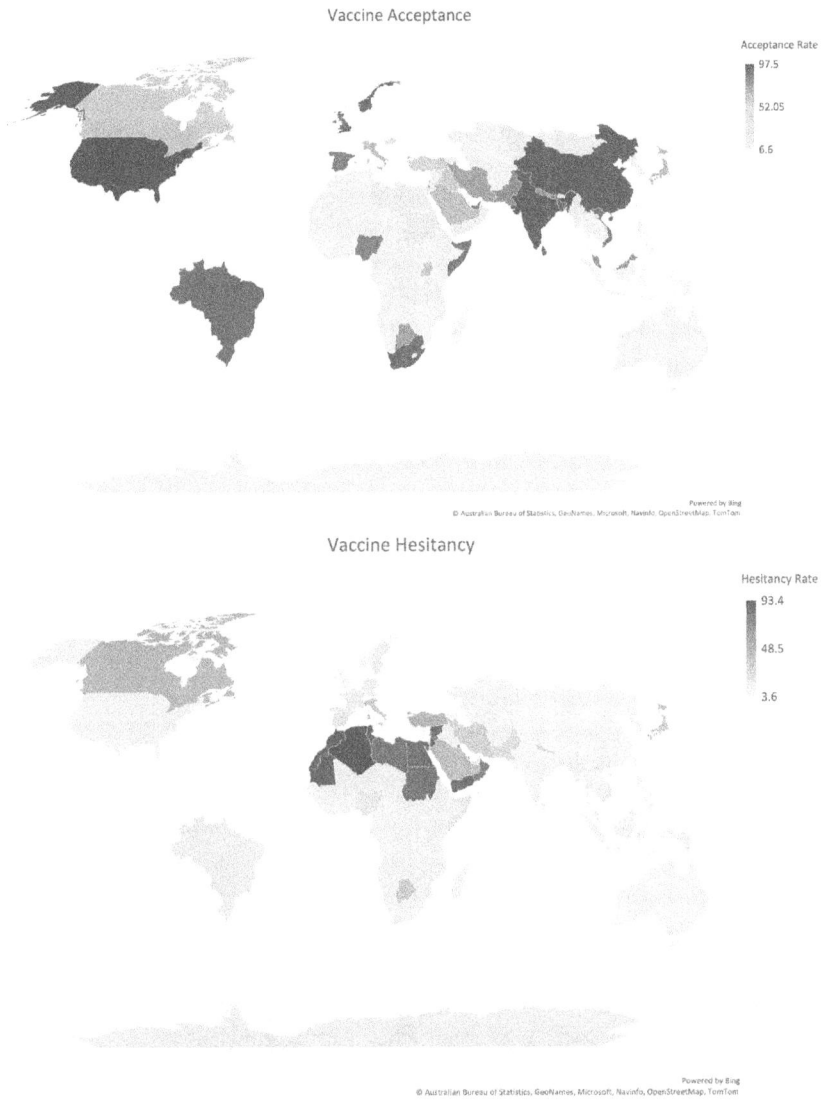

FIGURE 8.2 Vaccine acceptance rate (a) and vaccine hesitancy rate (b) across countries

Factors Linked with Vaccine Acceptance and Hesitancy

Across 54 studies, 125 factors were identified to be considerably linked with the acceptance/hesitancy of the COVID-19 vaccine. Nineteen factors repeatedly appeared in more than 15% of the studies, where 13 were demographic and six were psychological (see Figure 8.3). Gender was a prominent factor across studies; in 12 articles (22.22%), male gender was a substantial decisive factor for vaccine acceptance and hesitancy, whereas female gender was related to vaccine hesitancy

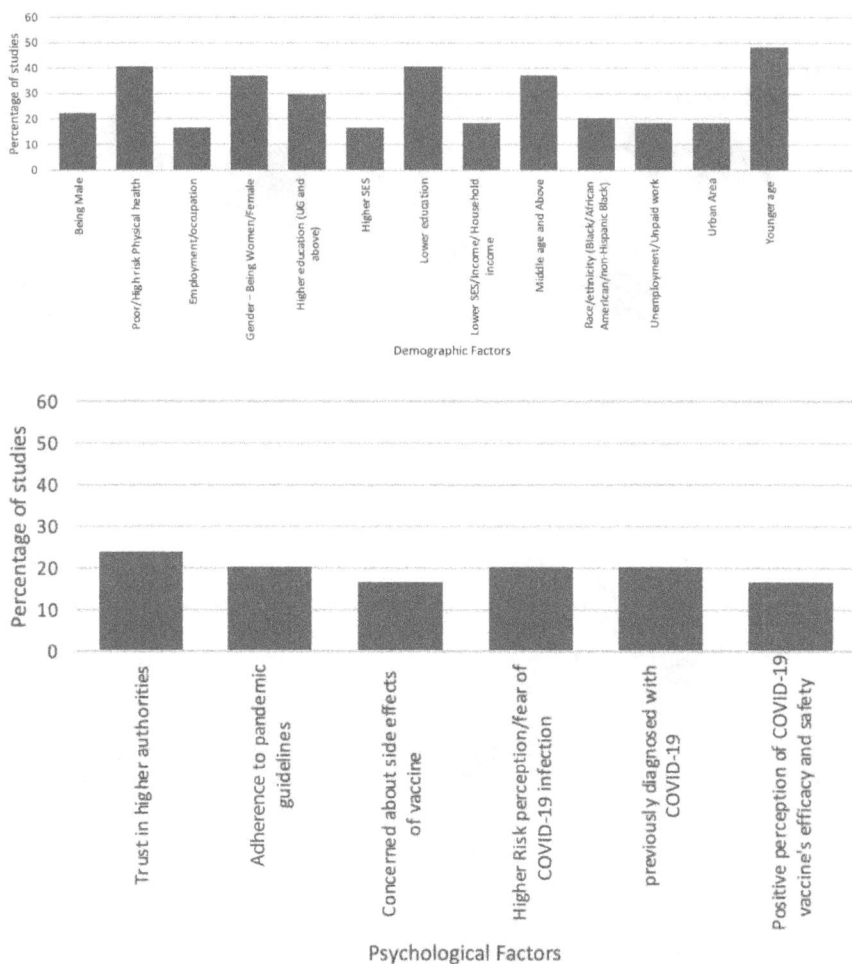

FIGURE 8.3 Important demographic factors (a) and psychological factors (b) associated with vaccine acceptance/hesitancy worldwide

in around 20 studies (37.04%). Education was revealed to be another significant determining factor linked with vaccine acceptance across studies. In 16 studies (29.63%), a higher degree of education (UG and above) was revealed to be a significant factor, whereas a lower level of education was found significant in 22 studies (40.74%). Age was another important demographic factor that substantially influenced vaccine acceptance and hesitancy across studies. Younger age was a significant determining factor in 26 studies (48.15%), whereas 20 studies (37.04%) reported middle age and above as a significant determining factor.

Furthermore, socio-economic status (SES) was found to be a significant determining factor across studies, where ten studies (18.52%) reported lower SES and nine studies (16.67%) reported higher SES to be a determining factor.

Additionally, employment or occupation was a significant determining factor in nine studies (16.67%), whereas unemployment or unpaid work was found in ten studies (18.52%). The urban residential area was significant in ten studies (18.52%) determining vaccine acceptance/hesitancy. Moreover, race/ethnicity, especially Black, African American, and non-Hispanic, was an important factor in 11 studies (20.37%). Poor physical health status or high risk of developing chronic diseases was also an important determining factor in 22 studies (40.74%).

Six psychological factors that repeatedly appeared in many studies were identified. Trust in higher authorities was found to be the highest repeating factor across 54 studies, which appeared to be a significant determining factor in 13 studies (24.07%), followed by adherence to pandemic guidelines, higher risk perception or fear regarding COVID-19, and having acquired COVID-19 previously which appeared in 11 studies (20.37%). In nine studies (16.67%), it was discovered that worries about the COVID-19 vaccine's possible side effects and its efficacy and safety were substantially related to the decision or desire to receive the vaccination.

Additionally, seven demographic and five psychological factors were identified, repeatedly appearing in about five to eight studies (9.26–14.81%). For instance being a smoker and having no health insurance were discovered to be linked to vaccination acceptance and hesitancy in five studies (9.26%). Living in a rural residential area and having a political orientation were discovered to be related to vaccination acceptance and hesitancy in six studies (11.11%). Religion, specifically Jewish and Catholic, was revealed to be significantly linked with vaccine acceptance/hesitancy in seven studies (12.96%). Moreover, having children in a household or big family size and race/ethnicity, such as being an Asian or Hispanic/Latino, were also found to be determining factors in eight studies (14.81%).

Mistrust in government, its agenda, and healthcare policies and faith in local leaders as a resource of COVID-19 knowledge were discovered to be important factors determining vaccine acceptance which were found significant in five studies (9.26%). Lower perceived seriousness of COVID-19 was revealed to be another significant factor determining vaccine acceptance/hesitancy in eight studies (14.81%), followed by the infection/death of a family member or admission to intensive care for COVID-19 as well as belief in myth/misinformation and conspiracy theories related to COVID-19 were also found to be significant factors associated with vaccine acceptance/hesitancy in seven studies (12.96%).

Discussion

Following a systematic review approach, the current chapter investigated the global acceptance and reluctance rates for the COVID-19 vaccination and related psychological and demographic factors. The results highlighted that the highest vaccine hesitancy was found in HICs (24.36%), followed by UMICs (19.80%), and the lowest vaccine hesitancy was found in the LMICs (16.50%). A similar pattern of results was obtained for vaccine acceptance, which was found to be the highest in LMICs (81.13%), followed by UMICs (80.89%), and the lowest acceptance rate was identified in HICs (69.48%).

Similar trends in vaccine acceptance were observed in another recently published yet highly influential study examining COVID-19 vaccine acceptance over 15 study samples in South America, Africa, Asia, the United States, and Russia (UMICs) (Solís Arce et al., 2021). The studies report that LMICs (80.3%) were more inclined to receive the COVID-19 vaccine than the United States (64.6%) and Russia (30.4%). Each LMIC sample's acceptance rate was stated to be greater than the acceptance rate of the United States and Russia. The average acceptance rate for vaccination across 24 LMICs in South America, Asia, and Africa was likewise shown to be much higher (80%) than in seven HICs in Europe (74%) and the United States (65%) in earlier research, which are in accordance with the current results (Mobarak et al., 2022). This disparity in COVID-19 vaccine acceptability corresponds to poorer pre-pandemic childhood vaccination trust in high-income nations (Mobarak et al., 2022; Solís Arce et al., 2021).

Several factors linked with the COVID-19 vaccine acceptance and hesitancy rates across 54 studies were identified, including demographic and psychological. Two of the highly influential factors were found to be the gender and age of the respondents. Female gender was related to vaccine hesitancy in 14 studies (25.93%), whereas it was associated with vaccine acceptance in six studies (11.11%). Male gender was found to be working as a promoter and a barrier to vaccine acceptance, depending on the context. For instance, in the US sample, the female gender was linked with higher hesitancy (King et al., 2021). In a recent study reporting UAE sample, interestingly, more women than men anticipated that the vaccination would lessen their concern about catching the coronavirus, that their doctor would recommend it, and that it would be free, widely available, and without significant side effects (Ahamed et al., 2021). The study found that females were more concerned about vaccination safety than males and required more information on vaccine safety and strong evidence from credible sources before they accept vaccination. These results are consistent with surveys in the UK and France, where being a female was linked with higher vaccine uncertainty and rejection (Paul et al., 2021; Schwarzinger et al., 2021). This could be because many clinical trials for COVID-19 vaccines excepted pregnant and nursing women, resulting in less assuring data for this subset of the population, which might influence vaccine acceptance in women who are in their reproductive age (Hesse, 2020).

Similarly, younger age (<35 years) was found to be a barrier to vaccine acceptance in most studies, that is 42.59%. However, most studies found people of middle age and above working as a promoter (22.22%). For instance Ahamed and colleagues (2021) highlighted that in the UAE sample, people over 35 years of age anticipated that the COVID-19 vaccine must protect them and their families. Thus, they were more inclined to accept the vaccine as they believed it should reduce the fear caused by corona infection and should make them feel safer. Interestingly, several motivational factors were also found to play a role, like social responsibility as a world citizen, national responsibility as a UAE resident, and duty towards maintaining the safety of the family members among participants above 35 years of age.

Level of education, employment, and socio-economic status (SES) were also revealed to be linked with rates of vaccine acceptance and hesitancy in many studies. Higher education (undergraduate and above) was always established to be a significant promoting factor for vaccine acceptance (29.63%). In contrast, a lower level of education was found to be a barrier towards vaccine acceptance in most studies (38.89%). An inverse relationship between vaccine hesitancy and educational attainment is often observed as it enables a more accurate knowledge of the disease's threat and vaccine benefit (Lenherr et al., 2014; Litaker et al., 2021). Lower household income was also a barrier to vaccine acceptance as it is a significant predictor for indecision regarding vaccination (Piltch-Loeb et al., 2022). In fact, participants with lesser education and income often have a higher distrust of vaccines (Shareef et al., 2022). Unemployment or unpaid work was found to be both a promoter and a barrier to vaccine acceptance in different contexts. In contrast, employment was found to be a promoter in about 11% of the studies.

Similarly, higher SES was a promoter of vaccine acceptance (16.67% of the studies), whereas lower SES worked as a barrier in all the studies (18.52%). Along with SES, residential areas influenced the decision to accept vaccination against COVID-19 in many studies. Living in urban areas was a promoter of vaccine acceptance in most of the studies (14.81%), whereas living in rural areas was a more complex factor working as a promoter in half and a barrier in the other half of the studies (5.56%).

Furthermore, race/ethnicity, especially being Black, non-Hispanic, Asian, African American, Hispanic/Latino in most of the studies and Native American in few studies, worked towards being a barrier to vaccine acceptance. For instance, in a longitudinal study of US adults by King and colleagues (2021), Black and Hispanic participants were more worried about safety than White adults. Another set of studies, however, reported higher vaccine hesitancy among Black adults in contrast to White adults in countries like the United States or where the Black population is not in the majority (Karpman et al., 2021; Khairat et al., 2022; Khubchandani et al., 2021; Olagoke et al., 2021; Viswanath et al., 2021). Moreover, poor physical health status, that is people with significant comorbidities, was a promoter of vaccine acceptance in 14 studies (25.93%) and a barrier in eight studies (14.81%).

Other than demographic factors, several psychological factors such as trust in higher authorities, adherence to pandemic guidelines, higher risk perception or apprehension of COVID-19, and positive perception of the efficacy and safety of its vaccine were also established to be significant promoters of vaccine acceptance in the bulk of studies (Shareef et al., 2022; Wafula et al., 2022). Worries concerning the COVID-19 vaccine's potential side effects were found to be a major significant factor associated with vaccine hesitancy across studies (Alqudeimat et al., 2021; King et al., 2021; Robertson et al., 2021). Mistrust in government, its agenda, and healthcare policies and credence in myth/misinformation and conspiracy theories about COVID-19 were also revealed to be significant barriers to vaccine acceptance in most of the studies. Efficient public health communications regarding the development of vaccines and their efficacy and safety could potentially resist the spread of misinformation (Lucia et al., 2021; Troiano & Nardi, 2021). The use of trusted traditional media, that is, TV or newspapers, further raises the probability of improving vaccine acceptance compared to social media sources, and it could be implemented as public-health intervention (Piltch-Loeb et al., 2022).

In conclusion, the current systematic review included 54 peer-reviewed studies and highlighted significant global demographic and psychological factors linked with vaccine acceptance and hesitancy. This study contributes significantly to the emerging scientific literature related to COVID-19 by providing cumulative evidence regarding the important factors that have the potential to alter the fate of any mass vaccination campaign. Therefore, the factors highlighted in the current review require significant attention from health authorities, governments, and policymakers and should be addressed while designing adequate policies and public health interventions in the current and future pandemics.

Limitations and Future Directions

In total, 125 factors appeared to have an important relationship with COVID-19 vaccine acceptance and hesitancy across 54 articles. The current chapter was limited to discussing the most prominent factors that repeatedly appeared in five or more studies. Several other factors, such as symptoms of anxiety and depression and marital status, were also found to be linked with vaccine acceptance and hesitancy in three studies (5.56%). White or Native Americans were also found to be quite hesitant to accept the COVID-19 vaccine, as reported in three studies (5.56%). Similarly, older age was revealed to be a significant promotor of COVID-19 vaccine acceptance, as reported in two studies (3.70%). The vaccine cost was another factor associated with the decision to be vaccinated, as reported by two studies (3.70%). Fear of dying, anticipated regret for not taking the vaccine, social distancing stress as well as the wish to get back to everyday life, and the desire to travel were discovered to be significant promoting factors for vaccine acceptance reported in one study (1.85%). The effects of living and housing conditions and political ideologies were less clear, and these are complex variables interacting with the willingness to be vaccinated against COVID-19 and should be explored in more detail in further studies. Moreover, the current study did not discuss the change in vaccine acceptance rates over time in distinct nations. It might be interesting to explore the longitudinal changes in vaccine acceptance and hesitancy rates in future studies and important factors that govern these changes over time.

Implications

Based on the results of the current systematic review, it has been found that low-middle-income countries (LMICs) have better acceptance rates and less non-acceptance rates than high-income countries (HICs). In light of these findings, it will be appropriate to ask if there is something to learn from the public health policies of these countries. We recommend reviewing the policies of countries such as China and India regarding accessibility, transparency, and handling the uncertainty of vaccine responses. With respect to accessibility, faith in government and public health experts and the execution of related health policies can be improved if vaccines are available within the public reach at an affordable cost or free of cost, including convenient access to citizens in rural places. Furthermore, information dissemination and awareness should target false beliefs in the public. Mediating agents such as public health officials or media representatives can be included in the network of public health communication, limiting social media sources. With respect to transparency, adequate information about clinical trials of vaccines and all possible risks of vaccination should be communicated to the public in the local language in layperson's terms to ensure the development of trust in the vaccines. Providing proper context and authentic sources that can be corroborated by other nodal points, such as community leaders or scientists from government-affiliated organisations, can make public health communication authentic and transparent.

Clearly, the range of factors identified in the current review indicates that vaccine-reluctant population might require different approaches, as vaccine hesitation can be handled by providing proper advice and information. However, the reluctant population might have certain disbeliefs. Moreover, gender was found to be a prominent factor in the current study, as it appears that women are more vulnerable during pregnancy if they are provided with proper advice/information, and they are more likely to accept the vaccine. But in the case of a community of people holding false beliefs about vaccines due to religion or lack of faith in the government, it demands different trust-building public health strategies by engaging religious leaders. Increasing vaccine acceptance among the general population based on evidence from the current review implies identifying sources of negative or unclear information and taking a plural approach to involve or develop credible organisations transparently to counter the effects of false information.

Acknowledgements

The researchers want to thank the book editors for their insightful comments throughout the early stages of the review.

Funding

The authors received no funding for the current systematic review.

Conflicts of Interest

The authors report no conflicts of interest.

Supplementary Materials

Each country's vaccine acceptance and hesitancy rate data can be found in the supplementary data file (see Table 8.3). Demographic and psychological factors linked with vaccine acceptance and hesitancy revealed in the 54 articles in the current systematic review are reported in Table 8.4 in the supplementary data file.

Additional information: The protocol was registered with PROSPERO (registration number: CRD42022369290) (Moher et al., 2009).

TABLE 8.3 Vaccine acceptance and non-acceptance rate data for various countries reported across 54 studies

Country	Vaccine Acceptance Rate (%)	Country	Vaccine Non-acceptance Rate (%)
Canada	56	Canada	43
Great Britain	83	Iran	27.9
Hungary	31	Italy	35.3
Iran	72.2	Japan	34.6
Iraq	56	Malaysia	17.92
Italy	64.6	Norway	4.6
Japan	65.5	Saudi Arabia	38
Malaysia	82.09	Singapore	11.4
Norway	95.3	Spain	15.1
Saudi Arabia	62	The UAE	15.2
Singapore	88.6	The UK	8.4
Spain	84.5	The USA	8
Switzerland	58.5	China	4.9
The UAE	84.2	South Africa	8.5
The UK	91.7	Botswana	31
The USA	97.5	Brazil	10.5
China	95.3	Malaysia	17.92
South Africa	91.5	Turkey	46
Botswana	73	Nigeria	14.71
Israel	74.1	Bangladesh	7.8
Brazil	89.5	India	4.9
Malaysia	82.09	Pakistan	21.4
Turkey	54	Somalia	13.6
Nigeria	85.29	Sri Lanka	7.5
Uganda	57.8	Vietnam	11.6
Bangladesh	92.2	Nepal	26
India	95.1	Australia	3.6
Pakistan	78.6	France	13
Somalia	88.5	Germany	13
Sri Lanka	92.4	Luxembourg	13
Vietnam	88.4	Spain	13
Nepal	74	Sweden	13
Australia	96.4	Algeria	93.4
Algeria	6.6	Bahrain	78.2
Bahrain	21.7	Egypt	82.9
Egypt	17	Jordan	81.5
Jordan	18.5	Kuwait	76.6
Kuwait	23.4	Lebanon	85.2
Lebanon	14.8	Libya	78.6
Libya	21.4	Mauritania	88.5
Mauritania	11.1	Morocco	88.6
Morocco	11.5	Oman	76
Oman	24	Palestine	79.8
Palestine	20.2	Qatar	71.3
Qatar	28.7	Sudan	78.7
Sudan	21.4	Syria	85.1
Syria	14.8	Tunisia	90.6
Tunisia	9.4	Yemen	84.9
Yemen	15.1		

TABLE 8.4 Demographic and psychological factors associated with vaccine acceptance and hesitancy identified in finally included 54 studies

Sr. No.	Authors/ Publication Year	Demographic Factors	Psychological Factors
1	Adzrago et al., 2022	1. Age 2. Gender identity 3. Sexual orientation 4. Race/ethnicity 5. Level of education completed 6. Marital status 7. Annual household income 8. Health insurance status 9. General physical health status	1. Social-distancing stress 2. Depression symptoms 3. Anxiety symptoms 4. Anxiety/depression 5. PTSD-5 qualifying status 6. Perceived likelihood of contracting COVID-19
2	Beca-Martínez et al., 2022	1. Gender 2. Age	1. Being concerned about COVID-19 2. People not wearing a face mask 3. Adherence to preventive behaviours such as using hydroalcoholic gel and other hand disinfectants 4. Using face masks following national recommendations 5. High confidence in scientists to address the challenges of the COVID-19 pandemic 6. High confidence in schools to address the challenges of the COVID-19 pandemic 7. High perceived probability of infection when going to a health centre (risk perception), and 8. Having a low self-efficacy
3	Bagasra et al., 2021	1. Race, 2. Latinx identity	1. Trust in the scientific community 2. Trust in government actions

(*Continued*)

TABLE 8.4 (Continued)

Sr. No.	Authors/ Publication Year	Demographic Factors	Psychological Factors
4	Ahiakpa et al., 2022	1. Occupation	1. Positive perception of the safety and effectiveness of the COVID-19 vaccines
5	King et al., 2021	1. Gender 2. Age 3. Race 4. Education 5. Urban/rural 6. Working outside of the home 7. Living in a state with a Republican governor 8. Living in a county with higher Trump support 9. Living in a county with a lower April COVID-19 death rate 10. History of a positive COVID-19 test versus no history 11. Having a high-risk health condition 12. Less worry about self or immediate family becoming seriously ill from COVID-19 13. Not having versus having received a past-year flu vaccine	1. Lack of worry about COVID-19 2. Never intentionally avoiding contact with others
6	Enders et al., 2022	1. Partisanship 2. Ideology 3. Trump's Approval	1. COVID Misinformation 2. COVID conspiracy beliefs 3. Science literacy 4. Narcissism 5. Conspiracy thinking 6. Trust in scientists

	Author/Year	Demographic factors	Psychological factors
7	Kumari et al., 2021	1. Age 2. Socio-economic status	NA
8	Ahamed et al., 2021	1. Gender 2. Age 3. Marital status	1. Trust in UAE Health Authority
9	Morales et al., 2022	1. Gender 2. Age 3. Type of building 4. Having children 5. Health insurance 6. Race	NA
10	Paul et al., 2021	1. Rural/urban 2. Education 3. Age	1. Belief in effectiveness of COVID-19 vaccine
11	Nguyen et al., 2021	1. Age 2. Race/ethnicity 3. Education status 4. Annual household income 5. Insurance status 6. Housing type	1. Previous COVID-19 diagnosis status
12	Oyekale, 2022	1. Zone 2. Rural/urban 3. Age	1. Perception of the financial threats posed by COVID-19 2. COVID-19 risk perception 3. COVID-19 prevention compliance

(Continued)

TABLE 8.4 (Continued)

Sr. No.	Authors/ Publication Year	Demographic Factors	Psychological Factors
13	Burger et al., 2022	1. Age 2. Housing 3. Religion	1. Trust in social media as a source of COVID-19 information 2. Trust in community leaders as a source of COVID-19 information
14	Kadoya et al., 2021	1. Gender 2. Age 3. University degree 4. Having children 5. Employed 6. Subjective health status	1. Future anxiety 2. Myopic view of the future
15	Ohlsen et al., 2022	1. Race/ethnicity	NA
16	Levin and Bradshaw, 2022	1. Political orientation	NA
17	Sekizawa et al., 2022	1. Age 2. Gender 3. Income 4. Education	1. Generalized trust 2. Moderately severe or severe levels of depression 3. Moderate or severe levels of generalized anxiety 4. Fear of COVID-19
18	Touré et al., 2022	1. Employment/occupation 2. Middle age and above 3. Higher education (UG and above)	1. Vaccine accessibility/ability to get the vaccine 2. Insufficient knowledge about the vaccine/no knowledge/insufficient data on the vaccine 3. Negative attitude towards vaccine 4. Subjective norms, and 5. People with a positive attitude towards vaccine

19	Wafula et al., 2022	1. Being women/female	1. Concern about COVID-19 infection/concerns about
		2. Region (Western, Northern)	the chances of getting COVID-19 in the future
		3. Being male	2. Concerned about the side effects of the vaccine, and
		4. Chronic diseases/physical diseases/underlying	3. Uncomfortable/not be able to breathe
		medical condition	
		5. Higher SES/higher income, and	
		6. Middle age and above	
20	Burch et al., 2022	1. Younger age	1. Higher risk perception/fear of COVID-19 infection
		2. Lower education	2. Previously diagnosed with COVID-19
		3. No health insurance	3. Perceived risk of vaccine 4. Perceived likelihood of
		4. Poor physical health or diagnosed physical health	contracting COVID-19/tested for COVID-19
		conditions (e.g. cancer, diabetes, or heart disease)	
		5. Being women/female	
		6. Chronic diseases/physical disease/underlying	
		medical condition	
		7. Lower SES/income/household income	
		8. Healthcare visits in the previous year, and	
		9. Years since the last healthcare visit	
		10. Prescription medication	

(Continued)

TABLE 8.4 (Continued)

Sr. No.	Authors/ Publication Year	Demographic Factors	Psychological Factors
21	Piltch-Loeb et al., 2022	1. Younger age 2. Race/Ethnicity – Black/African American/non-Hispanic Black/Arab ethnicity/Caucasians/mixed/non-Hispanic Whites, non-Hispanic Black 3. Lower education 4. No health insurance 5. Being women/female 6. Employment/occupation 7. Middle age and above 8. Being male 9. Higher education (UG and above) 10. Urban area 11. Unemployment/unemployed/unpaid work/loss of employment 12. Lower SES/Income/household income 13. Political orientation right and centre-right/living in Republican states/right-wing political ideology 14. Republican or Independent	1. Having a family member affected/died or admitted to intensive care for COVID-19 2. Previously diagnosed with COVID-19
22	Upenieks et al., 2021	1. Race/ethnicity – Black/African American/Non-Hispanic Black/Arab ethnicity/Caucasians/Mixed/Non-Hispanic Whites, non-Hispanic Black, 2. Lower education 3. Religion – Jewish-religiosity (religious affiliation, attendance, religious importance), Catholics or practices/Experiences/conservatism, 4. Higher education	1. Spirituality/trust in god/superiority of natural immunity/divine control beliefs 2. Having a family member affected/died or admitted to intensive care for COVID-19

23	Wong et al., 2021	1. Lower education 2. Being women/female 3. Middle age and above 4. Being male, 5. Higher education (UG and above)	1. Belief/positive perception of the safety and effectiveness of the COVID-19 vaccines 2. Vaccine's efficacy and accepting a COVID-19 vaccine with the duration of protection of no less than 12 months 3. Importance of vaccine's country of origin
24	Zarbo et al., 2022	1. Younger age 2. Lower education 3. Poor physical health or diagnosed physical health conditions (e.g. cancer, diabetes, or heart disease) 4. Employment/occupation, 5. Chronic diseases/physical disease/underlying medical condition, 6. Old age (above 75 years), 7. Higher education (UG and above), 8. Unemployment/unemployed/unpaid work/loss of employment 9. Lower SES/income/household income	1. Higher risk perception/fear of COVID-19 infection, 2. Adherence to preventive behaviours/influenza vaccine, 3. Trust in health authorities or govt. or science/medical/healthcare professionals/doctors/local public health officials (e.g. county health departments/CDC/WHO information), 4. Previously diagnosed with COVID-19, 5. Trust in social media as a source of COVID-19 information/trust of information, 6. Personal health engagement, 7. Negative attitude towards vaccine/scepticism towards vaccines/mistrust in vaccine benefits, 8. Resilience 9. Perceived risk of vaccine, and 10. Having a family member affected/died or admitted to intensive care for COVID-19
25	Shareef et al., 2022	1. Younger age 2. (Having) children/more households or big family size 3. Chronic diseases/physical disease/underlying medical condition 4. Being male, and 5. Urban area	1. Previously diagnosed with COVID-19, 2. Concerned side effects of vaccine, 3. Mistrust on government or distrust in healthcare policies, 4. Lack of efficacy of vaccine, and 5. Having a family member affected/died or admitted to intensive care for COVID-19

(Continued)

TABLE 8.4 (Continued)

Sr. No.	Authors/ Publication Year	Demographic Factors	Psychological Factors
26	Frankenthal et al., 2022	1. Younger age, 2. Race/ethnicity – Black/African American/Non-Hispanic Black/Arab ethnicity/Caucasians/mixed/non-Hispanic White, non-Hispanic Black, 3. Lower education, 4. Religion – Jewish-religiosity (religious affiliation, attendance, religious importance), Catholics or practices/experiences/conservatism. 5. Chronic diseases/physical disease/underlying medical condition, 6. Being male, and 7. Higher education	1. Previously diagnosed with COVID-19, 2. Insufficient knowledge about vaccine/no knowledge/insufficient data on the vaccine, 3. Concerned side effects of vaccine, 4. Lack of efficacy of vaccine, 5. No fear or worry about COVID-19 infection/believe less that COVID-19 is a serious illness/lower perceived seriousness of COVID-19/ever diagnosed with COVID-19, 6. Unemployment/loss of employment

(Continued)

27	Borga et al., 2022	1. Younger age,	1. Adherence to preventive behaviours/influenza vaccine

		1. Younger age,	1. Adherence to preventive behaviours/influenza vaccine
27	Borga et al., 2022	2. Lower education,	
		3. Poor physical health or diagnosed physical health conditions (e.g. cancer, diabetes, or heart disease),	
		4. Occupation – being retired,	
		5. Higher SES/higher income,	
		6. (Being) married,	
		7. (Having) children/more households or big family size,	
		8. Religion – Jewish-Religiosity (religious affiliation, attendance, religious importance), Catholics or practices/experiences/conservatism,	
		9. Middle age and above,	
		10. Chronic diseases/physical disease/underlying medical condition,	
		11. Higher education (UG and above),	
		12. Unemployment/unemployed/unpaid work/loss of employment,	
		13. Home ownership, and	
		14. Political orientation right and centre right/living in Republican states/right wing political ideology	

TABLE 8.4 (Continued)

Sr. No.	Authors/ Publication Year	Demographic Factors	Psychological Factors
28	Tlale et al., 2022	1. Lower education, 2. Poor physical health or diagnosed physical health conditions (e.g. cancer, diabetes, or heart disease), 3. Being women/female, 4. Religion —Jewish-Religiosity (religious affiliation, attendance, religious importance), Catholics or practices/experiences/conservatism, 5. Middle age and above, 6. Unemployment, unemployed/unpaid work/loss of employment, and 7. Non-comorbidities/no chronic diseases	1. Willingness to wear mask
29	Adu et al., 2022	1. (Having) children/more households or big family size, 2. Employment/occupation, 3. Being male, and 4. Material and social deprivation indices	1. More interpersonal contact/relationship/social network/friends

| 30 | Rogers et al., 2022 | 1. Younger age,
2. Race/ethnicity – Asians and Hispanics/Latinos/non-Black African/minority category/Black, Asian and mixed/White,
3. Lower education,
4. Occupation – being retired,
5. Higher SES/higher income,
6. Employment/occupation,
7. Middle age and above,
8. Chronic diseases/physical disease/underlying medical condition,
9. Unemployment//unemployed/unpaid work/loss of employment,
10. Not concerned at all of COVID-10,
11. Vaccines are still questionably safe,
12. Not enough information about COVID vaccine,
13. Do not know the type of vaccine authorized in their countries, and
14. Living conditions/single parent with children/ shared apartment | 1. Trust in health authorities or govt. or science/ medical/healthcare professionals/doctors/ local public health officials (e.g. county health departments/CDC/WHO information),
2. Concerned side effects of vaccine,
3. Beliefs such as "Will be very sick if I get COVID-19/I will feel very ill and uncomfortable/not be able to breathe",
4. Beliefs such as "I do not want to be in the hospital",
5. Afraid of dying,
6. Mistrust on government/mistrust in government's management of COVID-19 |
| 31 | Qunaibi et al., 2021 | 1. Non-comorbidities/no chronic diseases,
2. Living conditions/single parent with children/shared apartment,
3. Chronic diseases/physical disease/underlying medical condition,
4. Lower education,
5. Being women/female | 1. Adherence to preventive behaviours/influenza vaccine,
2. Higher risk perception/fear of COVID-19 infection,
3. Previously diagnosed with COVID-19,
4. Concerned side effects of vaccine,
5. Mistrust on government or distrust in healthcare policies,
6. Unemployment/loss of employment, and
7. Published studies |

(Continued)

TABLE 8.4 (Continued)

Sr. No.	Authors/ Publication Year	Demographic Factors	Psychological Factors
32	Szilagyi et al., 2021	1. Younger age, 2. Race/ethnicity – Black/African American/non-Hispanic Black/Arab ethnicity/Caucasians/mixed/non-Hispanic Whites, non-Hispanic Black, 3. Lower education, 4. Being women/female, 5. Middle age and above, 6. Chronic diseases/physical disease/underlying medical condition, 7. Lower SES/income/household income	1. Personal health engagement, 2. Trust in COVID-19 vaccine's efficacy and safety, development process for COVID-19 vaccines, 3. Concerned side effects of vaccine, 4. Adherence to preventive behaviours/influenza vaccine, 5. Trust in health authorities or government or science/medical/healthcare, professionals/doctors/local public health officials (e.g. county health departments/CDC/WHO information), 6. Trust in scientific or community leaders as a source of COVID-19 information
33	Yahia et al., 2021	1. Younger age, 2. Being male	1. Trust in COVID-19 vaccine's efficacy and safety, development process for COVID-19 vaccines
34	Stead et al., 2021	1. Younger age, 2. Race/ethnicity – Black/African American/non-Hispanic Black/Arab ethnicity/Caucasians/mixed/non-Hispanic White, non-Hispanic Black, 3. Middle age and above, 4. Higher education (UG and above), 5. Urban area, 6. Lower SES/income/household income	1. Previously diagnosed with COVID-19, 2. Trust in scientific or community leaders as a source of COVID-19 information, 3. Vaccine accessibility/ability to get a vaccine

| 35 | Wisniak et al., 2021 | 1. Younger age,
2. Lower education
3. Occupation (being retired),
4. Higher SES,
5. Middle age and above
6. Chronic diseases/physical disease/underlying medical condition,
7. Being male,
8. Higher education
9. Urban area,
10. Unemployment, unemployed/unpaid work/loss of employment,
11. Current/former smokers, and
12. Non-comorbidities/no chronic diseases | 1. (Lower) perceived likelihood of contracting COVID-19/tested for COVID-19,
2. Higher risk perception/fear of COVID-19 infection,
3. Previously diagnosed with COVID-19,
4. Desire to get back to normal, and 5. Desire to travel |
| 36 | Dambadarjaa et al., 2021 | 1. Younger age
2. Lower education,
3. Middle age and above,
4. Higher education (UG and above),
5. Urban area | 1. Belief/positive perception of the safety and effectiveness of the COVID-19 vaccines,
2. Trust in health authorities or government or science/medical/healthcare professionals/doctors/local public health officials (e.g. county health departments/CDC/WHO information),
3. Trust in social media as a source of COVID-19 information/trust of information,
4. Trust in scientific or community leaders as a source of COVID-19 information,
5. Concerned side effects of vaccine, and 6. Unemployment/loss of employment |

(Continued)

TABLE 8.4 (Continued)

Sr. No.	Authors/ Publication Year	Demographic Factors	Psychological Factors
37	Shah et al., 2022	1. Younger age, 2. Race/ethnicity – Black/African American/non-Hispanic Black/Arab ethnicity/Caucasians/mixed/non-Hispanic White, non-Hispanic Black 3. (Having) children/more households or big family size, 4. Current/former smokers, and 5. Current/former smokers, and 6. Elderly members residing in same house aged > 65 years	1. Higher self-efficacy, 2. More knowledge about COVID-19, 3. Perceived barriers (towards individual/government), 4. Perceived susceptibility towards individual risk, 5. Perceived response efficacy towards public health system, and 6. More knowledge about COVID-19
38	Goodwin et al., 2022	1. Being male, 2. Higher education (UG and above)	1. Adherence to preventive behaviours/influenza vaccine, 2. Perceived barriers (towards individual/government), 3. Subjective rated health/lower depression score, 4. Benefits of vaccine, 5. Anticipated regret, 6. Subjective norms, 7. Beliefs in a COVID-19 conspiracy/belief in misinformation/COVID-19 myth
39	Raffetti et al., 2022	1. Higher SES/higher income 2. Higher education (UG and above) 3. Political orientation right and centre right/living in Republican states/right wing political ideology	1. Experience of epidemics

40	Ebrahimi et al., 2021	1. Rural area, 2. (Having) children/more households or big family size, 3. Being male	1. Trust in social media as a source of COVID-19 information/trust of information, 2. Trust in scientific or community leaders as a source of COVID-19 information, 3. Perceived risk of vaccine, 4. Fear of significant others being infected, 5. Length of exposure to strict distancing protocols, 6. Adherence to pandemic mitigation protocol/guidelines
41	Moore et al., 2021	1. Lower household income (it can be added lower income place), 2. Rural area, 3. Middle age and above, 4. Being male 5. Urban area, 6. Lower SES/income/household income	1. Higher risk perception/fear of COVID-19 infection, 2. Previously diagnosed with COVID-19, 3. Concerned side effects of COVID-19 vaccine, 4. Importance of COVID-19 vaccine's country origin, 5. No fear or worry about COVID-19 infection/believe less than COVID-19 is a serious illness/lower perceived seriousness of COVID-19/ever diagnosed with COVID-19 6. Having a family member affected/died or admitted to intensive care for COVID-19, 7. Vaccine efficacy and accepting a COVID-19 vaccine with a duration of protection, of no less than 12 months
42	Kollamparambil et al., 2021	1. Race/ethnicity —Asians and Hispanics/Latinos/non-Black African/minority category/Black, Asian and mixed/White, 2. Lower education, 3. Being women/female, 4. Chronic diseases/physical, disease/underlying medical condition, and 5. Urban area	1. Higher self-efficacy, 2. Perceived susceptibility towards individual risk

(Continued)

TABLE 8.4 (Continued)

Sr. No.	Authors/ Publication Year	Demographic Factors	Psychological Factors
43	Okamoto et al., 2022	1. Younger age, 2. Being women/female, 3. Higher SES/higher income, 4. (Having) children/more households or big family size, 5. Employment/occupation, 6. Middle age and above, 7. Higher education, 8. Elderly members residing in same house aged > 65 years	1. Subjective rated health/lower depression score 2. Fear of significant others being infected, 3. Time preference
44	Ng et al., 2022	1. Religion – Jewish-Religiosity (religious affiliation, attendance, religious importance), Catholics or practices/experiences/conservatism 2. Middle age and above	1. Higher risk perception/fear of COVID-19 infection, 2. More interpersonal contact/relationship/social network/friends, 3. Trust in COVID-19 vaccine's efficacy and safety, development process for COVID-19 vaccines, 4. People with positive attitude towards vaccine

| 45 | Hawlader et al., 2022 | 1. Being women/female,
2. Rural area
3. Higher SES/higher income,
4. Employment/occupation,
5. Middle age and above,
6. Chronic diseases/physical disease/underlying medical condition,
7. Higher education (UG and above),
8. Urban area,
9. Cost of vaccine | 1. Trust in health authorities or govt. or science/medical/healthcare professionals/doctors/local public health officials (e.g. county health departments/CDC/WHO information),
2. Higher risk perception/fear of COVID-19 infection,
3. Concerned side effects of vaccine,
4. Risk of developing severe disease,
5. No fear or worry about COVID-19 infection/believe less that COVID-19 is a serious illness/lower perceived seriousness of COVID-19/ever diagnosed with COVID-19,
6. Trust in COVID-19 vaccine's efficacy and safety, development process for COVID-19 vaccines,
7. Having a family member affected/died or admitted to intensive care for COVID-19,
8. Immune to coronavirus, and 9. Big impact on life |
| 46 | Pérez-Bermejo et al., 2022 | 1. Lower education,
2. Being women/female
3. Middle age and above,
4. Higher education (UG and above),
5. Unemployment/unemployed/unpaid work/loss of employment, and
6. Subjective identification with low/poor class | NA |

(Continued)

TABLE 8.4 (Continued)

Sr. No.	Authors/ Publication Year	Demographic Factors	Psychological Factors
47	Seddig et al., 2022	1. Middle age and above, 2. Being male, 3. Immigrants	1. Higher risk perception/fear of COVID-19 infection, 2. Trust in health authorities or govt. or science/ medical/healthcare professionals/doctors/ local public health officials (e.g. county health departments/CDC/WHO information), 3. Negative attitude towards vaccine/scepticism towards vaccines/mistrust in vaccine benefit, 4. Personal attitudes, 5. Beliefs in a COVID-19 conspiracy/Belief in misinformation/COVID-19 myth
48	Eshel et al., 2022	NA	1. Perceived social standing (partial social integration)
49	Schmidtke et al., 2022	1. Younger age, 2. Race/ethnicity – Asians and Hispanics/Latinos/non-Black African/minority category/Black, Asian and mixed/White	1. Moral foundation of care, authority, 2. Moral foundation of liberty, 3. Plan to wait and see/don't believe I need it/others needs it more
50	Tram et al., 2021	1. Race/ethnicity – Black/African American/non-Hispanic Black/Arab ethnicity/Caucasians/mixed/non-Hispanic Whites, non-Hispanic Black, 2. Race/ethnicity – Asians and Hispanics/Latinos/non-Black African/minority category/Black, Asian, and mixed/White 3. Lower education, 4. Being women/female, 5. Middle age and above, 6. Lower SES/income/ household income, 7. Political orientation right and centre right/living in Republican states/right wing political ideology, and 8. Cost of vaccine	1. Concerned side effects of vaccine, 2. Mistrust on government or distrust in healthcare policies, 3. No fear or worry about COVID-19 infection/ believe less that COVID-19 is a serious illness/ lower perceived seriousness of COVID-19/ever diagnosed with COVID-19; trust in COVID-19 vaccine's efficacy and safety, development process for COVID-19 vaccines, 4. Benefits of vaccine, 5. Big impact on life, 6. Plan to wait and see/don't believe I need it/others need it more

51	Chen et al., 2022	1. Being women/female, 2. Higher SES/higher income, 3. Middle age and above, 4. Chronic diseases/physical disease/underlying medical condition, 5. Old age (above 75 years), 6. Higher education (UG and above), and 7. Urban area	1. Adherence to preventive behaviours/influenza vaccine 2. Having a family member affected/died or admitted to intensive care for COVID-19, 3. Beliefs in a COVID-19 conspiracy/belief in misinformation/COVID-19 myth, and 4. Perceived information overload
52	Karabela et al., 2021	NA	1. Adherence to preventive behaviours/influenza vaccine 2. Trust in health authorities or government or science/medical/healthcare professionals/doctors/local public health officials (e.g. county health departments/CDC/WHO information), 3. Not trusting social media, 4. Individuals who perceived conspiracy theories and belief factors as cause of COVID-19, 5. The perception that coronavirus comes from a human or divine source, 6. Coronavirus is caused by ecological/environmental problem

(Continued)

TABLE 8.4 (Continued)

Sr. No.	Authors/Publication Year	Demographic Factors	Psychological Factors
53	Wu et al., 2021	1. Race/ethnicity – Asians and Hispanics/Latinos/non-Black African/minority category/Black, Asian and mixed/White, 2. Lower education, 3. Religion – Jewish-Religiosity (religious affiliation, attendance, religious importance), Catholics or practices/experiences/conservatism, 4. Middle age and above, 5. Chronic diseases/physical disease/underlying medical condition, 6. Being male, 7. Married 8. Current/former smokers, and 9. Higher subjective social status	1. Mistrust on government or distrust in healthcare policies and 2. Subjective rated health/lower depression score
54	Gerretsen et al., 2021	1. Younger age 2. Race/ethnicity – Black/African American/non-Hispanic Black/Arab ethnicity/Caucasians/mixed/non-Hispanic Whites, non-Hispanic Black, 3. Being women/female 4. Employment/occupation 5. Lower SES/income/household income 6. Political orientation right and centre right/living in Republican states/right-wing political ideology, 7. Lower population density	1. Spirituality/trust in god/superiority of natural immunity/divine control beliefs 2. Negative attitude towards vaccine/scepticism towards vaccines/mistrust in vaccine benefit, 3. No fear or worry about COVID-19 infection/believe less that COVID-19 is a serious illness/lower perceived seriousness of COVID-19/ever diagnosed with COVID-19, 4. Concerns about commercial profiteering

Notes

1 Only vaccine hesitancy for subgroups in the sample size is provided.
2 Only the rate of already vaccinated population (31%) is provided.
3 Data on vaccinated population is also provided (36.6%).
4 Data on vaccinated population is also provided (39.4%).
5 Uptake of COVID-19 vaccine data provided (52.5%).
6 Out of 47.5% sample population who were not vaccinated, their hesitancy data was reported as follows: mean 5.56 (SD = 1.72) of Hesitancy Scale of 1 to 7.

References

Adu, P. A., Iyaniwura, S. A., Mahmood, B., Jeong, D., Makuza, J. D., Cua, G., Binka, M., Garcia, H. H., Ringa, N., Wong, S., Yu, A., Irvine, M. A., Otterstatter, M. C., & Janjua, N. Z. (2022). Association between close interpersonal contact and vaccine hesitancy: Findings from a population-based survey in Canada. *Frontiers in Public Health, 10.* https://doi.org/10.3389/fpubh.2022.971333

Adzrago, D., Sulley, S., Ormiston, C. K., Mamudu, L., & Williams, F. (2022). Differences in the Perceived Likelihood of Receiving COVID-19 Vaccine. *International Journal of Environmental Research and Public Health, 19*(21), 13723. https://doi.org/10.3390/ijerph192113723

Ahamed, F., Ganesan, S., James, A., & Zaher, W. (2021). Understanding perception and acceptance of Sinopharm vaccine and vaccination against COVID–19 in the UAE. *BMC Public Health, 21*(1). https://doi.org/10.1186/s12889-021-11620-z

Ahiakpa, J. K., Cosmas, N. T., Anyiam, F. E., Enalume, K. O., Lawan, I., Gabriel, I. B., Oforka, C. L., Dahir, H. G., Salisu, T., Nwobodo, M. A., Massawe, G. P., Obagha, A. S., Okeh, D. U., Karikari, B., Aderonke, S. O., Awoyemi, O. M., Aneyo, I., & Doherty, F. V. (2022). COVID-19 vaccines uptake: Public knowledge, awareness, perception and acceptance among adult Africans. *medRxiv (Cold Spring Harbor Laboratory).* https://doi.org/10.1101/2022.02.06.22270405

Alqudeimat, Y., Alenezi, D., AlHajri, B., Alfouzan, H., Almokhaizeem, Z., Altamimi, S., Al-mansouri, W., Alzalzalah, S., & Ziyab, A. H. (2021). Acceptance of a COVID-19 Vaccine and Its Related Determinants among the General Adult Population in Kuwait. *Medical Principles and Practice, 30*(3), 262–271. https://doi.org/10.1159/000514636

Bagasra, A., Doan, S., & Allen, C. C. R. (2021). Racial differences in institutional trust and COVID-19 vaccine hesitancy and refusal. *BMC Public Health, 21*(1). https://doi.org/10.1186/s12889-021-12195-5

Beca-Martínez, M. T., Romay-Barja, M., Ayala, A., Falcon-Romero, M., Rodriguez-Blazquez, C., Benito, A., & Forjaz, M. J. (2022). Trends in COVID-19 vaccine acceptance in Spain, September 2020–May 2021. *American Journal of Public Health, 112*(11), 1611–1619. https://doi.org/10.2105/ajph.2022.307039

Borga, L. G., Clark, A. G., D'Ambrosio, C., & Lepinteur, A. (2022). Characteristics associated with COVID-19 vaccine hesitancy. *Scientific Reports, 12*(1). https://doi.org/10.1038/s41598-022-16572-x

Burch, A. E., Lee, E., Shackelford, P. O., Schmidt, P., & Bolin, P. (2022). Willingness to vaccinate against COVID-19: Predictors of vaccine uptake among adults in the US. *Journal of Prevention, 43*(1), 83–93. https://doi.org/10.1007/s10935-021-00653-0

Burger, R., Köhler, T., Gołos, A., Buttenheim, A. M., English, R., Tameris, M., & Maughan-Brown, B. (2022). Longitudinal changes in COVID-19 vaccination intent among South

African adults: Evidence from the NIDS-CRAM panel survey, February to May 2021. *BMC Public Health, 22*(1). https://doi.org/10.1186/s12889-022-12826-5

Chen, X., Lee, W., & Lin, F. (2022). Infodemic, institutional trust, and COVID-19 vaccine hesitancy: A cross-national survey. *International Journal of Environmental Research and Public Health, 19*(13), 8033. https://doi.org/10.3390/ijerph19138033

Covidence Systematic Review Software, Veritas Health Innovation, Melbourne, Australia. Retrieved from www.covidence.org

Dambadarjaa, D., Altankhuyag, G., Chandaga, U., Khuyag, S., Batkhorol, B., Khaidav, N., Dulamsuren, O., Gombodorj, N., Dorjsuren, A., Singh, P. N., Nyam, G., Otganbayar, D., & Tserennadmid, N. (2021). Factors associated with COVID-19 vaccine hesitancy in Mongolia: A web-based cross-sectional survey. *International Journal of Environmental Research and Public Health, 18*(24), 12903. https://doi.org/10.3390/ijerph182412903

Dryhurst, S., Schneider, C., Kerr, J. M., Freeman, A. F., Recchia, G., Van Der Bles, A. M., Spiegelhalter, D., & Van Der Linden, S. (2020). Risk perceptions of COVID-19 around the world. *Journal of Risk Research, 23*(7–8), 994–1006. https://doi.org/10.1080/13669 877.2020.1758193

Ebrahimi, O. V., Johnson, M. J., Ebling, S., Amundsen, O. M., Halsøy, Ø., Hoffart, A., Skjerdingstad, N., & Johnson, S. U. (2021). Risk, trust, and flawed assumptions: Vaccine hesitancy during the COVID-19 pandemic. *Frontiers in Public Health, 9*. https://doi. org/10.3389/fpubh.2021.700213

Enders, A. M., Uscinski, J. E., Klofstad, C. A., & Stoler, J. (2022). On the relationship between conspiracy theory beliefs, misinformation, and vaccine hesitancy. *PLoS One, 17*(10), e0276082. https://doi.org/10.1371/journal.pone.0276082

Eshel, Y., Kimhi, S., Marciano, H., & Adini, B. (2022). Partial social integration as a predictor of COVID-19 vaccine rejection and distress indicators. *Frontiers in Public Health, 10*. https://doi.org/10.3389/fpubh.2022.900070

Frankenthal, D., Zatlawi, M., Karni-Efrati, Z., Keinan-Boker, L., Luxenburg, O., & Bromberg, M. (2022). COVID-19 vaccine hesitancy among Israeli adults before and after vaccines' availability: A cross-sectional national survey. *Vaccine, 40*(43), 6271–6276. https://doi.org/10.1016/j.vaccine.2022.08.070

Gerretsen, P., Kim, J., Caravaggio, F., Quilty, L. C., Sanches, M., Wells, S., Brown, E. D., Agic, B., Pollock, B. G., & Graff-Guerrero, A. (2021). Individual determinants of COVID-19 vaccine hesitancy. *DOAJ (DOAJ: Directory of Open Access Journals).* https://doi.org/10.1371/journal.pone.0258462

Goodwin, R., Ben-Ezra, M., Takahashi, M., Luu, L. a. N., Borsfay, K., Kovács, M., Hou, W. K., Hamama-Raz, Y., & Levin, Y. (2022). Psychological factors underpinning vaccine willingness in Israel, Japan and Hungary. *Scientific Reports, 12*(1). https://doi. org/10.1038/s41598-021-03986-2

Group, W. H. O. W. (2006). Nonpharmaceutical interventions for pandemic influenza, national and community measures. *Emerging Infectious Diseases, 12*(1), 88. https://doi. org/10.3201/eid1201.051371

Harada, N., Shigemura, J., Tanichi, M., Kawaida, K., Takahashi, S., & Yasukata, F. (2015). Mental health and psychological impacts from the 2011 Great East Japan Earthquake Disaster: A systematic literature review. *Disaster and Military Medicine, 1*(1). https:// doi.org/10.1186/s40696-015-0008-x

Hawlader, M. D. H., Rahman, M. L., Nazir, A., Ara, T., Haque, M. M. A., Saha, S., . . . Siddiquea, S. R. (2022). COVID-19 vaccine acceptance in South Asia: A multi-country study. *International Journal of Infectious Diseases, 114*, 1–10. https://doi.org/10.1016/j. ijid.2021.09.056

Hesse, M. (2020). Why might women be less eager to get the coronavirus vaccine? An investigation. *Washington Post*. Retrieved from https://www.washingtonpost.com/lifestyle/style/women-covid-vaccine-skeptical/2020/12/15/63551cac-3a61-11eb-9276-ae0ca72729be_story.html

Kadoya, Y., Watanapongvanich, S., Yuktadatta, P., Putthinun, P., Lartey, S. T., & Khan, M. S. R. (2021). Willing or Hesitant? A socioeconomic study on the potential acceptance of COVID-19 vaccine in Japan. *International Journal of Environmental Research and Public Health*, *18*(9), 4864. https://doi.org/10.3390/ijerph18094864

Karabela, Ş. N., Coşkun, F., & Hoşgör, H. (2021). Investigation of the relationships between perceived causes of COVID-19, attitudes towards vaccine and level of trust in information sources from the perspective of Infodemic: The case of Turkey. *BMC Public Health*, *21*(1). https://doi.org/10.1186/s12889-021-11262-1

Karpman, M., Kenney, G. M., Zuckerman, S., Gonzalez, D., & Courtot, B. (2021). Confronting COVID-19 vaccine hesitancy among nonelderly adults. *Robert Wood Johnson Foundation and Urban Institute*. Retrieved from https://www.urban.org/sites/default/files/publication/103713/confronting-covid-19-vaccine-hesitancy-among-nonelderly-adults_0_0.pdf

Khairat, S., Zou, B., & Adler-Milstein, J. (2022). Factors and reasons associated with low COVID-19 vaccine uptake among highly hesitant communities in the US. *American Journal of Infection Control*, *50*(3), 262–267. https://doi.org/10.1016/j.ajic.2021.12.013

Khubchandani, J., Sharma, S. K., Price, J. H., Wiblishauser, M., Sharma, M., & Webb, F. J. (2021). COVID-19 vaccination hesitancy in the United States: A rapid national assessment. *Journal of Community Health*, *46*(2), 270–277. https://doi.org/10.1007/s10900-020-00958-x

King, W. C., Rubinstein, M., Reinhart, A., & Mejia, R. (2021). Time trends, factors associated with, and reasons for COVID-19 vaccine hesitancy: A massive online survey of US adults from January-May 2021. *PLoS One*, *16*(12), e0260731. https://doi.org/10.1371/journal.pone.0260731

Kollamparambil, U., Oyenubi, A., & Nwosu, C. O. (2021). COVID19 vaccine intentions in South Africa: Health communication strategy to address vaccine hesitancy. *BMC Public Health*, *21*(1). https://doi.org/10.1186/s12889-021-12196-4

Kumari, A., Ranjan, P., Chopra, S., Kaur, D., Kaur, T., Upadhyay, A. D., Isaac, J., Kasiraj, R., Prakash, B., Kumar, P., Dwivedi, S. N., & Vikram, N. K. (2021). Knowledge, barriers and facilitators regarding COVID-19 vaccine and vaccination programme among the general population: A cross-sectional survey from one thousand two hundred and forty-nine participants. *Diabetes and Metabolic Syndrome: Clinical Research and Reviews*, *15*(3), 987–992. https://doi.org/10.1016/j.dsx.2021.04.015

Lenherr, N., Berndt, A., Ritz, N., & Rudin, C. (2014). *Aerococcus urinae*: A possible reason for malodorous urine in otherwise healthy children. *European Journal of Pediatrics*, *173*(8), 1115–1117. https://doi.org/10.1007/s00431-014-2348-9

Levin, J., & Bradshaw, M. (2022). Determinants of COVID-19 skepticism and SARS-CoV-2 vaccine hesitancy: Findings from a national population survey of U.S. adults. *BMC Public Health*, *22*(1). https://doi.org/10.1186/s12889-022-13477-2

Litaker, J. R., Tamez, N., Bray, C. L., Durkalski, W., & Taylor, R. P. (2021). Sociodemographic factors associated with vaccine hesitancy in Central Texas immediately prior to COVID-19 vaccine availability. *International Journal of Environmental Research and Public Health*, *19*(1), 368. https://doi.org/10.3390/ijerph19010368

Lucia, V. C., Kelekar, A., & Afonso, N. (2021). COVID-19 vaccine hesitancy among medical students. *Journal of Public Health*, *43*(3), 445–449. https://doi.org/10.1093/pubmed/fdaa230

Mobarak, A. M., Miguel, E., Abaluck, J., Ahuja, A., Alsan, M., Banerjee, A., Breza, E., Chandrasekhar, A. G., Duflo, E., Dzansi, J., Garrett, D. O., Goldsmith-Pinkham, P., Gonsalves, G., Hossain, M., Jakubowski, A., Kang, G., Kharel, A., Kremer, M., Meriggi, N. F., . . . Więcek, W. (2022). End COVID-19 in low- and middle-income countries. *Science*, *375*(6585), 1105–1110. https://doi.org/10.1126/science.abo4089

Moher, D., Liberati, A., Tetzlaff, J., & Altman, D. G. (2009). Preferred reporting items for systematic reviews and meta-analyses: The PRISMA statement. *PLOS Medicine*, *6*(7), e1000097. https://doi.org/10.1371/journal.pmed.1000097

Moore, D. C. B. C., Nehab, M. F., Camacho, K. G., Reis, A. T., De Fátima Junqueira-Marinho, M., Abramov, D. M., De Azevedo, Z. M. A., De Menezes, L. R., Salú, M. D. S., Da Silva Figueiredo, C. E., Moreira, M. E. L., Vasconcelos, Z., Carvalho, F. C., De Rezende De Mello, L., Correia, R. T. P., & Gomes, S. C., & Junior. (2021). Low COVID-19 vaccine hesitancy in Brazil. *Vaccine*, *39*(42), 6262–6268. https://doi.org/10.1016/j.vaccine.2021.09.013

Morales, D. X., Beltran, T. F., & Morales, S. A. (2022). Gender, socioeconomic status, and COVID-19 vaccine hesitancy in the US: An intersectionality approach. *Sociology of Health and Illness*, *44*(6), 953–971. https://doi.org/10.1111/1467-9566.13474

Ng, J.W.J, Vaithilingam, S., Nair, M., Hwang, L., & Musa, K. I. (2022). Key predictors of COVID-19 vaccine hesitancy in Malaysia: An integrated framework. *PLoS One*, *17*(5), e0268926. https://doi.org/10.1371/journal.pone.0268926

Nguyen, K. H., Nguyen, K., Corlin, L., Allen, J. D., & Chung, M. (2021). Changes in COVID-19 vaccination receipt and intention to vaccinate by socioeconomic characteristics and geographic area, United States, January 6 – March 29, 2021. *Annals of Medicine*, *53*(1), 1419–1428. https://doi.org/10.1080/07853890.2021.1957998

Ohlsen, E. C., Yankey, D., Pezzi, C., Kriss, J. L., Lu, P., Hung, M., Bernabe, M. a. B., Kumar, G. S., Jentes, E. S., Elam-Evans, L. D., Jackson, H. A., Black, C. L., Singleton, J. A., Ladva, C., Abad, N., & Rodriguez-Lainz, A. (2022). Coronavirus Disease 2019 (COVID-19) Vaccination coverage, intentions, attitudes, and barriers by race/ethnicity, language of interview, and nativity – national immunization survey adult COVID module, April 22 2021–January 29 2022. *Clinical Infectious Diseases*, *75*(Supplement_2), S182–S192. https://doi.org/10.1093/cid/ciac508

Okamoto, S., Kamimura, K., & Komamura, K. (2022). COVID-19 vaccine hesitancy and vaccine passports: A cross-sectional conjoint experiment in Japan. *BMJ Open*, *12*(6), e060829. https://doi.org/10.1136/bmjopen-2022-060829

Olagoke, A. A., Olagoke, O. O., & Hughes, A. M. (2021). Intention to vaccinate against the novel 2019 coronavirus disease: The role of health locus of control and religiosity. *Journal of Religion & Health*, *60*(1), 65–80. https://doi.org/10.1007/s10943-020-01090-9

Orita, M., Hayashida, N., Urata, H., Shinkawa, T., Endo, Y., & Takamura, N. (2013). Determinants of the return to hometowns after the accident at Fukushima Dai-ichi nuclear power plant: A case study for the village of Kawauchi. *Radiation Protection Dosimetry*, *156*(3), 383–385. https://doi.org/10.1093/rpd/nct082

Oyekale, A. S. (2022). Factors influencing willingness to be vaccinated against COVID-19 in Nigeria. *International Journal of Environmental Research and Public Health*, *19*(11), 6816. https://doi.org/10.3390/ijerph19116816

Paul, A., Sikdar, D., Mahanta, J., Ghosh, S., Jabed, M. A., Paul, S., Yeasmin, F., Sikdar, S., Chowdhury, B., & Nath, T. K. (2021). Peoples' understanding, acceptance, and perceived challenges of vaccination against COVID-19: A cross-sectional study in Bangladesh. *PLoS One*, *16*(8), e0256493. https://doi.org/10.1371/journal.pone.0256493

Paul, E., Steptoe, A., & Fancourt, D. (2021). Attitudes towards vaccines and intention to vaccinate against COVID-19: Implications for public health communications. *The Lancet Regional Health, 1,* 100012. https://doi.org/10.1016/j.lanepe.2020.100012

Pérez-Bermejo, M., Cloquell-Lozano, A., Moret-Tatay, C., & Pérez-Bermejo, M. (2022). Social vulnerability and COVID-19 vaccine in Spain. *International Journal of Environmental Research and Public Health, 19*(21), 14013. https://doi.org/10.3390/ijerph192114013

Piltch-Loeb, R., Silver, D., Kim, Y., Norris, H. C., McNeill, E. M., & Abramson, D. H. (2022). Determinants of the COVID-19 vaccine hesitancy spectrum. *PLoS One, 17*(6), e0267734. https://doi.org/10.1371/journal.pone.0267734

Porritt, K., Gomersall, J. S., & Lockwood, C. (2014). JBI's systematic reviews. *American Journal of Nursing, 114*(6), 47–52. https://doi.org/10.1097/01.naj.0000450430.97383.64

Qunaibi, E. A., Helmy, M., Basheti, I. A., & Sultan, I. (2021). A high rate of COVID-19 vaccine hesitancy in a large-scale survey on Arabs. *eLife, 10.* https://doi.org/10.7554/elife.68038

Raffetti, E., Mondino, E., & Di Baldassarre, G. (2022). COVID-19 vaccine hesitancy in Sweden and Italy: The role of trust in authorities. *Scandinavian Journal of Public Health, 50*(6), 803–809. https://doi.org/10.1177/14034948221099410

Robertson, E. V., Reeve, K., Niedzwiedz, C. L., Moore, J., Blake, M. L., Green, M. F., Katikireddi, S. V., & Benzeval, M. (2021). Predictors of COVID-19 vaccine hesitancy in the UK household longitudinal study. *Brain Behavior and Immunity, 94,* 41–50. https://doi.org/10.1016/j.bbi.2021.03.008

Rogers, B. G., Tao, J., Almonte, A., Toma, E., Nagel, K. I., Fain, R., Napoleon, S. C., Maynard, M. A., Murphy, M. C., Sarkar, I. N., & Chan, P. W. H. (2022). Statewide evaluation of COVID-19 vaccine hesitancy in Rhode Island. *PLoS One, 17*(6), e0268587. https://doi.org/10.1371/journal.pone.0268587

Santirocchi, A., Spataro, P., Costanzi, M., Doricchi, F., Rossi-Arnaud, C., & Cestari, V. (2022). Predictors of the intention to be vaccinated against COVID-19 in a sample of Italian respondents at the start of the immunization campaign. *Journal of Personalized Medicine, 12*(1), 111. https://doi.org/10.3390/jpm12010111

Schmidtke, K. A., Kudrna, L., Noufaily, A., Stallard, N., Skrybant, M., Russell, S. E., & Clarke, A. (2022). Evaluating the relationship between moral values and vaccine hesitancy in Great Britain during the COVID-19 pandemic: A cross-sectional survey. *Social Science & Medicine, 308,* 115218. https://doi.org/10.1016/j.socscimed.2022.115218

Schwarzinger, M., Watson, V., Arwidson, P., Alla, F., & Luchini, S. (2021). COVID-19 vaccine hesitancy in a representative working-age population in France: A survey experiment based on vaccine characteristics. *The Lancet. Public Health, 6*(4), e210–e221. https://doi.org/10.1016/s2468-2667(21)00012-8

Seddig, D., Maskileyson, D., Davidov, E., Ajzen, I., & Schmidt, P. (2022). Correlates of COVID-19 vaccination intentions: Attitudes, institutional trust, fear, conspiracy beliefs, and vaccine skepticism. *Social Science & Medicine, 302,* 114981. https://doi.org/10.1016/j.socscimed.2022.114981

Sekizawa, Y., Hashimoto, S., Denda, K., Ochi, S., & So, M. (2022). Association between COVID-19 vaccine hesitancy and generalised trust, depression, generalised anxiety, and fear of COVID-19. *BMC Public Health, 22*(1). https://doi.org/10.1186/s12889-021-12479-w

Shah, S., Gui, H., Chua, P. E. Y., Tan, J., Suen, L. K., Chan, S. W., & Pang, J. (2022). Factors associated with COVID-19 vaccination intent in Singapore, Australia and Hong Kong. *Vaccine, 40*(21), 2949–2959. https://doi.org/10.1016/j.vaccine.2022.03.062

Shareef, L. G., Al-Hussainy, A. H., & Hameed, S. (2022). COVID-19 vaccination hesitancy among Iraqi general population between beliefs and barriers: An observational study. *F1000Research, 11*, 334. https://doi.org/10.12688/f1000research.110545.2

Sheeran, P., Harris, P. C., & Epton, T. (2014). Does heightening risk appraisals change people's intentions and behavior? A meta-analysis of experimental studies. *Psychological Bulletin, 140*(2), 511–543. https://doi.org/10.1037/a0033065

Sjo"berg, L. (2000). Factors in risk perception. *Risk Analysis, 20*(1), 1–12. https://doi.org/10.1111/0272–4332.00001

Solís Arce, J. S., Warren, S. S., Meriggi, N. F., Scacco, A., McMurry, N., Voors, M., . . . Adeojo, O. (2021). COVID-19 vaccine acceptance and hesitancy in low-and middle-income countries. *Nature Medicine, 27*(8), 1385–1394. https://doi.org/10.1038/s41591-021-01454-y

Stead, M., Jessop, C., Angus, K., Bedford, H., Ussher, M., Ford, A., Eadie, D., MacGregor, A., Hunt, K., & MacKintosh, A. M. (2021). National survey of attitudes towards and intentions to vaccinate against COVID-19: Implications for communications. *BMJ Open, 11*(10), e055085. https://doi.org/10.1136/bmjopen-2021-055085

Szilagyi, P. G., Thomas, K. H., Shah, M. K., Vizueta, N., Cui, Y., Vangala, S., Fox, C. R., & Kapteyn, A. (2021). The role of trust in the likelihood of receiving a COVID-19 vaccine: Results from a national survey. *Preventive Medicine, 153*, 106727. https://doi.org/10.1016/j.ypmed.2021.106727

Takeda, S., Orita, M., Fukushima, Y., Kudo, T., & Takamura, N. (2016). Determinants of intention to leave among non-medical employees after a nuclear disaster: A cross-sectional study. *BMJ Open.* https://doi.org/10.1136/bmjopen-2016-011930

Thomson, A., Robinson, K., & Vallée-Tourangeau, G. (2016). The 5As: A practical taxonomy for the determinants of vaccine uptake. *Vaccine, 34*(8), 1018–1024. https://doi.org/10.1016/j.vaccine.2015.11.065

Tlale, L. D. N., Gabaitiri, L., Totolo, L. K., Smith, G., Puswane-Katse, O., Ramonna, E., Mothowaeng, B., Tlhakanelo, J. T., Masupe, T., Rankgoane-Pono, G., Irige, J. M., Mafa, F., & Kolane, S. (2022). Acceptance rate and risk perception towards the COVID-19 vaccine in Botswana. *PLoS One, 17*(2), e0263375. https://doi.org/10.1371/journal.pone.0263375

Touré, A., Traore, F. A., Camara, G., Magassouba, A. S., Barry, I., Kourouma, M. L., Sylla, Y., Conte, N. Y., Cisse, D., Dioubaté, N., Sidibe, S., Beavogui, A. H., & Delamou, A. (2022). Facilitators and barriers to COVID-19 vaccination among healthcare workers and the general population in Guinea. *BMC Infectious Diseases, 22*(1). https://doi.org/10.1186/s12879-022-07742-3

Tram, K. H., Saeed, S., Bradley, C., Fox, B., Eshun-Wilson, I., Mody, A., & Geng, E. (2021). Deliberation, dissent, and distrust: Understanding distinct drivers of coronavirus disease 2019 vaccine hesitancy in the United States. *Clinical Infectious Diseases, 74*(8), 1429–1441. https://doi.org/10.1093/cid/ciab633

Troiano, G., & Nardi, A. (2021). Vaccine hesitancy in the era of COVID-19. *Public Health, 194*, 245–251. https://doi.org/10.1016/j.puhe.2021.02.025

Upenieks, L., Ford-Robertson, J., & Robertson, J. (2021). Trust in god and/or science? Sociodemographic differences in the effects of beliefs in an engaged god and mistrust of the COVID-19 vaccine. *Journal of Religion & Health, 61*(1), 657–686. https://doi.org/10.1007/s10943-021-01466-5

Viswanath, K., Bekalu, M. A., Dhawan, D., Pinnamaneni, R., Lang, J., & McLoud, R. (2021). Individual and social determinants of COVID-19 vaccine uptake. *BMC Public Health, 21*(1). https://doi.org/10.1186/s12889-021-10862-1

Wafula, S. T., Mugume, I. B., Sensasi, B., Okware, S., Chimbaru, A., Nanyunja, M., Talisuna, A., Kabanda, R., Bakyaita, T., Wanyenze, R. K., & Byakika-Tusiime, J. (2022). Intention to vaccinate against COVID-19 and adherence to non-pharmaceutical interventions against COVID-19 prior to the second wave of the pandemic in Uganda: A cross-sectional study. *BMJ Open, 12*(6), e057322. https://doi.org/10.1136/bmjopen-2021-057322

Weinstein, N. D. (1988). The precaution adoption process. *Health Psychology, 7*(4), 355–386. https://doi.org/10.1037/0278-6133.7.4.355

WHO. (2020). Retrieved December 21, 2022, from www.who.int/news/item/31-12-2020-who-issues-its-first-emergency-use-validation-for-a-covid-19-vaccine-and-emphasizes-need-for-equitable-global-access

WHO. (2022). Retrieved December 21, 2022, from https://covid19.who.int/

Wisniak, A., Baysson, H., Pullen, N., Nehme, M., Pennacchio, F., Zaballa, M., Guessous, I., & Stringhini, S. (2021). COVID-19 vaccination acceptance in the canton of Geneva: A cross-sectional population-based study. *Schweizerische Medizinische Wochenschrift, 151*(4950), w30080. https://doi.org/10.4414/smw.2021.w30080

Wong, L. P., Alias, H., Danaee, M., Ahmed, J., Lachyan, A. S., Cai, C. Z., Lin, Y., Hu, Z., Tan, S. H. S., Lu, Y., Cai, G., Nguyen, D. K., Seheli, F. N., Alhammadi, F. A., Madhale, M., Atapattu, M., Quazi-Bodhanya, T., Mohajer, S., Zimet, G. D., & Zhao, Q. (2021). COVID-19 vaccination intention and vaccine characteristics influencing vaccination acceptance: A global survey of 17 countries. *Infectious Diseases of Poverty, 10*(1). https://doi.org/10.1186/s40249-021-00900-w

World Bank. Retrieved December 28, 2022, from https://datatopics.worldbank.org/world-development-indicators/the-world-by-income-and-region.html

World Health Organization Writing Group, Bell, D., Nicoll, A., Fukuda, K., Horby, P., Monto, A., Hayden, F., Wylks, C., Sanders, L., & van Tam, J. (2006). Non-pharmaceutical interventions for pandemic influenza, national and community measures. *Emerging Infectious Diseases, 12*(1), 88–94. https://doi.org/10.3201/eid1201.051371.

Wu, J., Li, Q., Tarimo, C. S., Wang, M., Gu, J., Wei, W., Ma, M., Zhao, L., Mu, Z., & Miao, Y. (2021). COVID-19 vaccine hesitancy among Chinese population: A large-scale national study. *Frontiers in Immunology, 12.* https://doi.org/10.3389/fimmu.2021.781161

Yahia, A. I. O., Alshahrani, A., Alsulmi, W. G. H., Alqarni, M. H., Abdulrahim, T. K. A., Heba, W., Alqarni, T. M., Alharthi, K. M., & Buhran, A. a. A. (2021). Determinants of COVID-19 vaccine acceptance and hesitancy: A cross-sectional study in Saudi Arabia. *Human Vaccines & Immunotherapeutics, 17*(11), 4015–4020. https://doi.org/10.1080/21645515.2021.1950506

Zarbo, C., Candini, V., Ferrari, C., D'Addazio, M., Calamandrei, G., Starace, F., Caserotti, M., Gavaruzzi, T., Lotto, L., Tasso, A., Zamparini, M., & De Girolamo, G. (2022). COVID-19 Vaccine hesitancy in Italy: Predictors of acceptance, fence sitting and refusal of the COVID-19 vaccination. *Frontiers in Public Health, 10.* https://doi.org/10.3389/fpubh.2022.873098

9

LEVERAGING DIGITAL HEALTH TECHNOLOGIES IN THE BACKDROP OF COVID-19

A Systematic Literature Review

Shruti Dua and Bhavya Chhabra

Introduction

The application of digital recording and capturing of physical health status, experiences, and narratives have paved the way for revolutionary advancements with the integrated real-time generation of new knowledge and insights (Perakslis & Ginsburg, 2021). This chapter alludes to digital health technology and its progress, indicating the advancing digital health interventions and how they have impacted humans' lifestyles and healthcare. This chapter elucidates the evolving digital health interventions during COVID and post-COVID times and their application for the emerging population. The primary objectives of this review chapter are to understand and assess the impact and utility of digital health technologies on patient outcomes and to identify successful practices, leading innovators, and current trends in deploying these technologies globally. We specifically aim to explore how digital health interventions have transformed healthcare, from enhancing medical accessibility and fostering patient-centric care to improving mental health and facilitating a shift from treatment-based to preventive healthcare. A vital aspect of the study is examining the digital health technologies implemented in the Indian context. Moreover, we aim to identify gaps in current knowledge and highlight areas where further research is needed, such as the long-term effectiveness of digital health interventions and their implications in diverse settings and populations.

Digital health, often known as digital healthcare, is a wide, multidisciplinary term encompassing ideas where technology and healthcare converge and amalgamate with evolving digitally mediated abilities (Abernethy et al., 2022). By merging software, hardware, and services, digital health brings digital transformations to the healthcare industry. The term 'digital health' refers to utilising digital information, data, and communication technologies to gather, disseminate, and analyse

DOI: 10.4324/9781003357209-12

health information to improve patient health and healthcare delivery (Solomon & Rudin, 2020).

Digital health technologies like the electronic health record, virtual visits, mobile health, wearable technology, digital therapeutics, artificial intelligence, cloud computing, and machine learning, paired with increasingly sophisticated health information systems, have transformed exponentially over the past decade (Abernethy et al., 2022; Labrique et al., 2018). For instance one can significantly benefit from using electronic health records (EHRs), mobile phones, and portable computers (also known as m-health). They can assist in maintaining track of patients in HIV programmes where the loss rate (patients who discontinue treatment) can be as high as 76% and support a health worker conducting clinical activities in the absence of medical doctors (Blaya et al., 2010; Pai et al., 2021). Since these technologies are becoming more common, they can enhance vital aspects of mental and physical wellness aspects, including access, outcomes, adherence, and research (Abernethy et al., 2022; Solomon & Rudin, 2020).

Concomitantly, these traditional healthcare models are being revamped and modernised more than ever, owing to the widespread adoption of Healthcare 4.0's digital technologies (Awad et al., 2021). Digital health technologies have revolutionised healthcare delivery and disease management across the globe, with countries like India and other nations adopting various tools for improving patient outcomes (WHO, 2019). Telemedicine has experienced rapid growth in India, supported by initiatives such as the National Telemedicine Network and eSanjeevani, which bridge the gap between rural and urban healthcare access (Suhas et al., 2022). Similarly, telehealth services have seen widespread adoption in the United States, driven by legislation like the Creating Opportunities Now for Necessary and Effective Care Technologies (CONNECT) for Health Act and the COVID-19 pandemic (Anderson et al., 2022). Electronic health records (EHRs) are becoming increasingly common in both countries, with India's National Digital Health Mission aiming to create a digital health ecosystem. At the same time, the United States has long-established EHR initiatives like the Meaningful Use programme (Pai et al., 2021). Mobile health (mHealth) applications have gained popularity worldwide for monitoring and managing chronic diseases, with both countries investing in this technology to address their unique healthcare needs (Asi & Williams, 2018; Fan & Zhao, 2022). Lastly, artificial intelligence (AI) is being integrated into healthcare systems to aid diagnostics and treatment planning, with countries like India, the United States, and the United Kingdom investing heavily in AI research and development (Davenport & Kalakota, 2019).

Every step of the patient care pathway is convalescing because of the upsurge of these digital healthcare technologies across global settings. Through this, swift diagnosis, prevention, and interventions are being efficiently embraced, eventually benefitting millions around the clock and almost daily (Asi & Williams, 2018; Howitt et al., 2012). Within medical logistics, advanced technologies like drones, precision to surgeries, rehabilitation, artificial intelligence, machine learning, virtual reality, robots, smart design with voice enablement, and mobile care – telemedicine (i.e. telementoring, tele-critical care, and targeted drug delivery) are being explored and leveraged for critical treatment (Asi & Williams, 2018; Awad et al., 2021). Such healthcare technologies are being extensively utilised in today's modern era to create a closed-loop system to help communicate remotely with one another, enabling seamless integration within the healthcare industry (Awad et al., 2021; Scott et al., 2020).

Digital health infrastructure aims to enable seamless interfaces and real-time interoperability of devices (Awad et al., 2021). Being cognizant of the future, there is an apparent and imperative need for a theoretical framework that can be used to regulate how technology is employed in behavioural modification; yet, the literature on the topic is sparse, recent, and heterogeneous (Choukou et al., 2023). Therefore, this work serves the scholastic literature on this matter.

Digital Health Technologies: Before the Unprecedented Times

Earlier, the promise of digital health was illusory despite noteworthy advancements made possible by significant investments (Golinelli et al., 2020). For instance digital interfaces in inpatient care systems were frequently cumbersome earlier in the day, and large amounts of health data are frequently hidden, unavailable, and challenging to combine in a relevant and effective way (Golinelli et al., 2020). Furthermore, clinical staff members struggled to comprehend the preferences and circumstances of patients and families that supported health improvement outside of the clinic with the help of digital tools (Abernethy et al., 2022; Golinelli et al., 2020).

Intriguingly, conversely, individual clinical encounters between practitioners and patients were historically assumed to be the essential basis of clinical practice (Abernethy et al., 2022). However, in recent times, this presumption has been dynamically challenged and rethought, owing to the phenomenal accelerated advancement of digital health technologies (Abernethy et al., 2022; Labrique et al., 2018). Their interconnected mobility, efficiency, productivity, virtuality, surveillance informatics, and the scalability of medical processes make them groundbreaking (Kulikowski, 2022; Labrique et al., 2018).

Adopting digital health technology to directly boost public health systems had been relatively poor before the pandemic; nevertheless, during the COVID-19 outbreak, this acceleration was unrelenting (Labrique et al., 2018; Petracca et al., 2020). Global pandemics date back to a significant history. They have dramatically increased over the past few decades, beginning with the Severe Acute Respiratory Syndrome (SARS) pandemic in 2003 and continuing with the Middle East Respiratory Syndrome (MERS), Ebola, and the arrival of the Zika virus in Latin America in 2015. These pandemics are intrinsically linked to contemporary socio-technical advancements and globalisation processes, specifically digital health technologies that have expedited patient care lately (Petracca et al., 2020). The Severe Acute Respiratory Syndrome Coronavirus-2 (SARS-CoV-2), a previously unidentified SARS virus variation, was responsible for the World Health Organization's declaration of a new pandemic in the early months of 2020. COVID-19 is an infectious disease that is brought on by SARS-CoV-2 (Tilahun et al., 2021). Concerning this, digital health technologies in the contemporary context have significantly improved patient outcomes for morbidity and mortality when used in practice (Zwack et al., 2023).

Virtually every area of human effort has transformed in the past several decades due to the rapid growth of the digital health ecosystem. The implications of these changes for human health and their potential benefits and drawbacks have been the subject of considerable speculation and will continue to be so over the years.

A Pandemic of Lockdown: Amid the Backdrop of the COVID-19 Era

The COVID-19 pandemic has brought to a renewed reliance on digital health technologies, which has been a common development, thereby embracing the digital health transformation (Golinelli et al., 2020; Petracca et al., 2020). Like other worldwide disasters in human history, the Corona Virus Disease of 2019 (COVID-19) pandemic is no exception. The Severe Acute Respiratory Syndrome (SARS)-CoV and the Middle East Respiratory Syndrome (MERS)-CoV are members of the same coronavirus family as COVID-19 (Nikolich-Zugich et al., 2020). The World Health Organization (WHO) announced the COVID-19 outbreak a pandemic on 11th March 2020 (WHO, 2020). It has been creating unheard-of health and economic disruptions that the world has witnessed. However, this new scenario also encourages switching to digital solutions across various companies and society.

Education is a case in point of this change, and, along with education, even healthcare is transforming. The pandemic is synonymous with a scenario of collective hardship, times of lockdown, and loss. Digital transformations are being favoured by the COVID-19 pandemic across many businesses and across different societies. Healthcare industry organisations have quickly embraced digital healthcare solutions and cutting-edge technological tools in response to the pandemic's initial phase (Golinelli et al., 2020).

Such healthcare technologies are being extensively used to mitigate coronavirus, and these have been upcoming ever since. The rich scholastic literature has established that integrating digital health technologies with the National Emergency Tele-Critical Care Network (NETCCN) has been enormously supportive during the COVID era and beyond (Scott et al., 2020). Receiving real-time patient and supply data and sharing essential care knowledge, NETCCN, with digital health technologies enable healthcare providers wherever they may be (Scott et al., 2020). Not only this, the advances in surveillance and digital apps have proved to be extremely efficient during unprecedented times, considering the mental and physical health of the patients (Labrique et al., 2018).

For instance an app named TraceTogether was deployed in Singapore to monitor COVID-19-infected individuals (Faorrazzi et al., 2020). Singaporean health officials could track people and notify them if they came in contact with someone infected with COVID-19 through Bluetooth signalling. Although implementing this patient-monitoring system in European nations would be prohibited by national data privacy rules, it may be useful for disease surveillance and outbreak management. Another instance where the CoronApp was developed and implemented on the basis of comparable principles was created in France (Fagherazzi et al., 2020). The software requires users to register and fill out information about their health status and if they are experiencing any symptoms. This data is tracked using a geolocation system, which is updated hourly, owing to the advancements making such work seamlessly possible (Fagherazzi et al., 2020).

While understanding the health effects of structural and functional changes in the human genome, such digital technologies have worked immaculately in today's time (Abernethy et al., 2022; Golinelli et al., 2020). The COVID Symptom Tracker app was created at King's College London with the intention of assisting patients in keeping track of their own symptoms. The software became so well-known that the United States also started utilising it. In addition to its personal advantages, the application may be used for epidemiological research on COVID-19 (Fagherazzi et al., 2020). Insightfully, these digital diagnostic tools that work in conjunction with the already established clinical, molecular, or serological diagnostic techniques, including AI-based diagnostic algorithms based on both imaging and clinical data, have appeared to be beneficial in the realms of COVID-19 (Fagherazzi et al., 2020; Golinelli et al., 2020).

When leveraged effectively and with precision, digital health solutions have the capacity to expedite the development of each of the fundamental tenets of a digitally aided learning health system.

Benefits of Leveraging Digital Health Technologies

The management of population health is evolving due to clinically led improvement, facilitated by new technology incorporating the social determinant factors and eHealth Literacy (Foley et al., 2021). The whole globe recognises that the healthcare industry is at least a decade behind other establishments and sectors when it comes to implementing information technology (Ibrahim et al., 2021). It is possible that it is even further behind in realising the benefits in both productivity and value, which have been witnessed elsewhere due to the application of information technology (Biggs et al., 2019). Failures in the introduction of information technology that has received a lot of public attention have increased the workload for frontline employees and have not brought about any cost savings (Imison et al., 2016).

The manpower and productivity in the healthcare sector are impacted by digital technologies like electronic health records, monitoring equipment, telehealth, wearable devices, electronic communications, cloud-based and web-based instruments, and data analytics (Imison et al., 2016). Becoming a digitally enabled healthcare provider requires re-evaluating tasks, revamping procedures, and maximising data-driven insights and improvement opportunities (Biggs et al., 2019). Where technological solutions have fallen short, new technologies have been layered on top of the old ones, generating extra work for healthcare workers (Perakslis & Ginsburg, 2021).

Digital health technologies, therefore, integrate clinical information decision support and knowledge management systems into standard workflows to improve care (Sutton et al., 2020). It allows real-time patient surveillance and robust analytics enabling proactive and focused care, lowering costs, and increasing results (Imison et al., 2016). It helps to develop information technology systems to unify and regulate care by helping providers collaborate to reduce costs and harms from poor communication and divided care (West, 2016).

According to the Digital Health Market Size, Share & Trends Report, 2030, the global digital health market was USD 211.0 billion in 2022 and is anticipated to grow by 18.6% from 2023 to 2030. The market growth is driven by increased smartphone adoption, 4G/5G internet connectivity, healthcare IT infrastructure development, the need to lower healthcare costs, chronic disease prevalence, and virtual care usability.

Methods

Literature Search/Locating Studies

The search was confined to English-language empirically published research papers in peer-reviewed journals. Original scholarly work incorporating digital health technologies after the onset of COVID-19 qualifies to be a part of this review. The present chapter excludes conference proceedings, dissertations, abstracts, methodological papers, editorials, and non-English publications. Table 9.1 depicts the inclusion and exclusion criteria for the evaluated papers.

We present the systematic literature review of the studies as the outbreak of COVID was embraced (2020 onwards to 2023) in the scope of digital health technologies. COVID-19 has made everyone exposed to technology, and people are becoming technology-friendly. Table 9.4 represents a summary of meta-analytic studies in the area of digital health interventions. Even though digital technology interventions started pre-COVID and post-COVID, there is a massive expansion

TABLE 9.1 Delimitations of the study: inclusion and exclusion criteria for the eligible articles

Inclusion Criteria	Exclusion Criteria
Empirical research papers on digital health technologies	Proceedings, abstracts
Examines interventions post the onset of COVID-19	Methodological papers, editorials
Written in English	Non-English publications
Published in peer-reviewed journals	Non-peer reviewed articles
Studying populations with clinical symptoms	

TABLE 9.2 Quality assessment of the included studies in a chronological order

	Study Screening Questions		Methodological Quality Criteria				
	S1 – Are there clear research questions?	S2 – Do the collected data allow addressing the research questions?	Q1 – Is the sampling strategy relevant to address the research question?	Q2 – Is the sample representative of the target population?	Q3 – Are the measurements appropriate	Q4 – Is the risk of non-response bias low?	Q5 – Is the statistical analysis appropriate to answer the research question?
1. Kolasa and Kozinski (2020)	Yes	Yes	Yes	Yes	?	Yes	Yes
2. Melia et al. (2020)	Yes	Yes	Yes	Yes	Yes	Yes	Yes
3. Patel et al. (2020)	Yes	Yes	Yes	Yes	Yes	Yes	Yes
4. Gilbey et al. (2020)	Yes	Yes	Yes	Yes	Yes	Yes	Yes
5. Peiris-John et al. (2020)	Yes	Yes	Yes	Yes	Yes	Yes	Yes
6. Van Rhoon et al. (2020)	Yes	Yes	Yes	Yes	Yes	Yes	Yes
7. Mosnaim et al. (2021)	Yes	Yes	Yes	Yes	Yes	Yes	Yes
8. Patel et al. (2021)	Yes	Yes	Yes	Yes	Yes	Yes	Yes
9. Wongvibulsin et al. (2021)	Yes	Yes	Yes	Yes	Yes	Yes	Yes
10. Sasseville et al. (2021)	Yes	Yes	Yes	Yes	Yes	Yes	Yes
11. Domhardt et al. (2021)	Yes	Yes	Yes	Yes	Yes	Yes	Yes
12. Mclaughlin et al. (2021)	Yes	Yes	Yes	Yes	Yes	Yes	Yes
13. Kitsiou et al. (2021)	Yes	Yes	Yes	Yes	Yes	Yes	Yes
14. Mbunge et al. (2022)	Yes	Yes	Yes	Yes	Yes	Yes	Yes
15. Marthick et al. (2021)	Yes	Yes	Yes	Yes	Yes	Yes	Yes
16. Akinosun et al. (2021)	Yes	Yes	Yes	Yes	Yes	Yes	Yes
17. Western et al. (2021)	Yes	Yes	Yes	Yes	Yes	Yes	Yes
18. Whitelaw et al. (2021)	Yes	Yes	Yes	Yes	Yes	Yes	Yes
19. Laranjo et al. (2021)	Yes	Yes	Yes	Yes	Yes	Yes	Yes
20. Kouvari et al. (2022)	Yes	Yes	Yes	Yes	Yes	Yes	Yes

21. Yao et al. (2022)	Yes	Yes	Yes	Yes	yes	Yes	Yes
22. Ridho et al. (2022)	Yes	Yes	Yes	Yes	Yes	Yes	Yes
23. Leach et al. (2022)	Yes	Yes	Yes	Yes	Yes	Yes	Yes
24. Singleton et al. (2022)	Yes	Yes	Yes	Yes	Yes	Yes	Yes
25. Morris et al. (2022)	Yes	Yes	Yes	Yes	Yes	Yes	Yes
26. Philippe et al. (2022)	Yes	Yes	Yes	Yes	Yes	Yes	Yes
27. Chen and Chan (2022)	Yes	Yes	Yes	Yes	Yes	Yes	Yes
28. Peyton et al. (2022)	Yes	Yes	Yes	Yes	Yes	Yes	Yes
29. Harith et al. (2022)	Yes	Yes	Yes	Yes	Yes	Yes	Yes
30. Manby et al. (2022)	Yes	Yes	Yes	Yes	Yes	Yes	Yes
31. Evans et al. (2022)	Yes	Yes	Yes	Yes	Yes	Yes	Yes
32. Choukou et al. (2023)	Yes	Yes	Yes	Yes	Yes	Yes	Yes
33. Goswami et al. (2023)	Yes	Yes	Yes	Yes	Yes	Yes	Yes
34. Ndayishimiye et al. (2023)	Yes	Yes	Yes	Yes	Yes	Yes	Yes
35. Lee et al. (2023)	Yes	Yes	Yes	Yes	Yes	Yes	Yes

of them across all sections of populations and different sectors. The meta-analytic findings present the positive impact of digital health interventions on the population, especially on people with clinical symptoms. It has shown a very impactful and positive future for a better lifestyle and well-being.

Search Strategy

The two independent, SD and BC of the current review conducted a systematic literature search using PsycINFO, PubMed, Web of Science, and Google Scholar databases to identify empirical studies on digital health technologies published since the COVID-19 outbreak. They applied PRISMA Guidelines to select eligible studies based on the predefined inclusion and exclusion criteria. The authors also screened the titles and abstracts followed by a full-text review for relevance. Any disagreements were resolved through discussion. The current research relies on a systematic search of the whole literature published from the onset of COVID-19 until 2023. Studies were independently selected in two stages by examining: (a) titles and abstracts and (b) full texts. Computer and manual sources were checked; the most recent search was conducted in 2023 by Lee et al., published on 6th January 2023, and the literature was again checked on 2nd March 2023 to ensure no research paper is missed for the systematic literature review. Witnessing the official announcement of COVID-19 as a global pandemic, the first paper that the authors selected that defined the inclusion criteria was published by Melia et al. on 15th January 2020. For the computer search, three main databases, Web of Science, PubMed through NCBI, and PsycINFO via EBSCOhost, were examined utilising the eligibility criteria. Google Scholar was also used to conduct extra searches, and additional records were also identified from other sources (snowballing method). The research was effectuated by using two clusters of search terms. 'Digital Health Technologies' was used as the first cluster. Given that various studies use different terminologies to refer to digital health technology (e.g. digital health intervention, digital health infrastructure, and the like) precisely, these terminologies were adopted to identify all potential papers. The term 'COVID-19' was central to the second search cluster. Table 9.3 depicts the combination of the employed search

TABLE 9.3 Search terms used in the current review

Digital health technology*, OR	COVID-19, OR
Digital health intervention*, OR	Pandemic, OR
Digital health infrastructure*, OR	Post-pandemic, OR
Digital health ecosystem*, OR	Disaster, OR
Digital health ecosphere*, OR	Epidemic, OR
eHealth, OR	Widespread disease, OR
electronic health record, OR	Fast replicating disease, OR
	Global dilemma, OR
	Clinical symptoms, OR
	2020–2023, OR

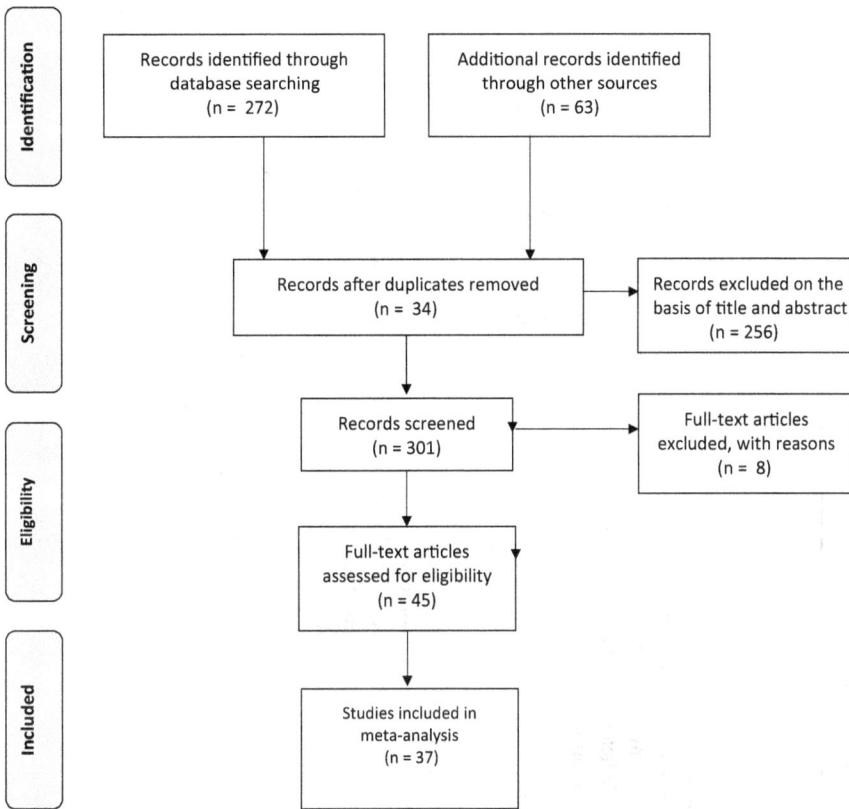

FIGURE 9.1   Flowchart of PRISMA review

terms. There were no geographical or cultural constraints. The bibliographical references of the published studies included in the present paper were manually and carefully checked for any additional suitable studies.

The search yielded 272 possible publications from three databases. Google Scholar and other sources yielded an additional 63 publications. After removing 34 duplicates, 301 papers were evaluated on the basis of the title and abstract, with 256 articles being excluded. The total number of papers covered in the present evaluation is 37, spanning the years from the outbreak of COVID-19 to March 2023 (see Figure 9.1).

Data Extraction and Analysis

Data extraction was performed by both the authors, using a standardised data extraction form to collect relevant information such as study design, population, intervention, comparison, and outcomes. They systematically conducted the quality assessment of the included studies, showcased in the quality assessment of the included studies' table (Table 9.4). The assessment evaluated potential

TABLE 9.4 Summary of meta-analysis studies on digital health interventions

Authors	Year	Number of Studies Included	Sample	Focus Area	Main Conclusion
Kolasa and Kozinski	2020	n = 11	General population	Digital health solutions and decision-makers' pricing and reimbursement framework.	Ensuring scientific rigour for digital health solution evaluation and comparison.
Melia et al.	2020	n = 7	Youth	Testing mobile health (mHealth) tools for suicide prevention.	The apps reduce depression, psychological distress, and self-harm in high-risk individuals and increase coping self-efficacy.
Patel et al.	2020	n = 24	General population	Identifying, assessing, and synthesising qualitative literature on service users' perspectives and interactions of digital health interventions for depression, anxiety, and somatoform disorders.	Personalized digital health interventions are needed.
Gilbey et al.	2020	n = 38	Young people with diverse sexuality	Evidence-based digital health interventions for LGBTIQ+ youth and their efficacy, acceptability, and feasibility.	Need of the digital health interventions for mental and physical health issues, with special targeted interventions for LGBTIQ+ population.
Peiris-John et al.	2020	n = 11	Adolescents	Integrating digital health interventions into secondary school health and well-being with adolescents and health providers.	Accessibility to large-scale youth health survey for better implementation.
Van Rhoon et al.	2020	n = 37	General population	Identifying technology-driven diabetes prevention interventions.	Integrating digital features with behaviour change techniques
Mosnaim et al.	2021	n = 121	Older population	Evaluating the acceptability and efficacy of digital asthma interventions and their potential for monitoring asthma patients.	Digital health interventions offer asthma disease treatment personalisation.
Patel et al.	2021	n = 53	Clinical population	Treatment of obesity through digital health interventions.	Digital health interventions promotes self-monitoring for effective weight loss.

Author	Year	n	Population	Objective	Findings
Wongyibulsin et al.	2021	n = 31	Clinical population	Investigating digital technology interventions for cardiac rehabilitation.	Digital technologies have the potential in mitigating cardiac rehabilitation.
Sasseville et al.	2021	n = 35	Clinical population	Exploring the prevention, detection, and management of chronic mental health problems.	Digital technologies help people in preventing and managing chronic mental health illnesses.
Domhardt et al.	2021	n = 19	Clinical population	Evaluating the efficacy of internet- and mobile-based interventions for different psychological and disease-related outcomes in children and adolescents with chronic medical conditions.	There is limited evidence on improving mental and health-related outcomes among children with chronic medical conditions.
Mclaughlin et al.	2021	n = 19	Adult population	Describing the association between digital health interventions and adult physical activity or sedentary behaviour.	Consistent positive relationship between digital health intervention engagement and physical activity outcomes.
Manyazewal et al.	2021	n = 52	General population	Exploring the impact of digital health technology on clinical and public health practices.	Digital health technology has shown positive results in tackling major clinical and public health backlogs and strengthening health systems.
Kitsiou et al.	2021	n = 25	Clinical population	Evaluating the effects of mobile health interventions on patients with heart failure.	Mobile health interventions reduce mortality but might not reduce all-cause hospitalizations in patients with heart failure.
Mbunge et al.	2022	n = 24	General population	Identifying the potential of virtual healthcare services and digital health technologies.	Digital health technologies have the potential to bridge the digital divide in rural areas and in development of sustainable strategies.
Marthick et al.	2021	n = 20	Clinical population	Evaluating digital health interventions among cancer patients.	Digital health interventions are helpful and effective for supportive care of patients with cancer; however, it needs more research.
Akinosun et al.	2021	n = 25	Clinical population	Identifying the effectiveness of digital technology in determining behaviour change in patients with cardiovascular disease.	Digital interventions are effective in improving healthy behavioural factors.

(Continued)

TABLE 9.4 (Continued)

Authors	Year	Number of Studies Included	Sample	Focus Area	Main Conclusion
Western et al.	2021	n = 19	General population	Exploring digital interventions' efficacy in promoting physical activity in low socio-economic populations.	Digital interventions were not effective enough in targeting physical activity in people of low socio-economic status.
Snoswell et al.	2021	n = 17	Clinical population	Examining the quality of life for patients with asthma using interactive telehealth interventions.	A positive change in the quality of life was observed by the implementation of telehealth interventions for individuals with asthma.
Whitelaw et al.	2021	n = 29	Clinical population	Determining the barriers and facilitators of digital health technology for cardiac patients.	There are a multiple n umber of barriers and facilitators for using the digital health technology in cardiovascular care.
Laranjo et al.	2021	n = 28	General population	Exploring the effectiveness of physical activity interventions involving digital health technology through automated and continuous self-monitoring and feedback.	Interventions using apps and trackers are effective in promoting physical activity, and future studies should explore different intervention components on long-term engagement and effectiveness.
Kouvari et al.	2022	n = 9	Children and adolescents	Examining the effect of technology-based interventions on overweight and obesity treatment in children and adolescents.	Enhancement in weight loss among overweight or obese children and adolescents and improvement of a healthy lifestyle and well-being.
Yao et al.	2022	n = 41	General population	Identifying the inequities in healthcare services through the adoption of digital health technologies.	There are certain limitations in the application of digital health technologies in healthcare services.

Study	Year	n	Population	Aim	Findings
Ridho et al.	2022	n = 16	Clinical population	Efficacy of digital health technology in the treatment of patients with tuberculosis.	The development of digital health technology interventions with personalized feedback is for beneficial effect on medication for patients with tuberculosis.
Leach et al.	2022	n = 19	Clinical population	Exploring trends in digital health interventions in co-occurring disorders in criminal justice settings.	There is limited literature on digital health interventions for criminal justice populations diagnosed with disorders.
Singleton et al.	2022	n = 36	Clinical population	Evaluating the effectiveness of digital interventions for breast cancer patients.	Improvement in quality of life, distress, self-efficacy, and fatigue among patients with breast cancer.
Morris et al.	2022	n = 54	Clinical population	Examining digital technologies to support rural oncology care.	Rural cancer survivors value digital care, so social and behavioural determinants of health and technology must be considered.
Philippe et al.	2022	n = 304	General population	Assessing the state of digital health interventions for the treatment of mental health conditions.	Digital interventions are safer than in-person treatment. However, their applications in mental health need more research.
Chen and Chan	2022	n = 34	General population	Examining the effectiveness of digital health interventions in preventing unintentional injuries, violence, and suicide.	Digital health interventions reduce unintentional injury, violence, and suicide in at-risk populations; however, more research is needed to understand successful interventions.
Peyton et al.	2022	n = 5	General population	Exploring digital health interventions and parental outcomes.	There is no high-quality evidence that digital health interventions can improve parents' mental health literacy.
Harith et al.	2022	n = 7	Youth	Evaluating the efficacy of digital health interventions on university students.	Digital mental health interventions help university students overcome mental health problems, current issues, and barriers.
Manby et al.	2022	n = 25	Clinical population	Effectiveness of eHealth interventions for HIV patients.	Use of eHealth interventions in the improvement of HIV management behaviours.

(Continued)

TABLE 9.4 (Continued)

Authors	Year	Number of Studies Included	Sample	Focus Area	Main Conclusion
Evans et al.	2022	n = 17	Pregnant women	Evaluating remotely delivered digital interventions to support pregnant women with symptoms of anxiety during pregnancy.	Remote digital interventions help pregnant women in disclosing their anxiety symptoms with greater anonymity and help them feel more confident.
Choukou et al.	2023	n = 7	Clinical population	Assessing digital health technology to help healthcare providers and family caregivers to care for patients with cognitive impairment.	High scope of digital health technology for the treatment of patients with cognitive impairment.
Goswami et al.	2023	n = 15	Clinical population	Investigating the use of digital health interventions for minority ethnic population suffering from cardiovascular disease and type 2 diabetes.	Using digital health interventions positively supports minority ethnic populations to help them manage their cardiovascular disease and type 2 diabetes.
Ndayishimiye et al.	2023	n = 46	General population	Exploring the use of digital health technologies to support primary healthcare during COVID-19.	Digital health technology during COVID-19 was essential for primary healthcare delivery and has a great future.
Lee et al.	2023	n = 231	Clinical population	Assessing the digital health for cancer patients.	Positive outcomes of digital health interventions for cancer care.

sources of bias, including selection, performance, detection, attrition, and reporting biases. The authors also performed a narrative synthesis to summarise the findings, given the heterogeneity of the included studies. Studies were selected independently by both the authors. Author one extracted data in standardised tables, which were then verified by author two. The objective was to assess the frequency of data extraction errors and their potential impact on the results of systematic reviews of interventions. Moreover, the effect of different extraction methods (e.g. independent data extraction by the two authors versus verification by the second author) and later the results were evaluated together. This thorough approach aimed to ensure the accuracy and reliability of the review's findings.

Best Practices: The Indian Scenario

In order to transform India into a knowledge economy with mobile access to information, government, and services, the Government of India (GoI) commenced the 'Digital India' campaign in 2015. Over the past few years, the nation has surpassed all other nations in the world's digital adoption rate. India has grown into a significant player in the technological world. The quick upsurge of digital permeation, coupled with the outstanding space technology accomplishments of the Indian Space Research Organization (ISRO), and the emergence of India-trained CEOs heading the most appreciated technological businesses in the world are all evidence of this (Ranganathan, 2020).

However, the state of healthcare in India is still far from being ideal. Compared to what the World Health Organization (WHO) suggests as the ideal number of physicians, nurses, medical technicians, and healthcare facilities needed to serve the population, it falls significantly short of the target (Ranganathan, 2020).

Federated National Health Information System: India's Plot

The Indian Ministry of Health and Family Welfare (MoHFW) has started implementing policy measures to digitise healthcare. A 'Federated National Health Information System' is presented as a thorough architectural framework published in January 2020. It suggests tying together systems from primary, secondary, and tertiary care value chains inside private and public health providers' organisations. This is consistent with the National Health Policy's 2017 goal, which is to develop an integrated health information system for all parties involved in the health system to increase effectiveness, transparency, and citizen satisfaction (Ranganathan, 2020).

Ayushman Bharat Digital Mission (ABDM)

The mission seeks to create the framework to sustain the nation's integrated digital health infrastructure. It would bridge the distance between the various healthcare ecosystem stakeholders via advanced digital solutions and digital highways.

Many such revolutionary best practices in digital infrastructure are being adopted and implemented in India. These facilities are equipped to provide the finest healthcare solutions to people from all states in the country, drawing inspiration from the Western world.

Future Recommendations

In order to maintain continuous readiness, such healthcare capabilities should be updated and tested frequently between disasters (Scott et al., 2020). More analysis and research into digital technologies, specifically their long-term usefulness, are required as more unique technologies become available and more people participate in remote healthcare monitoring. Additionally, it should be considered to adopt developing technologies that have been assessed and/or verified into clinical practice as therapy and preventative modalities (Zwack et al., 2023). Most imperatively, research should be accelerated in this domain, emphasising the popular digital health technologies that could be further recommended for many patient requirements (of all ages) and purposes. This entails adherence, lifestyle, and patient involvement, which are crucial factors in determining a holistic patient's health in today's era.

Limitations

Given the astounding results of digital health technologies, it is also very critical to recognise some brewing ethical limitations. These technologies can potentially alter the personal freedom of choice, values, and obligations arising in relationships between medical professionals and their patients during a clinical encounter (Kulikowski, 2022). The often exaggerated claims made today by digital health technologies about '*resolving and deciphering*' clinical problems with proficient algorithms and data primarily devalue the role of the clinical judgements inherently fundamental in personal clinical encounters and consider them to be precisely insignificant (Kulikowski, 2022).

Most intriguing, the over-dependence on data and machine learning and such oversimplified models pose pressing concerns about how inclusivity, equity, safety, and bias are handled in such practical systems. In the real and the ideal world, the ethical obligations of individual patients and practitioners intertwine with communities. They are central to how clinical encounters evolve with and in the future of digital health (Kulikowski, 2022).

Conclusion

With everything gathered, it is imperative to be cognizant of the digital health innovation that aims to support patients and surveillance; enhance outcomes; and encourage early diagnoses, prevention, and therapies (Abernethy et al., 2022;

Golinelli et al., 2020). However, there has been and will continue to be considerable speculation about such implications for holistic human health and the positive and negative repercussions of such digital health changes beyond human endeavours (Abernethy et al., 2022; Arigo et al., 2019).

As a responsible community, one must consciously continue to work towards bracing and training the workforce of the twenty-first century for a better digital health ecosystem, mindfully working towards advancing such methods with the desire for rigour and the need to support ethical practices for promoting healthy behaviour. For a fully embracing digital health, the concerned authorities, public–private partnerships, and robust academic–industry collaborations must ensure the ethical and just use of data, facilitating the near-real-time gathering, storing, protecting, and sharing of correct datasets with the derived insights (Arigo et al., 2019). In addition, based on the generated actionable intelligence, such digital solutions must continue to ensure revolutionary improvements in medical treatment and in specific matters with patient security (Abernethy et al., 2022; Kulikowski, 2022).

Realising and envisaging a seamless, healthier future through digital health that ascertains quality and equitable care for all will require a promising investment in evidence-based research, more clinical and field investigations, and a deeper commitment from all the respective stakeholders.

Digital health solutions have proven to be effective in addressing chronic mental and physical health challenges, fostering self-monitoring, and delivering personalised care for various demographics. These innovations resolve clinical and public health bottlenecks, close the digital gap, and enhance access to health services. Nonetheless, further research is required to comprehend their effectiveness in specific scenarios, such as cancer patient support, mental health initiatives, and programmes for vulnerable groups. Although certain limitations exist, digital health technology has played a crucial role in healthcare provision, particularly during the COVID-19 crisis, and holds immense potential for future advancements.

References

Akinosun, A. S., Polson, R., Diaz-Skeete, Y., De Kock, J. H., Carragher, L., Leslie, S., . . . Gorely, T. (2021). Digital technology interventions for risk factor modification in patients with cardiovascular disease: Systematic review and meta-analysis. *JMIR mHealth and uHealth*, *9*(3), e21061. https://doi.org/10.2196/21061

Anderson, J. T., Bouchacourt, L. M., Sussman, K. L., Bright, L. F., & Wilcox, G. B. (2022). Telehealth adoption during the COVID-19 pandemic: A social media textual and network analysis. *Digital Health*, *8*, 20552076221090041. https://doi.org/10.1177/20552076221090041

Arigo, D., Jake-Schoffman, D. E., Wolin, K., Beckjord, E., Hekler, E. B., & Pagoto, S. L. (2019). The history and future of digital health in the field of behavioral medicine. *Journal of Behavioral Medicine*, *42*, 67–83.

Asi, Y. M., & Williams, C. (2018). The role of digital health in making progress toward Sustainable Development Goal (SDG) 3 in conflict-affected populations. *International Journal of Medical Informatics*, *114*, 114–120.

Awad, A., Trenfield, S. J., Pollard, T. D., Ong, J. J., Elbadawi, M., McCoubrey, L. E., . . . Basit, A. W. (2021). Connected healthcare: Improving patient care using digital health technologies. *Advanced Drug Delivery Reviews, 178,* 113958.

Biggs, J. S., Willcocks, A., Burger, M., & Makeham, M. A. (2019). Digital health benefits evaluation frameworks: Building the evidence to support Australia's National Digital Health Strategy. *Medical Journal of Australia, 210,* S9–S11.

Blaya, J. A., Fraser, H. S., & Holt, B. (2010). E-health technologies show promise in developing countries. *Health Affairs, 29*(2), 244–251.

Chen, M., & Chan, K. L. (2022). Effectiveness of digital health interventions on unintentional injury, violence, and suicide: Meta-analysis. *Trauma, Violence, & Abuse, 23*(2), 605–619. https://doi.org/10.1177/1524838020967

Choukou, M. A., Olatoye, F., Urbanowski, R., Caon, M., & Monnin, C. (2023). Digital health technology to support health care professionals and family caregivers caring for patients with cognitive impairment: Scoping review. *JMIR Mental Health, 10,* e40330.

Davenport, T., & Kalakota, R. (2019). The potential for artificial intelligence in healthcare. *Future Healthcare Journal, 6*(2), 94–98. https://doi.org/10.7861/futurehosp.6-2-94

Domhardt, M., Schröder, A., Geirhos, A., Steubl, L., & Baumeister, H. (2021). Efficacy of digital health interventions in youth with chronic medical conditions: A meta-analysis. *Internet Interventions, 24,* 100373. https://doi.org/10.1016/j.invent.2021.100373

Evans, K., Rennick-Egglestone, S., Cox, S., Kuipers, Y., & Spiby, H. (2022). Remotely delivered interventions to support women with symptoms of anxiety in pregnancy: Mixed methods systematic review and meta-analysis. *Journal of Medical Internet Research, 24*(2), e28093. https://doi.org/10.2196/28093

Fagherazzi, G., Goetzinger, C., Rashid, M. A., Aguayo, G. A., & Huiart, L. (2020). Digital health strategies to fight COVID-19 worldwide: Challenges, recommendations, and a call for papers. *Journal of Medical Internet Research, 22*(6), e19284.

Fan, K., & Zhao, Y. (2022). Mobile health technology: A novel tool in chronic disease management. *Intelligent Medicine, 2*(1), 41–47.

Foley, K., Freeman, T., Ward, P., Lawler, A., Osborne, R., & Fisher, M. (2021). Exploring access to, use of and benefits from population-oriented digital health services in Australia. *Health Promotion International, 36*(4), 1105–1115.

Gilbey, D., Morgan, H., Lin, A., & Perry, Y. (2020). Effectiveness, acceptability, and feasibility of digital health interventions for LGBTIQ+ young people: Systematic review. *Journal of Medical Internet Research, 22*(12), e20158. https://doi.org/10.2196/20158

Golinelli, D., Boetto, E., Carullo, G., Nuzzolese, A. G., Landini, M. P., & Fantini, M. P. (2020). Adoption of digital technologies in health care during the COVID-19 pandemic: Systematic review of early scientific literature. *Journal of Medical Internet Research, 22*(11), e22280.

Goswami, A., Poole, L., Thorlu-Bangura, Z., Khan, N., Hanif, W., Khunti, K., Gill, P., Sajid, M., Blandford, A., Stevenson, F., Banerjee, A., & Ramasawmy, M. (2023). The use of digital health interventions for cardiometabolic diseases among South Asian and Black Minority Ethnic Groups: Realist review. *Journal of Medical Internet Research, 25,* e40630. https://doi.org/10.2196/40630

Harith, S., Backhaus, I., Mohbin, N., Ngo, H. T., & Khoo, S. (2022). Effectiveness of digital mental health interventions for university students: An umbrella review. *PeerJ, 10,* e13111. https://doi.org/10.7717%2Fpeerj.13111

Howitt, P., Darzi, A., Yang, G. Z., Ashrafian, H., Atun, R., Barlow, J., . . . Wilson, E. (2012). Technologies for global health. *The Lancet, 380*(9840), 507–535.

Ibrahim, H., Liu, X., Zariffa, N., Morris, A. D., & Denniston, A. K. (2021). Health data poverty: An assailable barrier to equitable digital health care. *The Lancet Digital Health, 3*(4), e260–e265. https://doi.org/10.1016/S2589-7500(20)30317-4

Imison, C., Castle-Clarke, S., Watson, R., & Edwards, N. (2016). *Delivering the benefits of digital health care* (pp. 5–6). Nuffield Trust.

Kitsiou, S., Vatani, H., Paré, G., Gerber, B. S., Buchholz, S. W., Kansal, M. M., . . . Creber, R. M. M. (2021). Effectiveness of mobile health technology interventions for patients with heart failure: Systematic review and meta-analysis. *Canadian Journal of Cardiology, 37*(8), 1248–1259. https://doi.org/10.1016/j.cjca.2021.02.015

Kolasa, K., & Kozinski, G. (2020). How to value digital health interventions? A systematic literature review. *International Journal of Environmental Research and Public Health, 17*(6), 2119. https://doi.org/10.3390/ijerph17062119

Kouvari, M., Karipidou, M., Tsiampalis, T., Mamalaki, E., Poulimeneas, D., Bathrellou, E., . . . Yannakoulia, M. (2022). Digital health interventions for weight management in children and adolescents: Systematic review and meta-analysis. *Journal of Medical Internet Research, 24*(2), e30675. https://doi.org/10.2196/30675

Kulikowski, C. A. (2022). Ethics in the history of medical informatics for decision-making: Early challenges to digital health goals. *Yearbook of Medical Informatics, 31*(1), 317–322.

Labrique, A. B., Wadhwani, C., Williams, K. A., Lamptey, P., Hesp, C., Luk, R., & Aerts, A. (2018). Best practices in scaling digital health in low and middle income countries. *Globalization and Health, 14*, 1–8.

Laranjo, L., Ding, D., Heleno, B., Kocaballi, B., Quiroz, J. C., Tong, H. L., . . . Bates, D. W. (2021). Do smartphone applications and activity trackers increase physical activity in adults? Systematic review, meta-analysis and metaregression. *British Journal of Sports Medicine, 55*(8), 422–432. http://dx.doi.org/10.1136/bjsports-2020-102892

Leach, R., Carreiro, S., Shaffer, P. M., Gaba, A., & Smelson, D. (2022). Digital health interventions for mental health, substance use, and co-occurring disorders in the criminal justice population: A scoping review. *Frontiers in Psychiatry, 12*, 2455. https://doi.org/10.3389/fpsyt.2021.794785

Lee, K., Kim, S., Kim, S. H., Yoo, S. H., Sung, J. H., Oh, E. G., . . . Lee, J. (2023). Digital health interventions for adult patients with cancer evaluated in randomized controlled trials: Scoping review. *Journal of Medical Internet Research, 25*, e38333. https://doi.org/10.2196/38333

Manby, L., Aicken, C., Delgrange, M., & Bailey, J. V. (2022). Effectiveness of ehealth interventions for HIV prevention and management in sub-Saharan Africa: Systematic review and meta-analyses. *AIDS and Behavior, 26*(2), 457–469. https://doi.org/10.1007/s10461-021-03402-w

Manyazewal, T., Woldeamanuel, Y., Blumberg, H. M., Fekadu, A., & Marconi, V. C. (2021). The potential use of digital health technologies in the African context: A systematic review of evidence from Ethiopia. *NPJ Digital Medicine, 4*(1), 125. https://doi.org/10.1038/s41746-021-00487-4

Marthick, M., McGregor, D., Alison, J., Cheema, B., Dhillon, H., & Shaw, T. (2021). Supportive care interventions for people with cancer assisted by digital technology: Systematic review. *Journal of Medical Internet Research, 23*(10), e24722. https://doi.org/10.2196/24722

Mbunge, E., Batani, J., Gaobotse, G., & Muchemwa, B. (2022). Virtual healthcare services and digital health technologies deployed during coronavirus disease 2019 (COVID-19)

pandemic in South Africa: A systematic review. *Global Health Journal*. https://doi. org/10.1016/j.glohj.2022.03.001

Mclaughlin, M., Delaney, T., Hall, A., Byaruhanga, J., Mackie, P., Grady, A., . . . Wolfenden, L. (2021). Associations between digital health intervention engagement, physical activity, and sedentary behavior: Systematic review and meta-analysis. *Journal of Medical Internet Research, 23*(2), e23180. https://doi.org/10.2196/23180

Melia, R., Francis, K., Hickey, E., Bogue, J., Duggan, J., O'Sullivan, M., & Young, K. (2020). Mobile health technology interventions for suicide prevention: Systematic review. *JMIR mHealth and uHealth, 8*(1), e12516. https://doi.org/10.2196/12516

Morris, B. B., Rossi, B., & Fuemmeler, B. (2022). The role of digital health technology in rural cancer care delivery: A systematic review. *The Journal of Rural Health, 38*(3), 493–511. https://doi.org/10.1111/jrh.12619

Mosnaim, G., Safioti, G., Brown, R., DePietro, M., Szefler, S. J., Lang, D. M., . . . Merchant, R. K. (2021). Digital health technology in asthma: A comprehensive scoping review. *The Journal of Allergy and Clinical Immunology: In Practice, 9*(6), 2377–2398. https://doi. org/10.1016/j.jaip.2021.02.028

Ndayishimiye, C., Lopes, H., & Middleton, J. (2023). A systematic scoping review of digital health technologies during COVID-19: A new normal in primary health care delivery. *Health and Technology*, 1–12. https://doi.org/10.1007/s12553-023-00725-7

Nikolich-Zugich, J., Knox, K. S., Rios, C. T., Natt, B., Bhattacharya, D., & Fain, M. J. (2020). SARS-CoV-2 and COVID-19 in older adults: What we may expect regarding pathogenesis, immune responses, and outcomes. *Geroscience, 42*, 505–514. https://doi. org/10.1007/s11357-020-00193-1

Pai, M. M., Ganiga, R., Pai, R. M., & Sinha, R. K. (2021). Standard electronic health record (EHR) framework for Indian healthcare system. *Health Services and Outcomes Research Methodology, 21*(3), 339–362.

Patel, M. L., Wakayama, L. N., & Bennett, G. G. (2021). Self-monitoring via digital health in weight loss interventions: A systematic review among adults with overweight or obesity. *Obesity, 29*(3), 478–499. https://doi.org/10.1002/oby.23088

Patel, S., Akhtar, A., Malins, S., Wright, N., Rowley, E., Young, E., . . . Morriss, R. (2020). The acceptability and usability of digital health interventions for adults with depression, anxiety, and somatoform disorders: Qualitative systematic review and meta-synthesis. *Journal of Medical Internet Research, 22*(7), e16228. https://doi.org/10.2196/16228

Peiris-John, R., Dizon, L., Sutcliffe, K., Kang, K., & Fleming, T. (2020). Co-creating a large-scale adolescent health survey integrated with access to digital health interventions. *Digital Health, 6*, 2055207620947962. https://doi.org/10.1177/2055207620947962

Perakslis, E., & Ginsburg, G. S. (2021). Digital health – The need to assess benefits, risks, and value. *JAMA, 325*(2), 127–128.

Petracca, F., Ciani, O., Cucciniello, M., & Tarricone, R. (2020). Harnessing digital health technologies during and after the COVID-19 pandemic: Context matters. *Journal of Medical Internet Research, 22*(12), e21815.

Peyton, D., Goods, M., & Hiscock, H. (2022). The effect of digital health interventions on parents' mental health literacy and help seeking for their child's mental health problem: Systematic review. *Journal of Medical Internet Research, 24*(2), e28771. https://doi. org/10.2196/28771

Philippe, T. J., Sikder, N., Jackson, A., Koblanski, M. E., Liow, E., Pilarinos, A., & Vasarhelyi, K. (2022). Digital health interventions for delivery of mental health care: Systematic and comprehensive meta-review. *JMIR Mental Health, 9*(5), e35159. https://doi. org/10.2196/35159

Ranganathan, S. (2020, April). Towards a holistic digital health ecosystem in India. *Observer Research Foundation.* https://www.orfonline.org/research/towards-a-holistic-digital-health-ecosystem-in-india-63993

Ridho, A., Alfian, S. D., van Boven, J. F., Levita, J., Yalcin, E. A., Le, L., . . . Pradipta, I. S. (2022). Digital health technologies to improve medication adherence and treatment outcomes in patients with tuberculosis: Systematic review of randomized controlled trials. *Journal of Medical Internet Research, 24*(2), e33062. https://doi.org/10.2196/33062

Sasseville, M., LeBlanc, A., Boucher, M., Dugas, M., Mbemba, G., Tchuente, J., . . . Gagnon, M. P. (2021). Digital health interventions for the management of mental health in people with chronic diseases: A rapid review. *BMJ Open, 11*(4), e044437. http://dx.doi.org/10.1136/bmjopen-2020-044437

Scott, B. K., Miller, G. T., Fonda, S. J., Yeaw, R. E., Gaudaen, J. C., Pavliscsak, H. H., . . . Pamplin, J. C. (2020). Advanced digital health technologies for COVID-19 and future emergencies. *Telemedicine and e-Health, 26*(10), 1226–1233.

Singleton, A. C., Raeside, R., Hyun, K. K., Partridge, S. R., Di Tanna, G. L., Hafiz, N., . . . Redfern, J. (2022). Electronic health interventions for patients with breast cancer: Systematic review and meta-analyses. *Journal of Clinical Oncology, 40*(20), 2257–2270. https://doi.org/10.1200/JCO.21.01171

Snoswell, C. L., Rahja, M., & Lalor, A. F. (2021). A systematic review and meta-analysis of change in health-related quality of life for interactive telehealth interventions for patients with asthma. *Value in Health, 24*(2), 291–302. https://doi.org/10.1016/j.jval.2020.09.006

Solomon, D. H., & Rudin, R. S. (2020). Digital health technologies: Opportunities and challenges in rheumatology. *Nature Reviews Rheumatology, 16*(9), 525–535.

Suhas, S., Kumar, C. N., Math, S. B., & Manjunatha, N. (2022). E-Sanjeevani: A pathbreaking telemedicine initiative from India. *Journal of Psychiatry Spectrum, 1*(2), 111–116. https://doi.org/10.4103/jopsys.jopsys_8_21

Sutton, R. T., Pincock, D., Baumgart, D. C., Sadowski, D. C., Fedorak, R. N., & Kroeker, K. I. (2020). An overview of clinical decision support systems: Benefits, risks, and strategies for success. *NPJ Digital Medicine, 3*(1), 17. https://doi.org/10.1038/s41746-020-0221-y

Tilahun, B., Gashu, K. D., Mekonnen, Z. A., Endehabtu, B. F., & Angaw, D. A. (2021). Mapping the role of digital health technologies in prevention and control of COVID-19 pandemic: Review of the literature. *Yearbook of Medical Informatics, 30*(1), 026–037.

Van Rhoon, L., Byrne, M., Morrissey, E., Murphy, J., & McSharry, J. (2020). A systematic review of the behaviour change techniques and digital features in technology-driven type 2 diabetes prevention interventions. *Digital Health, 6,* 2055207620914427. https://doi.org/10.1177/2055207620914427

West, D. M. (2016). How 5G technology enables the health internet of things. *Brookings Center for Technology Innovation, 3*(1), 20.

Western, M. J., Armstrong, M. E., Islam, I., Morgan, K., Jones, U. F., & Kelson, M. J. (2021). The effectiveness of digital interventions for increasing physical activity in individuals of low socioeconomic status: A systematic review and meta-analysis. *International Journal of Behavioral Nutrition and Physical Activity, 18*(1), 1–21. https://doi.org/10.1186/s12966-021-01218-4

Whitelaw, S., Pellegrini, D. M., Mamas, M. A., Cowie, M., & Van Spall, H. G. (2021). Barriers and facilitators of the uptake of digital health technology in cardiovascular care: A systematic scoping review. *European Heart Journal-Digital Health, 2*(1), 62–74. https://doi.org/10.1093/ehjdh/ztab005

Wongvibulsin, S., Habeos, E. E., Huynh, P. P., Xun, H., Shan, R., Porosnicu Rodriguez, K. A., . . . Martin, S. S. (2021). Digital health interventions for cardiac rehabilitation:

Systematic literature review. *Journal of Medical Internet Research, 23*(2), e18773. https://doi.org/10.2196/18773

World Health Organization. (2019). *Digital health for the end TB strategy*. Retrieved from www.who.int/tb/areas-of-work/digital-health/en/

World Health Organization. (2020). WHO Director-General's opening remarks at the media briefing on COVID-19 – 11 March 2020. Retrieved from https://www.who.int/director-general/speeches/detail/who-director-general-s-opening-remarks-at-the-media-briefing-on-covid-19---11-march-2020

Yao, R., Zhang, W., Evans, R., Cao, G., Rui, T., & Shen, L. (2022). Inequities in health care services caused by the adoption of digital health technologies: Scoping review. *Journal of Medical Internet Research, 24*(3), e34144. https://doi.org/10.2196/34144

Zwack, C. C., Haghani, M., Hollings, M., Zhang, L., Gauci, S., Gallagher, R., & Redfern, J. (2023). The evolution of digital health technologies in cardiovascular disease research. *NPJ Digital Medicine, 6*(1), 1.

10

EFFICACY OF DIGITAL INFRASTRUCTURE PROVIDING PSYCHOLOGICAL SUPPORT AMONG GLOBAL ADULT POPULATION DURING THE COVID-19 PANDEMIC

A Systematic Review

Ravi Shanker Datti, Nidhi Mishra,
Maneela Sirisety and Ashutosh Tewari

Introduction

One of the major crises in any healthcare system is the non-availability of treatment services to the target population who need these services or interventions to reduce the healthcare burden. To address this concern, researchers and practitioners have adopted one of the solutions, "digital health innovations using health informatics", and revolutionised clinical and research practices (Brewer et al., 2020). Currently, psychological services using digital infrastructure are being used to reach out to communities that need psychological support and to engage them equally. These digital health technologies and other stakeholders like healthcare service providers and digital tools create a robust ecosystem for patient care. With the advent of mobile health technologies, it is evident that the services for mental health problems have seen growth in health-based applications delivering interventions using these technologies (Lecomte et al., 2020).

Consequently, the investment costs and infrastructure around mental health are lower due to the unique potential these health technologies have, which can create access to care even in lower-income nations (Rudd & Beidas, 2020). Though health informatics made a considerable ground in terms of providing services, still there is a considerable gap providing these services in the mental health settings. These gaps have further widened due to digital divides and inequities. Furthermore, these digital health infrastructures' success depends on user acceptance, engagement, and stepped-care models (Linardon et al., 2022).

The digital infrastructure has created an opportunity to provide psychological services to meet therapists anytime and anywhere due to their unique properties at both the hardware and software levels. At the hardware level, these can be related to the wireless technologies, connectivity, and sensors used to capture health

DOI: 10.4324/9781003357209-13

parameters and compactness. From a software perspective, these can be applications built and the ease of sharing health informatics between the stakeholders (Torous et al., 2021). These advancements have proliferated across different users. However, a 2018 survey on mobile phone ownership data reported that in emerging economies, only 45% owned a smartphone (Silver, 2020). Despite a digital divide and inequity, it is still viable to consider the number of people who would have access to these digital technologies or technologies that support these devices (Torous et al., 2021). Routes to deliver psychological services can be in the form of telehealth and mobile health (mHealth), which is an emerging area revolutionising health promotion. Healthcare delivery through mHealth using sophisticated digital technologies like mobile apps, health monitors, text messages, and sensors that help track and record health parameters in wearable devices provided an unprecedented opportunity to reach and engage communities in synchronous and asynchronous environments (Steinhubl et al., 2015). These technologies can foster mental healthcare in ways that can reach the target population. Primarily, they have ways of capturing rich health data that can be helpful in monitoring, diagnosis, and prognosis of the health condition.

Further, the advancement of machine learning has helped practitioners and service providers develop insights and predict the health behaviours of users. Finally, analysing the big data of health informatics gave a broad scope for interventions to be delivered through these routes via apps, virtual therapies, personalised protocols, emergency care, and clinical care (Timakum et al., 2022; Torous et al., 2021). It allowed an unprecedented growth in digital health services for mental healthcare, substantially impacting the population that needed these psychological services, especially during the COVID-19 pandemic. The major challenge that practitioners face is trying to deliver their health services through available routes, and few have the technical know-how to deliver them. Further, how effective these services can be using these technologies is still being explored.

The pandemic of COVID-19 hastened the acceptance of digital healthcare. As a reaction to it, many healthcare facilities and clinical services were rolled back or even ceased (Ting et al., 2020). During the pandemic, across the globe, high priority was given to restricting the spread of COVID-19. Lockdown restrictions led to many challenges for the stakeholders to deliver the required services to the target population. Concerns regarding patient health safety and patients with pre-existing diseases became another challenge. Postponing mental healthcare services or restricting the services is not a viable choice in the long run. Healthcare practitioners started offering their services through digital routes to meet the challenge. To say the same was true in the case of mental health services is still contentious. However, mental health services did address the unwarranted changes or disruptions by adopting video or teleconferencing at the synchronous level (Ganjali et al., 2022). In the asynchronous modes, these psychological services have been catered to during the pandemic through guided and unguided formats such as online mental health resources (Richardson et al., 2020). Despite these changes and adaptations, many countries needed comprehensive readiness within healthcare systems (Mohammadpour et al., 2021). It could be because they need more infrastructure and technical know-how to enable digital care delivery. Thus, services provided under these digital health technologies need to be delivered with a sense of caution. Consequently, the impetus could be whether digital health technologies have improved the service provision and the challenges in implementing these healthcare provisioning systems.

Therefore, this study attempts to systematically review how effective these digital infrastructures were in providing psychological support during the COVID-19 pandemic to the adult population. The objective of this systematic examination had three main goals: (a) to identify the effects of digital intervention on psychological health; (b) to identify the risk and protective factors associated with receiving digital therapeutic support; and (3) to identify the implications and barriers and to understand the structure of these findings.

Method

The systematic review was carried out by following PRISMA guidelines and registered with PROSPERO (registration number: CRD42022370432).

Eligibility Criteria

The inclusion criteria were: (a) participants who are older than 18 years; (b) participants who are diagnosed with or observed to have a psychological problem; (c) studies that show the effect of a psychological intervention provided through online platforms when compared to the control group; and (d) randomised controlled trials. The exclusion criteria were: (a) papers with no full-text availability; (b) papers published in languages other than English; (c) protocols and pilot studies; and (d) studies conducted before the pandemic.

Information Sources and Search Strategy

The studies included in the review were searched from seven online sources, which include Scopus, PubMed, APA PsycINFO, EBSCO, ProQuest, the Cochrane Central Register of Controlled Trials (CENTRAL), and Wiley Library, between December 2019 and August 2022. Both published and unpublished studies are included during this stage to remove publication bias. All the searches are reassessed before the final analysis. The search terms were Telehealth, mHealth, eHealth, Videoconferencing, Mobile Applications, Mental Health Services, Mental Health Therapy, and Psychotherapy. A detailed search strategy is presented in Table 10.1.

TABLE 10.1 Search strategy used and the number of results generated

Sl. No.	Database	Number of Results	Search Strategy
1	Scopus	546	(("Telehealth" OR "mHealth" OR
2	PubMed	132	"eHealth" OR "Videoconferencing"
3	APA PsycInfo	123	OR "Mobile Applications" OR
4	EBSCO	325	"Smartphone") AND ("Mental Health
5	ProQuest	112	Services" OR "Mental Health therapy"
6	CENTRAL	485	OR "Psychotherapy") AND ("RCT" OR
7	Wiley	531	"Randomized trial*" OR "Randomized
			controlled trial" OR "Randomised
			controlled trial"))

Note: The search strategy was limited by the studies published in the English language between December 2019 and August 2022.

Selection of Studies (PICO)

The selection of studies is made with the help of the PICO (Population, Intervention, Control, and Outcomes) criteria. Only studies published in the English language are considered. Two reviewers (R.D., M.S.) independently screened the records, and the disagreements were solved through discussion.

Population

Participants older than 18 years and with psychological concerns were included.

Intervention/Control

This systematic review did not focus on specific psychological interventions but rather on the efficacy of psychological treatment received by adults via digital infrastructure compared to the waitlist control group (who either did not receive any support initially or received support differently from the intervention group). Here, the psychological treatment includes, but is not limited to, cognitive behavioural therapy, dialectical behavioural therapy, acceptance therapy, and other evidence-based therapies. The digital infrastructure includes telephone-based therapy, web-based therapy, therapies using digital applications, chat-based therapy, and mobile health applications.

Outcomes

The description of the results includes the following:

1 Effect of digital intervention on psychological health
2 The risk and protective factors associated with receiving digital therapeutic support
3 Researchers' recommendations along with the implications

Type of Studies

This review exclusively included randomised controlled trials.

Data Extraction

Two researchers (N.M., A.T.) did the data extraction process independently. All papers retrieved by the search strategy are screened for relevance, and those irrelevant are discarded. The eligible studies were noticed using the predefined inclusion and exclusion criteria. The disagreements were resolved through consensus after thorough discussions.

From the studies identified, the following information is extracted and presented in Table 10.2: (a) author and year of publication; (b) study population, including mean age (with range) and psychological condition; (c) intervention, including the type of the intervention, attrition, and duration to follow-up; and (d) study outcomes, including the effect of digital psychological intervention received. Two researchers (R.D., M.S.) have analysed the study characteristics.

Assessment of Risk of Bias

The Cochrane Risk of Bias tool for Randomised Trials (RoB 2.0) was used to assess the risk of bias in parallel-group and crossover trials. The studies were evaluated for risk of bias (low, some, or high concerns) arising from the randomisation process, effects of assignment to intervention and adherence to the intervention, missing data, measurement of outcome, and selection of results reported in the study. The risk of bias was evaluated by two independent researchers (R.D., M.S.), and any disputes were resolved through consensus with the assistance of a third researcher (N.M.).

Data Analysis

The review considers narrative synthesis to understand and explain the studies included for review. The results were synthesised on the basis of the similarities and differences emerging from the studies included for review. They are comparing different psychological supports (therapies and training) provided through different mediums (videoconferencing, mobile apps, and materials); comparing similar psychological interventions and problems; and comparing synchronous and asynchronous modes of psychological support.

The heterogeneity in the outcomes arising from the variations in the therapeutic protocols used during the intervention was also observed. These variations can be due to the session plans considered by these studies (such as structured or unstructured and the number of sessions). Conclusions were made by examining the quantitative measurement such as effect sizes.

TABLE 10.2 Descriptive details of the included studies

Authors (Year)	Age M [range]	Diagnosis	Therapy (n)	Attrition (%)	Treatment Length	Follow-up	Summary of relevant findings	*Quality Appraisal
Al-Refae et al. (2021)	25.2 [18–66]	Depression, anxiety, stress	Mindfulness and self-compassion-based cognitive mobile app (serene) (78) versus WLC (87)	Active arm: 38 Waitlist control: 26	Four weeks	None	There were notable differences between groups in terms of decisiveness (d = 0.34), depressive symptoms (d = −0.43), and self-compassion (d = 0.6), showing improvements in common humanity, self-kindness, mindfulness, reductions in isolation, overidentification, and self-judgement. The intervention group demonstrated a moderate decrease in anxiety symptoms (d = −0.47) and stress (d = −0.52) within the group.	Some concerns

Study	Age	Condition	Intervention	Sample	Duration	Follow-up	Results	Quality
Al-Alawi et al. (2021)	28.5 [range not reported]	Anxiety and depression	The therapist-guided online CBT and ACT (22) versus a newsletter delivered via email that provided self-help information and strategies for coping with distress related to COVID-19 (24).	Active arm: 26 Waitlist control: 20	Six weeks	None	Both study groups experienced a decrease in levels of anxiety and depression. However, the intervention group had a more significant reduction in symptoms than the control group (p = .049 vs. p = .02, respectively)	Low
Ben-Zeev et al. (2021)	37.9 [18–78]	Bipolar disorder, major depressive disorder, schizophrenia or schizoaffective disorder	CORE app (daily activities aimed at re-evaluating dysfunctional beliefs) (154) versus WLC (161)	Active arm: 58.4 Waitlist control: 51.1	30 days	30 days	The intervention group demonstrated significant effects on the RSES (d = 0.64), RAS (d = 0.58), and BDI-II (d = 0.58), a moderate effect on SDS (d = 0.44), and a negligible effect on GAD-7 (d = 0.20). Similar results were observed when the waitlist control group received CORE after 30 days.	Low

(Continued)

TABLE 10.2 (Continued)

Authors (Year)	Age M [range]	Diagnosis	Therapy (n)	Attrition (%)	Treatment Length	Follow-up	Summary of relevant findings	*Quality Appraisal
Catuara-Solarz et al. (2022)	40.0 [30–50]	Anxiety and stress	Foundations app (comprises interventions and psychoeducational content) (95) versus WLC (95)	Active arm: 22.1 Waitlist control: 34.7	Four weeks	None	The intervention group showed improvements in anxiety, resilience, sleep, and well-being measures compared to the control group within two weeks of using the app, and these effects became more pronounced at week 4.	Some concerns
Chang et al. (2022)	21.3 [range not reported]	Anxiety, depression, stress. Individuals with no psychological problems are also considered.	Online Isha Upa Yoga (326) versus WLC (352)	Active arm: 65 (week 4) and 89 (week 12) Waitlist control: 55 (week 4) and 87 (week 12)	Four weeks	12 weeks	By the fourth week, the intervention group demonstrated a significant decrease in stress levels (d = .27) and an improvement in well-being (d = .32). After the study, both the intervention and control group showed improvements in well-being, anxiety, depression, stress, and positive and negative affect.	High

Study	Age	Disorder	Intervention	Sample	Duration	Follow-up	Findings	Risk
Linardon et al. (2022)	28.9 [range not reported]	Eating disorder	Transdiagnostic cognitive behavioural therapy delivered through a mobile app (197) versus WLC (195)	Active arm: 51.2 (post-treatment) and 65.4 (follow-up) Waitlist control: 20 (post-treatment) and 67 (follow-up)	Four weeks	Eight weeks	Participants in the intervention group showed significant reductions in ED psychopathology at the post-test, and the symptoms remained stable during follow-up compared to the control group.	Some concerns
Maroti et al. (2022)	I: 43.3 [23–64]; C: 42.5 [26–62]	Somatic symptom disorder	Internet-administered emotional awareness and expression therapy (I-EAET) (37) versus WLC (37)	Active arm: 8 (post-treatment) and 11 (follow-up) Waitlist control: 3 (post-treatment) and 8 (follow-up)	Ten weeks	Four months	The intervention group significantly reduced somatic symptoms at both the post-treatment and follow-up stages compared to controls. Though the effects were not sustained at the follow-up stage, at the post-treatment stage, a significant reduction in pain, insomnia, depression, and anxiety levels was observed among the intervention group. The benefits of the intervention were partially due to emotional processing.	Some concerns

(*Continued*)

TABLE 10.2 (Continued)

Authors (Year)	Age M [range]	Diagnosis	Therapy (n)	Attrition (%)	Treatment Length	Follow-up	Summary of relevant findings	*Quality Appraisal
Sun et al. (2022)	22.2 [range not reported]	Depression and anxiety	Mindfulness-based mobile health (57) versus social support-based mHealth (57)	Active arm: 9 (post-intervention) and 9 (follow-up) Waitlist control: 9 (post-treatment) and 18 (follow-up)	One-month	Two months	Promising results are observed in young adults with depression when they received both mindfulness and social support via mHealth. However, mindfulness-based mHealth has shown to be particularly effective in reducing anxiety (p = .024, with a between-group effect size of d = 0.72).	Low
Thombs et al. (2021)	55 [range not reported]	Systemic sclerosis patients with at least mild anxiety and depression	Videoconference-based group intervention (86) versus WLC (86)	Active arm: 10 (post-intervention) and 13 (follow-up) Waitlist control: 4 (post-treatment) and 12 (follow-up)	Three times a week for four weeks (90 minutes each session)	Six weeks	Immediately after the intervention, there were no significant improvements in anxiety or other mental health outcomes. However, six weeks after the intervention, a decrease in anxiety and depression symptoms was observed.	Some concerns

Note: ACT, Acceptance and Commitment Therapy; BDI-II, Beck Depression Inventory-Second Edition; CBT, Cognitive Behavioral Therapy; GAD-7, Generalised Anxiety Disorder-7; n, number of participants; RAS, Recovery Assessment Scale; RSES, Rosenberg Self-Esteem Scale; SDS, Sheehan Disability Scale; WLC, Waitlist Control; *, Quality appraisal conducted using RoB 2.0.

Attrition (if not provided by the author in the article) is calculated using the formula: Number of participants without observed outcome data in the analysis/total number of participants × 10.

Results

Study Selection

Upon searching different databases systematically, 424 studies were found initially. Three hundred and four studies were screened against title and abstract after removing 120 duplicates. After applying inclusion and exclusion criteria, 149 studies were assessed for full-text eligibility, and nine were selected for review after applying inclusion and exclusion criteria. The PRISMA flow chart illustrates the study selection process (see Figure 10.1).

Study Characteristics

Designs

All the studies considered for the review are randomised controlled trials with two groups. Seven of the studies observed the intervention group with a waitlist control group, and two of them analysed the intervention group with the group receiving treatment differently from the intervention group.

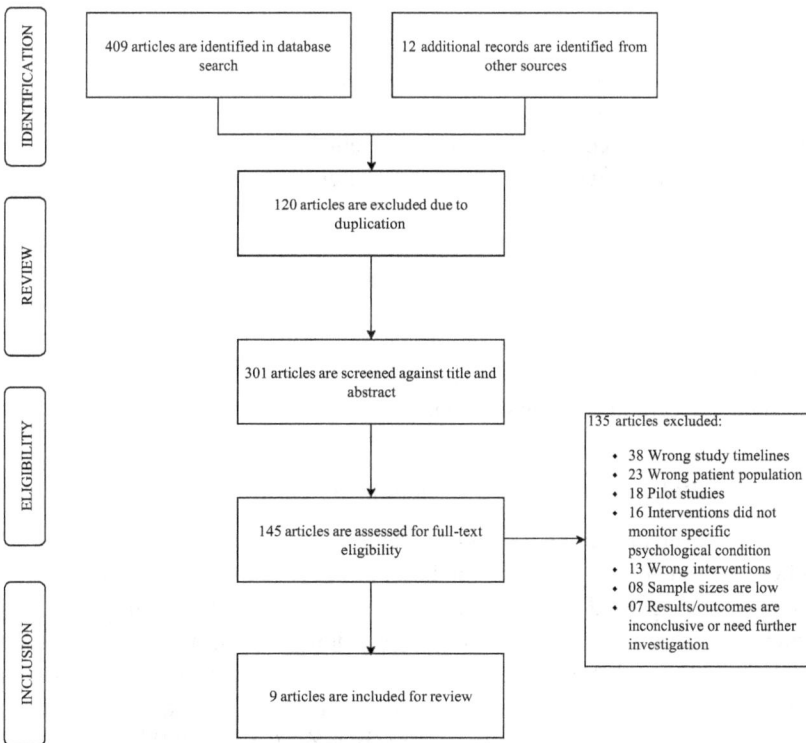

FIGURE 10.1 PRISMA flow chart showing the selection of studies at different stages

Samples

Participants numbering 2,147, oscillating between 46 and 679 participants with an average age of 33.5 years, were analysed in the nine studies selected for the systematic review. In all the studies, the percentage of the female population (ranging from 53% to 94%) was higher as compared to the males (ranging from 6% to 47%). The most common diagnosis observed were depression (n = 6), anxiety (n = 6), and stress (n = 3).

Interventions (Including Control Group)

Before being randomly allocated to intervention and control groups, all the participants were assessed for psychological problems such as depression, anxiety, and stress. Different interventions (such as cognitive behavioural therapy and app-based exercises) are incorporated by every study, though there is a similarity in the type of diagnosis. Though most studies (n = 7) have comparison groups as a waiting list, one study considered psychological support provided through newsletters via email, and another study considered psychological support provided through social support-based mobile health as the comparison groups.

Outcomes

Though the follow-ups varied from study to study (none to 12 weeks), a treatment period of four weeks was typical for all the studies. Every study assessed intervention effectiveness by comparing primary, baseline, and follow-up scores obtained when the participants were asked to answer different standard scales.

Risk of Bias

The risk of bias was low for both reporting (100%) and selection (100%) bias. On the other hand, the performance bias was with some concern in 33%, the attrition bias was with some concern in 22%, and the detection bias was high in 11% and with some concern in 33%, as shown in Figure 10.2.

Effect of Digital Intervention on Psychological Health

The effect of the digital intervention is analysed by looking at the findings of the studies and categorising them on the basis of the psychological problem the participants are diagnosed with. Those randomised controlled trials that considered participants who were shown to have depression, anxiety, or stress have shown that digital intervention, which is provided either by the therapist or through an app or in a group, has significantly improved the participants' mental health (Mohammed Al-Alawi et al., 2021; Sun et al., 2022; Ben-Zeev et al., 2021; Catuara-Solarz

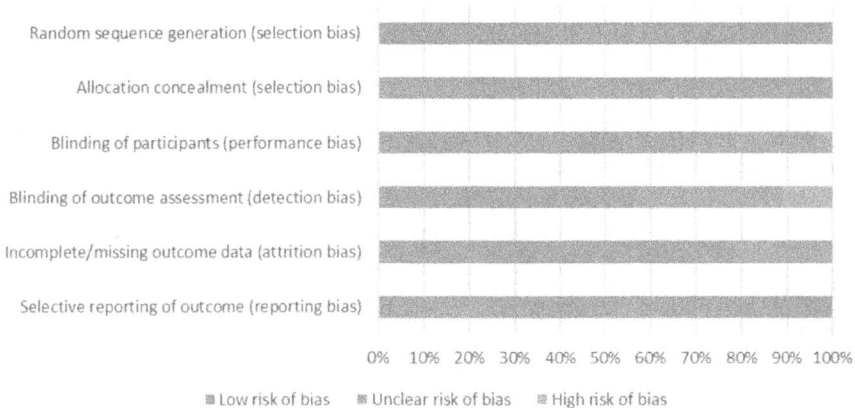

Random sequence generation (selection bias)

Allocation concealment (selection bias)

Blinding of participants (performance bias)

Blinding of outcome assessment (detection bias)

Incomplete/missing outcome data (attrition bias)

Selective reporting of outcome (reporting bias)

0% 10% 20% 30% 40% 50% 60% 70% 80% 90% 100%

■ Low risk of bias   ▨ Unclear risk of bias   ▨ High risk of bias

FIGURE 10.2   Analysis of risk of bias in the studies

et al., 2022; Chang et al., 2022; Thombs et al., 2021; Mohammed Al-Refae et al., 2021). However, these results were observed in different periods. Some interventions have observed a change immediately after the intervention. In contrast, a videoconference-based group intervention and an app-based intervention have seen better results during follow-ups (four weeks after the intervention).

The RCTs that considered participants diagnosed with eating disorders and somatic symptom disorders showed that digital interventions are effective whether provided through a mobile app or internet administration (Linardon et al., 2022; Maroti et al., 2022). However, the participants in the intervention group for somatic symptom disorder showed that the effects were not sustained till the follow-up stage. Conducting between- and within-group comparisons are not feasible with this review study as there are more differences than commonalities being observed.

The Risk and Protective Factors Associated with Receiving Digital Therapeutic Support

Protective factors identified from the review are presented in this section. One of the studies found that therapist-guided online therapy allows personalised treatment just like offline and is effective compared to self-help materials [Mohammed Al-Alawi et al., 2021]. On the other hand, Linardon et al. (2022) noted that app-based interventions showed results similar to that of a therapist-guided online intervention. This emphasises that an app developed by following principles, keeping the users in mind, and evaluating it rigorously can yield a good outcome. [Linardon et al., 2022; Sun et al., 2022]. A study [Ben-Zeev et al., 2021] showed that smartphone apps could be used transdiagnostically (for severe mental illnesses like bipolar disorder and schizophrenia). Mohammed Al-Refae et al. (2021) highlighted that the app modules (which are easy to refer to whenever needed) could promote self-compassion and help individuals identify and deal with negative thought patterns. This helps the individuals to gain self-insight and helps them with existing and new challenges that might emerge in the future. Apps also provide flexibility to individuals, where they can work towards their betterment at their own pace and take advantage of different app features to stay focused and on track [Catuara-Solarz et al., 2022]. A study by Thombs et al. (2021) showed that when this online support takes place in groups, it yields better results due to group cohesion.

Coming to the risk factors, it was found that high attrition rates and the inability to get sustained attention from the participants can result in low app retention and the effectiveness of the intervention [Linardon et al., 2022; Ben-Zeev et al., 2021; Chang et al., 2022]. Stalling the waitlist control group from receiving treatment may result in frustration, treatment assumptions, and an inability to explore alternative treatment options [Ben-Zeev et al., 2021]. Personalising the app depending on sociodemographic and symptom differences is only feasible when the app is tested and updated across different countries [Catuara-Solarz et al., 2022]. When participants are exposed to interventions that are not usual (i.e. online intervention instead offline), there is a possibility of participants taking the intervention negatively, resulting in negative intervention effects [Maroti et al., 2022]. Though all interventions are conducted in a controlled setting, and the effectiveness is checked, the results cannot be generalised as it was performed only on a certain population [Al-Alawi et al., 2021; Thombs et al., 2021]. Digital interventions are always restricted by factors like participants' education, access to the internet, and other culture-specific problems [Mohammed Al-Alawi et al., 2021].

Recommendations and Implications

Studies have recommended that the app care model (low cost and intensity) can be used as a treatment in the stepped-care model and as add-on support for those who receive offline therapist guidance, helping reduce the treatment gap. An app and e-guided self-help can also be welcoming for users who are apprehensive about taking or providing help [Linardon et al., 2022; Mohammed Al-Alawi et al., 2021; Sun et al., 2022]. During COVID-19, when providing/receiving health services became difficult, clinically tested apps could help individuals with severe mental illnesses [Ben-Zeev et al., 2021; Sun et al., 2022] and potential pandemic-related isolation effects [Mohammed Al-Refae et al., 2021]. Regarding implications, studies have noted that to reduce the gap between science-to-service delivery and provide mental health support to every individual, despite the barriers, disseminating evidence-based digital health intervention is necessary [Ben-Zeev et al., 2021]. Therapists should be trained to provide online and formal face-to-face therapy so that digital therapy efficacy increases and gets more abundant and accepted [Al-Alawi et al., 2021]. The researchers need to plan long-term studies to check the effectiveness of the intervention [Catuara-Solarz et al., 2022; Mohammed Al-Alawi et al., 2021; Sun et al., 2022]. It is necessary to understand why participants drop out to create effective apps or online interventions [Chang et al., 2022].

Discussion

Principal Findings

This review systematically evaluated the efficacy of digital psychological intervention among the adult population worldwide using evidence-based therapies, validated instruments, and scales. Though there are existing systematic reviews (Lau et al., 2021; Oliveira et al., 2021) that have evaluated different digital interventions to the extent considered, this could be the first review that has considered most of the digital infrastructure available to treat psychological concerns without limiting the diagnosis type and checked its efficacy. For the current review, we have identified nine studies that checked the effectiveness of digital psychological interventions. The interventions focused here are evidence-based treatment strategies like acceptance and commitment therapy, cognitive behavioural therapies, mindfulness, group therapies, self-help modules, and problem-solving strategies to treat psychological issues like depression, anxiety, stress, bipolar disorder, schizophrenia, and eating disorders. All the studies included are randomised control trials, where seven out of nine studies used a waitlist control group, five out of nine studies were app-based, six out of nine studies conducted follow-up, and the average treatment length was one month. No trial compared the face-to-face mode of therapy with digital.

Overall, these studies indicated that (a) psychological support obtained through digital infrastructures, such as app-based and video conference-based, maybe is acceptable and appropriate mode of intervention for the target population, given the individual has access to and knowledge of the tool; (b) during COVID-19, digital interventions have helped both the practitioners and the therapy-seekers; and (c) though there are some mixed responses in the efficacy of this mode of intervention, digital infrastructure can act as add-on support and can be used in the stepped-care model. Our review findings are consistent with the previous review findings, suggesting that digital support is effective and appropriate for adults with psychological concerns (Oliveira et al., 2021; Zakhour et al., 2020).

Quality of the Evidence

All the nine studies included in the review have considered a good number of participants in both experimental (ranging from 22 to 326) and (waitlist) control groups (24 to 352). All the studies randomly selected the participants and allocated them to groups. A reasonable explanation was provided by those studies that had not blinded the participants and outcome assessors regarding the intervention received. There are no highly notable methodological limitations observed in these studies. However, many of the studies showed high attrition rates. Despite some concerns, the studies included have shown the intervention's efficacy through randomisation, having a waitlist control group, and calculating the outcomes by taking measurements during the preliminary, baseline, and follow-up stage.

Limitations of the Review

This systematic review did not consider many relevant studies due to wrong study timelines, particularly those published before the COVID-19 pandemic. It is observed that most of the studies published during 2020–21 were registered and conducted during 2018–19 or prior. Moreover, generalisability is restricted due to this review's broad inclusion criteria and the latest technological advancements. Despite the condition that the review is to encompass as many studies as possible that focus on psychological issues as the primary outcome, a significant number of these studies either did not focus on psychological issues or combined them with physiological conditions. Studies that focused exclusively on physiological conditions were not considered for this review.

Additionally, the authors could not determine the baseline severity of symptoms of the psychological conditions due to the diversity of outcome measures utilised. The review looked at a specific range of digital infrastructure that effectively provides psychological interventions or services to the intended population, emphasising the effectiveness of self-help programmes and smartphone applications that require minimal supervision. Research evaluating these interventions is inconclusive.

Implications and Future Directions

In addition to the limitations above, this review observed some insights and future directions. First, extensive randomised controlled trials should examine statistical and clinical changes in psychological interventions delivered through digital infrastructure. Second, scholars and policymakers need to examine the effectiveness of these digital infrastructures, especially with new emerging telehealth and mHealth treatments, that is internet-based interventions and mobile applications. Third, future research could examine the efficacy of these digital infrastructures on psychological conditions across diverse populations and geographical locations to overcome digital inequity. The cost-effectiveness of implementing these psychological services through digital mode has to be documented so that the viability of implementing them would give policymakers a clear picture to consider them or not. Future research also needs to explore whether these interventions were developed using digital infrastructures that are in acceptance by the study populations and should consider digital inequity when rolling out such interventions or services. Finally, the review provides a good scope and promises that digital infrastructure can significantly reduce psychological conditions. However, one should be cautious in establishing these preliminary findings as viable options. Researchers need to test them more rigorously before they accept the efficacy of these digital interventions.

Other Information

Registration and Protocol

The systematic review was registered in PROSPERO by the corresponding author [R.D.] with the title "Efficacy of digital infrastructure providing psychological support among the global adult population during the COVID-19 Pandemic: a systematic review" and registration number CRD42022370432. The protocol was amended four times before publishing the review in the book chapter. The amendments were made in different sections with comments received from the PROSPERO team and during different review stages.

The protocol can be accessed using the registration number: CRD42022370432.

Support

The study received no funding.

Competing Interests

The authors declare no potential conflict of interest.

Availability of Data, Code, and Other Materials

The data generated during the review can be availed from the corresponding author [R.D.] upon reasonable request.

References

Al-Alawi, M., McCall, R. K., Sultan, A., Al Balushi, N., Al-Mahrouqi, T., Al Ghailani, A., Al Sabti, H., Al-Maniri, A., Panchatcharam, S. M., & Al Sinawi, H. (2021). Efficacy of a six-week-long therapist-guided online therapy versus self-help internet-based therapy for COVID-19-induced anxiety and depression: Open-label, pragmatic, randomized controlled trial. *JMIR Mental Health, 8*(2), e26683. https://doi.org/10.2196/26683

Al-Refae, M., Al-Refae, A., Munroe, M., Sardella, N. A., & Ferrari, M. (2021). A self-compassion and mindfulness-based cognitive mobile intervention (Serene) for depression, anxiety, and stress: Promoting adaptive emotional regulation and wisdom. *Frontiers in Psychology, 12*, 648087. https://doi.org/10.3389/fpsyg.2021.648087

Ben-Zeev, D., Chander, A., Tauscher, J., Buck, B., Nepal, S., Campbell, A., & Doron, G. (2021). A smartphone intervention for people with serious mental illness: Fully remote randomized controlled trial of CORE. *Journal of Medical Internet Research, 23*(11), e29201. https://doi.org/10.2196/29201

Brewer, L. C., Fortuna, K. L., Jones, C., Walker, R., Hayes, S. N., Patten, C. A., & Cooper, L. A. (2020). Back to the future: Achieving health equity through health informatics and digital health. *JMIR mHealth and uHealth, 8*(1), e14512. https://doi.org/10.2196/14512

Catuara-Solarz, S., Skorulski, B., Estella-Aguerri, I., Avella-Garcia, C. B., Shepherd, S., Stott, E., Hemmings, N. R., Ruiz de Villa, A., Schulze, L., & Dix, S. (2022). The efficacy of "foundations" a digital mental health app to improve mental well-being during COVID-19: Proof-of-principle randomized controlled trial. *JMIR mHealth and uHealth, 10*(7), e30976. https://doi.org/10.2196/30976

Chang, T. F. H., Ley, B. L., Ramburn, T. T., Srinivasan, S., Hariri, S., Purandare, P., & Subramaniam, B. (2022). Online Isha Upa Yoga for student mental health and well-being during COVID-19: A randomised control trial. *Applied Psychology Health and Well-being, 14*(4), 1408–1428. https://doi.org/10.1111/aphw.12341

Ganjali, R., Jajroudi, M., Kheirdoust, A., Darroudi, A., & Alnattah, A. (2022). Telemedicine solutions for clinical care delivery during COVID-19 pandemic: A scoping review. *Frontiers in Public Health, 10*, 937207. https://doi.org/10.3389/fpubh.2022.937207

Lau, N., Colt, S. F., Waldbaum, S., O'Daffer, A., Fladeboe, K., Yi-Frazier, J. P., McCauley, E., & Rosenberg, A. R. (2021). Telemental health for youth with chronic illnesses: Systematic review. *JMIR Mental Health, 8*(8). https://doi.org/10.2196/30098

Lecomte, T., Potvin, S., Corbière, M., Guay, S., Samson, C., Cloutier, B., Francoeur, A., Pennou, A., & Khazaal, Y. (2020). Mobile apps for mental health issues: Meta-review of meta-analyses. *JMIR mHealth and uHealth, 8*(5), e17458. https://doi.org/10.2196/17458

Linardon, J., Shatte, A., Rosato, J., & Fuller-Tyszkiewicz, M. (2022). Efficacy of a transdiagnostic cognitive-behavioral intervention for eating disorder psychopathology delivered through a smartphone app: A randomised controlled trial. *Psychological Medicine, 52*(9), 1679–1690. https://doi.org/10.1017/S0033291720003426

Maroti, D., Lumley, M. A., Schubiner, H., Lilliengren, P., Bileviciute-Ljungar, I., Ljótsson, B., & Johansson, R. (2022). Internet-based emotional awareness and expression therapy for somatic symptom disorder: A randomised controlled trial. *Journal of Psychosomatic Research, 163*, 111068. https://doi.org/10.1016/j.jpsychores.2022.111068

Mohammadpour, M., Zarifinezhad, E., Ghanbarzadegan, A., Naderimanesh, K., Shaarbafchizadeh, N., & Bastani, P. (2021). Main factors affecting the readiness and responsiveness of healthcare systems during epidemic crises: A scoping review on cases of SARS, MERS, and COVID-19. *Iranian Journal of Medical Sciences, 46*(2), 81–92. https://doi.org/10.30476/ijms.2020.87608.1801

Oliveira, C., Pereira, A., Vagos, P., Nóbrega, C., Gonçalves, J., & Afonso, B. (2021). Effectiveness of mobile app-based psychological interventions for college students: A systematic review of the literature. *Frontiers in Psychology, 12*. https://doi.org/10.3389/fpsyg.2021.647606

Richardson, C. G., Slemon, A., Gadermann, A., McAuliffe, C., Thomson, K., Daly, Z., Salway, T., Currie, L. M., David, A., & Jenkins, E. (2020). Use of asynchronous virtual mental health resources for COVID-19 pandemic-related stress among the general population in Canada: Cross-sectional survey study. *Journal of Medical Internet Research, 22*(12), e24868. https://doi.org/10.2196/24868

Rudd, B. N., & Beidas, R. S. (2020). Digital mental health: The answer to the global mental health crisis? *JMIR Mental Health, 7*(6), e18472. https://doi.org/10.2196/18472

Silver, L. (2020). Smartphone ownership is growing rapidly around the world, but not always equally. *Pew Research Center*. Retrieved December 10, 2022, from www.pewresearch.org/global/2019/02/05/smartphone-ownership-is-growing-rapidly-around-the-world-but-not-always-equally/

Steinhubl, S. R., Muse, E. D., & Topol, E. J. (2015). The emerging field of mobile health. *Science Translational Medicine, 7*(283), 283rv3. https://doi.org/10.1126/scitranslmed. aaa3487

Sun, S., Lin, D., Goldberg, S., Shen, Z., Chen, P., Qiao, S., Brewer, J., Loucks, E., & Operario, D. (2022). A mindfulness-based mobile health (mHealth) intervention among psychologically distressed university students in quarantine during the COVID-19 pandemic: A randomised controlled trial. *Journal of Counseling Psychology, 69*(2), 157–171. https://doi.org/10.1037/cou0000568

Thombs, B. D., Kwakkenbos, L., Levis, B., Bourgeault, A., Henry, R. S., Levis, A. W., Harb, S., Tao, L., Carrier, M. E., Bustamante, L., Duchek, D., Dyas, L., El-Baalbaki, G., Ellis, K., Rice, D. B., Wurz, A., Nordlund, J., Gagarine, M., Turner, K. A., Østbø, N., . . . Scleroderma Patient-centered Intervention Network Investigators. (2021). Effects of a multi-faceted education and support programme on anxiety symptoms among people with systemic sclerosis and anxiety during COVID-19 (SPIN-CHAT): A two-arm parallel, partially nested, randomised, controlled trial. *The Lancet. Rheumatology, 3*(6), e427–e437. https://doi.org/10.1016/S2665-9913(21)00060-6

Timakum, T., Xie, Q., & Song, M. (2022). Analysis of E-mental health research: Mapping the relationship between information technology and mental healthcare. *BMC Psychiatry, 22*(1), 57. https://doi.org/10.1186/s12888-022-03713-9

Ting, D. S. W., Lin, H., Ruamviboonsuk, P., Wong, T. Y., & Sim, D. A. (2020). Artificial intelligence, the internet of things, and virtual clinics: Ophthalmology at the digital translation forefront. *The Lancet, 2*(1), e8–e9. https://doi.org/10.1016/S2589-7500(19)30217-1

Torous, J., Bucci, S., Bell, I. H., Kessing, L. V., Faurholt-Jepsen, M., Whelan, P., Carvalho, A. F., Keshavan, M., Linardon, J., & Firth, J. (2021). The growing field of digital psychiatry: Current evidence and the future of apps, social media, chatbots, and virtual reality. *World Psychiatry: Official Journal of the World Psychiatric Association (WPA), 20*(3), 318–335. https://doi.org/10.1002/wps.20883

Zakhour, S., Nardi, A. E., Levitan, M., & Appolinario, J. C. (2020). Cognitive-behavioral therapy for treatment-resistant depression in adults and adolescents: A systematic review. *Trends in Psychiatry and Psychotherapy, 42*(1), 92–101. https://doi. org/10.1590/2237-6089-2019-0033

INDEX

Note: Page numbers in *italics* indicate a figure and page numbers in **bold** indicate a table on the corresponding page.

For Product Safety Concerns and Information please contact our EU
representative GPSR@taylorandfrancis.com
Taylor & Francis Verlag GmbH, Kaufingerstraße 24, 80331 München, Germany

www.ingramcontent.com/pod-product-compliance
Lightning Source LLC
Chambersburg PA
CBHW060240220326
41598CB00027B/3997

9 781032 412757